PHARMACEUTICAL ANALYSIS

We pay homage with reverence to the
late Prof. P.Parimoo

- Publishers

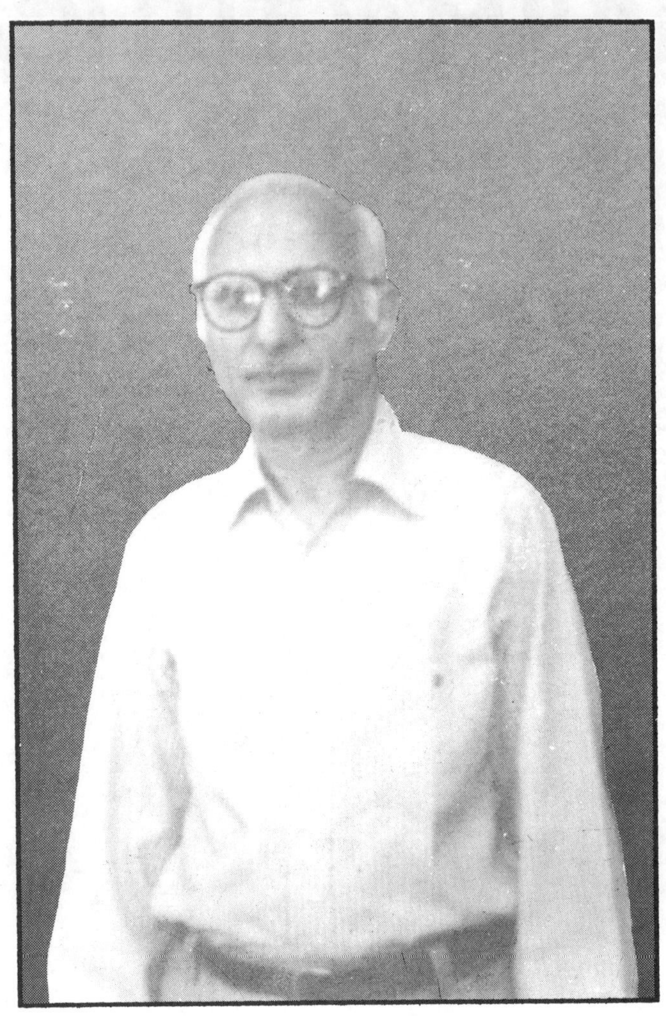

Prof. P. PARIMOO
1938 - 1998

"All great men rose in excellence because of their unswerving devotion to the ideal to which they dedicated themselves"

- Mahabharata

PHARMACEUTICAL ANALYSIS

P. PARIMOO MS., Ph.D
Professor of Pharmaceutical Chemistry
Birla Institute of Technology & Science
PILANI (Raj.), INDIA

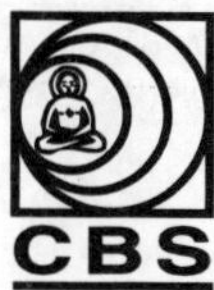

CBS Publishers & Distributors Pvt Ltd

New Delhi • Bengaluru • Chennai • Kochi • Kolkata • Lucknow • Mumbai
Hyderabad • Jharkhand • Nagpur • Patna • Pune • Uttarakhand

Pharmaceutical Analysis

ISBN: 978-81-239-0627-0

First Edition **1998**
Reprint 1999, 2004, 2005, 2006, 2007, 2008, 2009, 2012, 2018, 2019, 2020, **2025**

Published by **Satish Kumar Jain** and produced by **Varun Jain** for

CBS Publishers & Distributors Pvt Ltd

4819/XI Prahlad Street, 24 Ansari Road, Daryaganj, New Delhi 110 002, India.
Ph: 011-23266838, 23289259 Website: www.cbspd.com
e-mail: delhi@cbspd.com

Corporate Office: 204 FIE, Industrial Area, Patparganj, Delhi 110 092
Ph: 011-4934 4934 Fax: 011-4934 4935
e-mail: publishing@cbspd.com; publicity@cbspd.com

Branches

- **Bengaluru:** Seema House 2975, 17th Cross, KR Road, Banasankari 2nd Stage, Bengaluru 560 070, Karnataka, India
  Ph: +91-80-26771678/79 Fax: +91-80-26771680 e-mail: bangalore@cbspd.com
- **Chennai:** 18/8B, Subbarayan Street, Shenoy Nagar, Chennai 600 030, Tamil Nadu, India
  Ph: +91-44-42032115, 26681266 e-mail: chennai@cbspd.com
- **Kochi:** 42/1325, 1326, Power House Road, Opp KSEB, Power House, Ernakulum Kochi 682 018, Kerala, India
  Ph: +91-484-4059061-65,67 Fax: +91-484-4059065 e-mail: kochi@cbspd.com
- **Kolkata:** 147, Hind Ceramics Compound, 1st Floor, Nilgunj Road, Belghoria, Kolkata-700056, West Bengal, India
  Ph: +033-25633055, 033-25633056 e-mail: kolkata@cbspd.com
- **Lucknow:** Basement, Khushnuma Complex, 7 Meerabai Marg (Behind Jawahar Bhawan), Lucknow-226001, UP, India
  Ph: +0522-4000032 e-mail: tiwari.lucknow@cbspd.com
- **Mumbai:** PWD Shed, Gala no 25/26, Ramchandra Bhatt Marg, Next to JJ Hospital Gate no. 2, Opp. Union Bank of India, Noorbaug, Mumbai-400009, Maharashtra, India
  Ph: 022-66661880/89 e-mail: mumbai@cbspd.com

Representatives

- Hyderabad 0-9885175004
- Patna 0-9334159340
- Jharkhand 0-9811541605
- Pune 0-9664372571
- Nagpur 0-8692091830
- Uttarakhand 0-9716462459

Printed at Mudrak, Noida, UP, India

Preface

IN the last decade or so there has been improvement in the syllabi for courses on pharmaceutical analytical chemistry and pharmaceutical analysis at B-Pharm level. Some of the Pharmacy departments as well as colleges of pharmacy have been able to acquire and expose their senior level students to some of the sophisticated analytical instruments. However, at this juncture it may become needless to say that a few advanced centres in Pharmaceutical Sciences in the country have been holding workshops on advanced instrumental methods of analysis for the M-Pharm and Ph.D. level students. With the increased awareness as well as wide spread use of drug analysis and quality control techniques it has become necessary to have an up-dated instructional material available for both pharmacy colleges as well as for drug industry in this country. Consequently in the preparation of this text book an effort has been made to unify and select material that would satisfy differing needs and at the same time keep the book to a reasonable size.

The subject material has been arranged in the form of various sections to include variety of techniques that are available under chemical, physico-chemical and instrumental methods and in the process the book will also serve the purpose of advanced students at M-Pharm and Ph.D. level.

Section 1 comprises the classical methods of analysis which are meant for the 1st year level syllabus in Pharmaceutical analysis.

The section comprising chapters 8 and 9 will be useful of practical experiments covered in Pharmacognosy at different levels in B-Pharm course.

The chapters 10, 12 and 13 can be utilized for practical work in pharmaceutical chemistry at 3rd year level.

The section under spectroscopy is dealt in great depth and is meant for 4th year level as well as M-Pharm level students. It covers a wide variety of methods for both quantitative analysis and problems on structure elucidation.

The chapter on particle size determination and differential thermal analysis can be utilized for practical work in physical pharmacy course.

The chapters which deal with NMR and mass spectroscopy, ORD, radiochemical, GLC and HPLC methods have also been covered in great detail and should prove very useful for M-Pharm and Ph.D. level students.

Unsolved problems on quantitative analysis and structure elucidation have not been included in the present format of the text book but a fair number of known spectras as well as simple experiments have been incorporated in each chapter for practice purpose to provide a working knowledge of analysis and control. These exercises can be easily performed during a practical period for most of the pharmacy courses in India.

Many colleges may not have all the laboratory equipment to derive the benefit of this practical course, but the lack of such equipment should not become a deterrent to understanding the use of drug analysis and quality control.

Although as a graduate student I took courses in analytical methods and radioisotopes but it was through teaching such a course and doing research in drug analysis, synthesis and phytochemical work that motivated me to unify and publish this textual material. As almost all of the present analytical instruments contain electronic circuitry and are also interfaced with computers, therefore terminology on these subjects have been attached in the form of appendix rather than as separate chapters.

I also wish to thank authorities at B.I.T.S., for giving me an opportunity to be in-charge of Central Analytical Laboratory facilities as well as in-charge of the course "Instrumental Methods of Analysis" for several years.

It is hoped that both students and pharmacy teachers in India will find this textual material comprehensive, effective and easy to adopt for theory and practical work on the subject of Pharmaceutical analysis.

The author wishes to express thankfulness to companies for making use of diagrams from their catalogues and books since a variety of models are available to choose from in the international market.

Pilani, 1998 **P. Parimoo**

Selected References

1. Beckett, A.H and Stenlake, J.B., Practical Pharmaceutical Chemistry Part I & II, Athlone Press, London, 3rd Ed., 1976.
2. Conners, K.A., A text book of Pharmaceutical Analysis, 2nd Ed., John Wiley., N.Y., 1975.
3. Gearian, J.E. and Grabowski, B.F., Methods of Drug Analysis, Lea & Febiger, Philadelphia, 1969.
4. Chatten, L.G., Pharmaceutical Chemistry, Vol I & II, Marcel Dekker Incs. N.Y., 1969.
5. Higuchi, T. and Brockman-Hanssen, E., Pharmaceutical Analysis., John Wiley., N.Y., 1961.
6. Knevel, A.M and DiGangi, F.E., Jenkins Quantitative Pharmaceutical Chemistry. McGraw Hill, N.Y., 1977.
7. Florey, K., Analytical Profiles of Drug Substances, (several volumes) Academic Press, N.Y., 1972-1993.
8. Wilson, C.L. and Wilson, D.W., Comprehensive Analytical Chemistry, vol. I-IV, Elsvier Publishing company, N.Y., 1975.
10. Vogel, A.I., Text Book of Quantitative Analysis, 3rd ed., Longman, N.Y., 1972.
11. Pickering, W.F., Modern Analytical Chemistry, Marcel Dekker, N.Y., 1971.
12. Fritz, J.S. and Shenk, G.H., Quantitative Analytical Chemistry, 3rd ed., Allyn & Bacon, Boston, 1974.
13. Belcher, R., New Methods of Analytical Chemistry, 2nd ed, John Wiley, N.Y., 1966.
14. American Society for Testing Materials, ASTM Book of Standards, 7 Vol., Philadelphia, U.S.A., 1952.
15. Koltoff., I. M. and Elving, P.J., Treatise on Analytical Chemistry (various volumes) Intersciences, N.Y., 1959.
16. Skoog, D.A. and West, D.M. Fundamentals of Analytical Chemistry, 3rd ed, Holt, N.Y., 1976.
17. Flagg, J.F., Organic Reagents used in Gravimetric and volumetric Analysis, Interscience, N.Y., 1948.
18. Koltoff, I.M., Acid-Base Indicators; Macmillan, N.Y., 1937.

19. Welcher, F.J., Organic Analytical Reagents, (Four volumes), D. Von Nostrand Co. Inc, Princeton, N.J., 1948.
20. Cox, H.E., Chemical Analysis of Foods, Churchill, London, 1938.
21. Hamilton, L.F. and Simpson, S.G., Calculation of Analytical Chemistry, 7th ed, McGraw-Hill, N.Y., 1969.
22. Young, R.S., Industrial Inorganic Analysis, John Wiley, N.Y., 1953.
23. Willard, H.H, Merritt, L.L. and Dean, J.A., Instrumental Methods of Analysis, 6th ed, CBS Publishers and Distributors, New Delhi, 1986.
24. Ewing, G.W., Instrumental Methods of Chemical Analysis, 5th ed, McGraw-Hill, N.Y., 1988.
25. Dyer, J.R., Applications of Absorption Spectroscopy of Organic Compounds, Prentice-Hall, N.Y., 1965.
26. Silverstein, R.M. and Bassler, G.C., Spectrometric Identification of Organic Compounds, 4th ed, John Wiley, N.Y., 1981.
27. Skoog, D.A. and West, D.M., Principles of Instrumental Analysis, Hold Rinehart, N.Y., 1985.
28. Snell, F.D. and Snell, C.T., Colourimetric Methods of Analysis (Several volumes) D. Van Nostrand Co., N.Y., 1948-1971.
29. Elwell, W.T. and Gidley, J.A.F., Atomic Absorption Spectrophotometry, 2nd rev. ed, Pergamon Press, N.Y., 1966.
30. Dean, J.A. , Flame Photometry, McGraw-Hill, N.Y., 1960.
31. Sand, H.J.S., Electrochemical Analysis, Blackie, London, 1946.
32. Milner, G.W.C., Principles and Applications of Polarography, Longmans N.Y., 1957.
33. Lingane, J. J., Electroanalytical Chemistry, McGraw-Hill, N.Y., 1958.
34. Koltoff, I. M. and Ligane, J. J., Polarography, 2 vol, Interscience, N.Y., 1952.
35. Radley, J.A. and Grant, J., Fluorescence Analysis in Ultraviolet light, D. Van Nostrand Co., N. J., 1954.
36. Winefordner, J.D., Luminescence Spectrometry in Analytical Chemistry, John Wiley Inc, N.Y., 1972.
37. Elvitch, F. R. Fluorimetric Techniques in Clinical Chemistry, Little Brown & Co, Boston, 1973.
38. Bobbit, J. M., Introduction to Chromatography, D. Van Nostrand Co, N.Y., 1968
39. Cassiday, H. G., Fundamentals of Chromatography, Interscience, N.Y., 1957.
40. Lederer, E and Lederer, M., Chromatography, D. Van Nostrand Co., Princeton, N.J., 1957.
41. Mc Nair, H. M. and Bonelli, E. J., Basic Gas Chromatography, 5th ed, Varian Aerograph, california, 1969.
42. Stahl, E., Thin-Layer Chromatography, A Laboratory Manual Hand Book, 2nd ed, Springer-Verlag, N.Y., 1969.
43. Randerath, K., Thin Layer Chromatography, translated by D.D. Libman, 2nd ed, Academic Press, N.Y., 1966.
44. Brown, P. R., High Pressure Liquid Chromatography, Academic Press, N.Y., 1972.
45. Mackenzie, R.C., Differential Thermal Analysis, Academic Press, London, Vol 1 (1970), Vol 2, 1972.
46. Lambie, D.A., Techniques for use of Radioisotopes in Analysis, D. Van Nostrand, N.Y., 1964.
47. Overman, R. T. and Clerk, H. M., Radioisotope Techniques, McGraw-Hill, N.Y., 1960.
48. Glick, D., Methods of Biochemical Analysis, Vol 1-22, John wiley, N.Y., 1974.
49. Horwitz, W., Official Methods of Analysis of Association of Official Analytical Chemists, 12th ed, Association of Official Analytical Chemists, Washington, 1975.

50. Nakanishi, K., Infrased Absorption Spectroscopy, Holden-Dey Inc., San Francisco, 1962.
51. Bhacca, N.S., and Williams, D.H., Applications of NMR Spectroscopy in Organic Chemistry, Holden-Dey Inc., San Francisco, 1964.
52. Budzikiewiez, H., C. Djerassi and D.H. Williams, Interpretation of Mass Spectra of Organic Compounds, Holden-Dey Inc; San Francisco, 1964.
53. Artwick, B.A., Microcomputer Interfacing, Prentice-Hall, Englewood Cliffs, N.J., 1980.
54. G.D. Christian and J.E. O'Reilly, Instrumental Analysis, 2nd ed, Allyn and Bacon, Inc., Newton, Massachusetts, U.S.A., 1986.
55. Indian Pharmacopoeia, 1985, Vol I & II, Govt. of India, Ministry of Health and Family Welfare, Published by the Controller of Publications, Delhi.
56. Clark's Isolation and Identification of Drugs, 2nd ed, A.C. Moffat, The Pharmaceutical Press, London, 1986.
57. British Pharmacopoeia, 1988, Vol. I & II, Her Majesty's Stationary Office, London.
58. The United States Pharmacopoeia, 1990, 22nd ed.., United States Pharmaceutical Convention, Inc, 12601 Twinbrook Parkway, Rockville, MD.
59. The International Pharmacopoeia, 3rd ed (Reprint), Vol I, II & III (Quality specifications), CBS Publishers & Distributors, New Delhi, 1991.

Contents

SECTION-C : GENERAL PHYSICAL METHODS OF ANALYSIS

SECTION-D : ELECTROCHEMICAL METHODS OF ANALYSIS

SECTION-E : SPECTROSCOPIC METHODS OF ANALYSIS

SECTION-H : MISCELLANEOUS TYPES OF INSTRUMENTAL METHODS OF ANALYSIS

APPENDICES

SECTION-A
GENERAL INFORMATION

1

Tools and Techniques of Drug Analysis

1.1 General

The aim of this chapter is to build an awareness in an analyst about the basic requirements common for drug analysis and or quality control for pharmaceuticals. Some of these are concerned with general laboratory operations like weighing the sample, treatment of the sample, apparatus involved, errors, accuracy etc, while others deal with handling of the sophisticated instruments like the spectrophotometers etc.

1.2 Laboratory Note Book

It is necessary to maintain faithfully and carefully a notebook in which all data on a particular analysis is recorded. Although the type of notebook selected can be specified by an instructor, but a hard bound notebook is satisfactory. The data concerning each analysis can be entered in the following order: (i) Date (ii) objective (iii) Experimental Method/Procedure (iv) Reaction/Equations (v) Calculations (vi) Results (vii) conclusions.

All the items concerning each analysis should be clear and neatly written in ink and recorded immediately. One should never record any data for an analysis on loose sheets of paper. The objective should be clearly specified and procedure described systematically. All reactions concerning the analysis should be described and equations should be balanced.

Conclusions regarding an analysis in terms of success or any errors etc. should be indicated.

Any numerical data should be written in the form of tables.

1.3 Sampling And Samples

In a pharmaceutical analysis course, generally the students are supplied with samples which are ready for drying and weighing or in a solution form ready for the subsequent work. Therefore, one does not have to worry with the operation of sampling. However, one should be concerned about the origin of the samples and how samples are obtained.

In an analysis one is faced with two types of situations :

(i) either to determine the composition of the pure substance; or

(ii) to determine the average composition of a mass of material.

Therefore, it is important to have a representative sample. It is not possible to make fixed rules for sampling because it will depend on the nature of the material and the quantity from which a representative sample is to be made. So in general, whenever it is possible one should obtain a sample from each package or containers. If only a single package is offered, the contents should be thoroughly mixed and then a small portion from this mixture is taken for final analysis. Once a sample is acquired, it should be spread on a watch glass and dried in an oven at the specified temperature to correct for any absorbed moisture. It should then be transferred to a weighing bottle and kept in a desiccator.

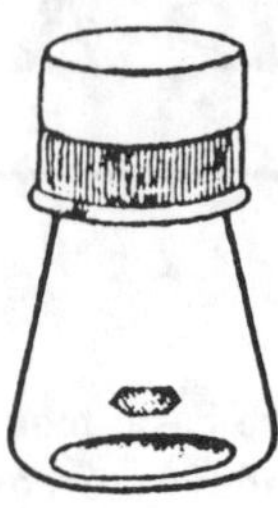

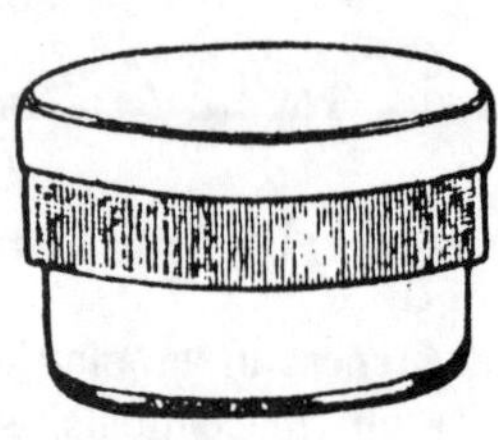

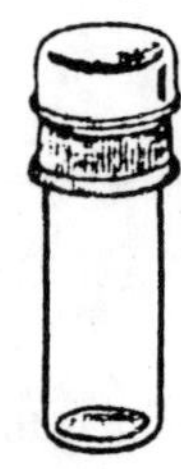

Fig. 1.1. Weighing bottle

1.4 Apparatus

(i) Weighing Bottles: The weighing of samples which are liquids and volatile or hygroscopic in nature is done in a small glass container provided with a stopper.

However, solid samples may be weighed on a watch glass or directly in a conical flask to save time for analysis.

(ii) *Volumetric Flasks:* These are measuring flasks usually pear shaped, flat bottomed with a long neck. The neck of the flask has a single graduation mark around it indicating a specified volume that it can hold at 25° . The neck of the flask is made narrow and long so that the final adjustment for the height of the liquid can be done by dropwise addition of the contents of the flask.

For convenience, the samples are first dissolved in a beaker with small amounts of the solvent and then transferred to the volumetric flask using a funnel and a glass rod. The remainder of the solvent is then added

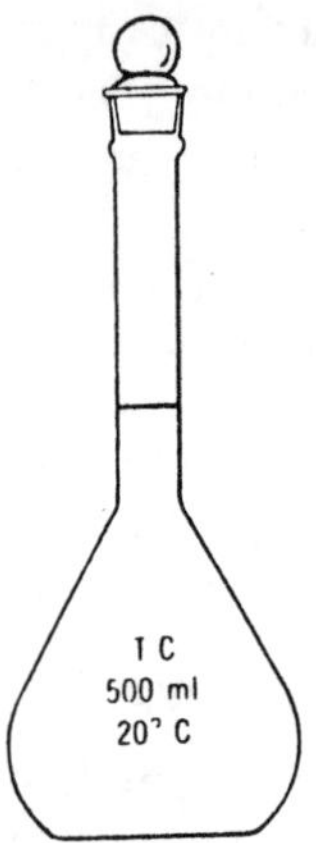

Fig. 1.2 Volumetric flask

slowly and finally volume adjusted at the mark by dropwise addition of the liquid. The volumetric flasks are manufactured in two types of tolerances, grade A and grade B respectively.

(iii) Burettes: A burette is a narrow graduated glass tube provided with a stop cock so that very accurate volumes of liquids can be delivered in experiments involving quantitative estimations. They are made in varying capacity from 1 ml up to 100 ml and as usual in two specifications i.e. grade A and grade B. They are graduated in millilitres and tenths of millilitres and readings can be recorded to the nearestof 0.02 ml.

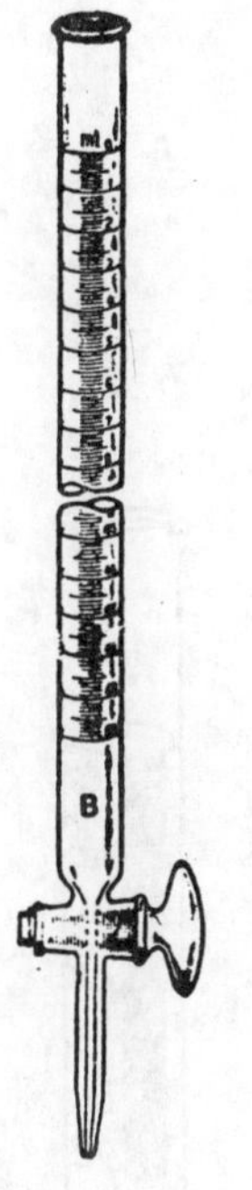

Fig. 1.3(a) Burette

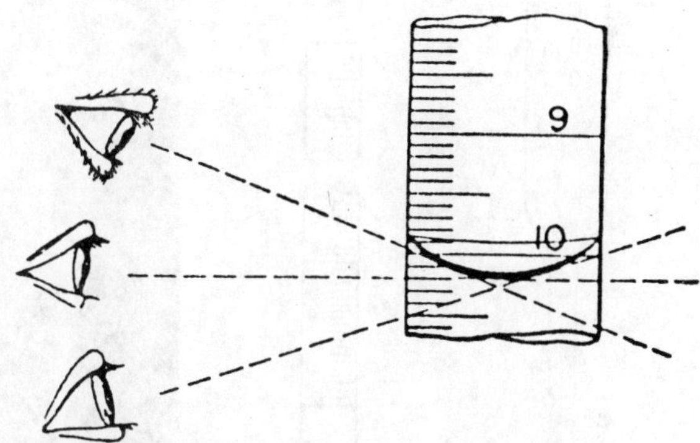

Fig. 1.3(b) Effect of parallax in reading buretts. Only when the eye is on a level with the meniscus will the reading give no parallactic error.

For accurate work, burette should be always cleaned before use and rinsed with the concerned titrant. The stop-cock should be properly greased and any air bubbles and leakage checked before starting with a titration. The burette must be read at the eye level in order to avoid errors in reading the meniscus.

(iv) *Pipettes*: The purpose of pipettes is to deliver specified volumes of liquids in quantitative determinations. There are three types of pipettes available namely:

(a) transfer pipettes (b) graduated pipettes and

(c) automatic pipettes.

The transfer pipettes have one single graduation mark around its body and its purpose is to deliver a specific volume of liquid under specified conditions. The capacity and temperature at which it was graduated and delivery time are also stated on the bulb of the pipette. This applies for water and aqueous solutions. As usual they are available in grade A and grade B specifications.

The graduated pipettes have completely graduated stems and are meant to deliver very small quantities of solutions even smaller than 1 ml. However, they do not give very exact volumes of liquids.

With the advances in technology various types of automatic pipettes are now available. They can deliver very accurate quantities of solutions even in microlitre capacities. They are usually piston driven and can also be used to deliver corrosive and toxic liquids.

(v) Measuring Cylinders: These are graduated vessels meant to transfer liquids when only approximate volumes are needed. They are available as stoppered or unstoppered and are available in capacities from 5 ml up to 2 litres. The smaller cylinders up to 100 ml capacity are usually graduated in millilitres or fractions of a millilitre while those of larger capacity are graduated in units of 2, 5, 10, 20, 20, etc ml as per the size.

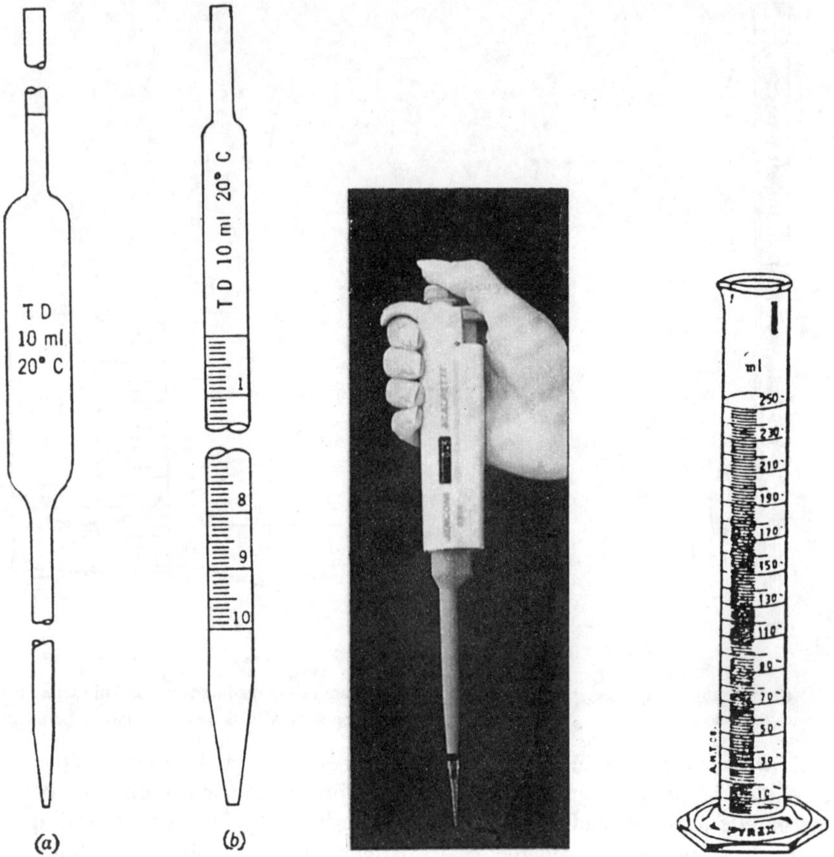

Fig. 1.4 (a) Transfer Pipette, (b) Measuring Pipette (c) Automatic Pipette

Fig. 1.5 Measuring Cylinder

(vi) *Apparatus for Filtration*: Various types of filtering apparatus are available for laboratory work in general and for gravimetric work in particular. These being (a) Sintered glass and sintered silica crucibles. (b) Gooch crucibles of porcelein or silica containing asbestos filter mats and (c) filter paper.

The sintered glass type of crucibles are commonly used now because they are convenient. They are available in various degrees of porosity numbers like 1, 2, 3, 4 etc. which indicate the decrease in pore size with increase in number i.e. No.3 crucible will be good for medium size particles while No.4 will be suitable for fine precipitates. They cannot be heated above 400°C.

Both Gooch and sintered crucibles have the advantage that filtration and washing can be done rapidly and neatly. They can be heated directly. Gooch crucibles require a soft rubber collar for a support when ready for filtration.

For the gravimetric work, Whatman No. 40, 41 or 42 filter papers are used because these have very small ash values.

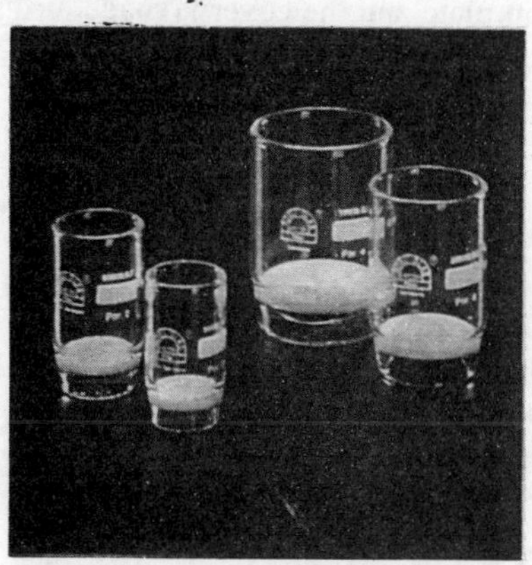
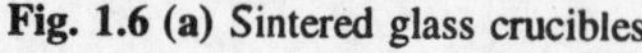

Fig. 1.6 (a) Sintered glass crucibles

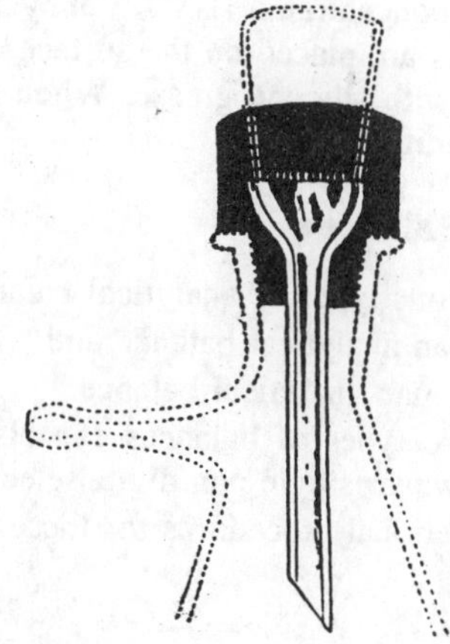

Fig. 1.6 (b) Gooch crucible assembly for filtration

No. 40 retains medium size particles and has medium speed while
No. 41 filter paper has fast speed and retains course particles,
No. 42 has slow speed and retains fine particles.

(vii) *Wash Bottles*: For use in pharmaceutical analysis wash bottles are prepared from flat-bottomed flasks of 500 ml capacity fitted with smoothly bent tubes and a jet on a rubber stopper as shown in the diagram. Now a days wash bottles made of poly-ethylene are available in various sizes and are convenient to use.

(viii) *Desiccator*: It consists of large glass vessel usually round in shape and provided with an airtight

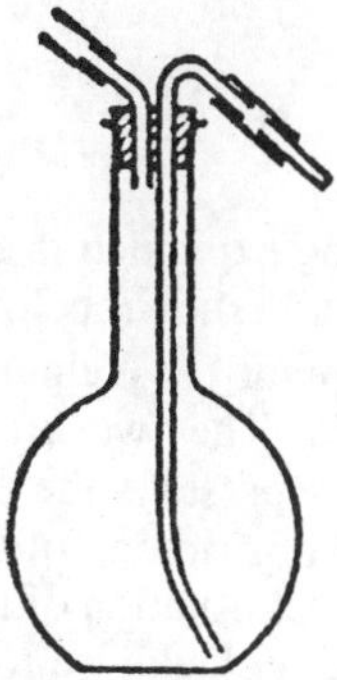

Fig. 1.7 Wash bottle for distilled water.

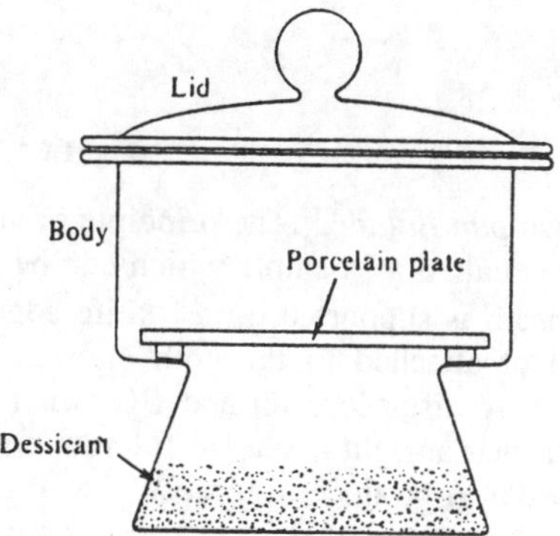

Fig. 1.8 Common form of desiccator.

cover. The cover may be provided with a side-arm stop-cock so that it can be attached to a vacuum pump and evacuated when needed.

The purpose of a desiccator is to provide a dry atmosphere for substances that might be affected by moisture or carbon dioxide. A desiccator partitioned into two portions or compartments which are usually separated by a perforated porcelein plate. The lower portion or compartment is filled with a dehydrating agent such as concentrated H_2SO_4 , anhydrous $CaCl_2$, P_2O_5, KOH pellets, silica gel etc. The crucibles or other apparatus are placed on the surface of the perforated porcelein plate and the cover is made airtight by coating it with silicone grease. When the desiccator is not in use, it should be either kept closed or in a clean condition.

1.5 Use of Balances

Although various types of analytical balances are available the two common ones are :

(a) two-pan analytical balance and

(b) single-pan analytical balance.

Both these types of balances can also be obtained in the form such that they can be electrically operated. However single-pan digital electronic balances are also available now.

The operational procedures for these two types of balances are described below.

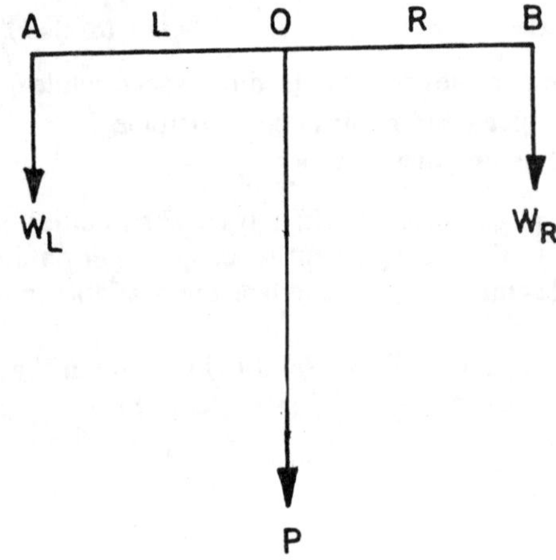

Fig. 1.9 "Two pan Balance Principle"

(a) *Two-pan Balance*: The principle of an analytical balance can be explained in terms of a "lever". The lever is called a "beam" which can be represented by the line A B shown below.

The beam is supported on a "knife edge" at its fulcrum i.e. at point O. Weights or objects can be suspended or attached to the both ends of the beam i.e. W_L & W_R. The two arms of the lever are represented by distances AO and BO which are equal. The line OP represents the "Pointer" which is rigidly attached at right angles to fulcrum and observes the horizontal positioning of the beam. A weight W_L attached at A produces a force $W_L \times L$ tending to cause counterclock rotation of the beam. Similarly, a weight W_R attached at B results in a force $W_R \times R$ tending to cause a clockwise rotation of the beam. When the forces causing clockwise and anticlockwise rotation equal other, the beam will be in a stationary horizontal position or oscillating back and forth about an equilibrium position in which state we can say that $W_L \times L = W_R \times R$.

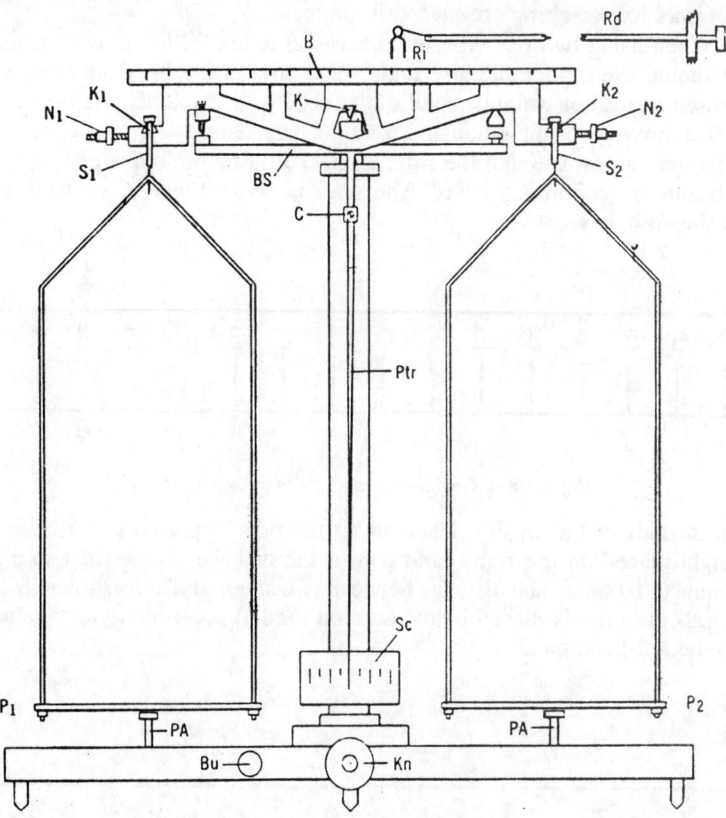

Fig. 1.10 Diagram of equal-arm rider balance. B, beam; K, central knife edge; P_1, P_2, pans, supported by stirrups S_1, S_2, with bearings resting on terminal knife edges K_1, K_2 ; N_1, N_2, nuts for adjusting horizontal equilibrium; Kn, knob to control beam support BS; PA, pan arrests, operated by button Bu; Ptr, pointer, which moves across scale Sc when beam is in motion; C, "bob" to adjust center of gravity; Ri, rider, placed on beam by operation of rod Rd.

The various components and their functions of a rider type two-pan balance are described below. The balance case is mounted on three brass legs which in some cases are placed in glass cups backed with rubber to prevent from slipping. The front legs are used to adjust the height and level the balance; the rear is of permanent length. The balance beam is mounted upon an upright in the centre on the top of which is an inlaid agate plate. The centre of the beam is placed on a steel or agate knife-edge on which are suspended the stirrups i.e. stirrups rest upon the corresponding knife-edges. The balance pans are attached to the stirrups. A pointer is attached to the Centre of the beam and as the beam oscillates the pointer moves in front of the scale near the base of the column. At the base of the column either in front or rear is fixed a spirit level. Within the upright is a mechanism which is controlled by a knob at the front of the balance case and is arranged in such a way as to raise the entire beam slightly just above the level at which knife-edges are in contact with the agate plates. A small weight or bob is attached to the pointer or to the beam by means of which the centre of gravity of the beam is regulated so that desired sensitivity of the balance is obtained. The sensitivity is factory regulated and rarely requires adjustments. At the bottom of the balance pans are two pan arrests which are operated by a knob from the front of the case. The arrests exert a very slight upward pressure upon the pans and minimise the displacement of the beam when objects for weighing are placed in the pans.

Use of a Rider: When using two-pan type of balances in the order to get very accurate weighings to the 4th decimal one should use a rider and also understand how to use it. A rider has a weight of 10 mg or 5 mg and can be used instead of weights smaller than 0.01 g. It is manipulated from outside by means of a sliding hook which moves over the graduated beam of the balance. Various types of graduated beams designed by manufacturers are in use and the rider is placed on the graduated scale of the beam. Three types of graduated beams are commonly noted. The scale is divided into 20 or 10 equal parts as in Fig 1.10 (a) (b) and (c) shown below.

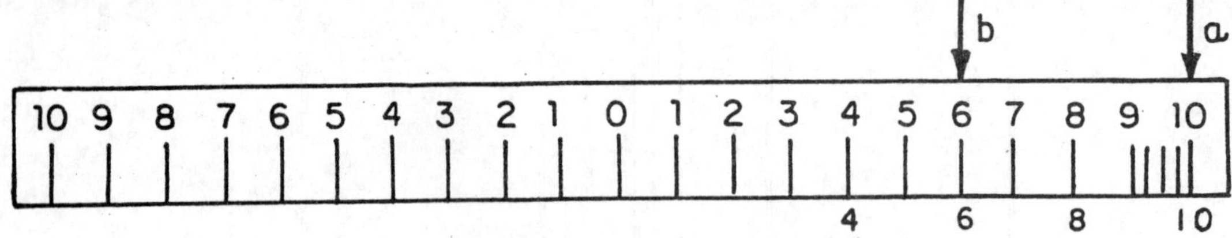

Fig. 1.10(a). Graduated beam of a two pan balance

When the beam is graduated as in Fig. 1.10a and if the rider is placed at "a" the effect is equal to that of a 0.01 g weight placed on the right hand pan of the balance. If the rider is placed at "b", the effective weight is equal to 0.006 g. The distance between two small divisions shown in scale A represents a weight of 0.0002 g. If the rider is placed below zero on the left hand section of the scale the effective weight is applied to the left-hand pan.

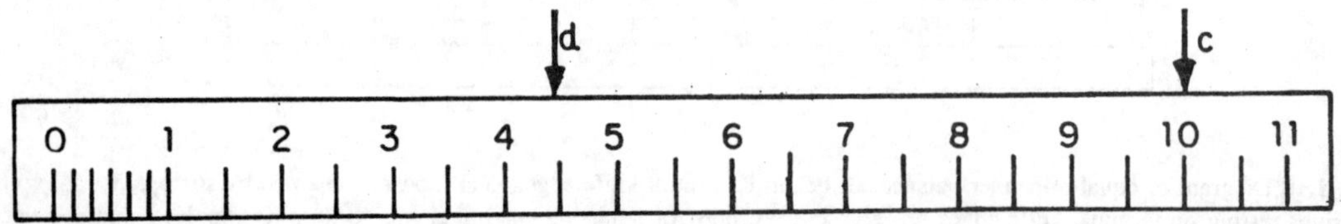

Fig. 1.10(b). Graduated beam of two pan balance.

A second type of graduated scale is shown is Fig. 1.10 b above. A 5 mg rider is used for such type of scale. In this case the zero position of the rider is on the beam at division zero and not on the hook itself. Thus the effective weight of the rider is always on the right-hand pan. If the rider is placed on position 'C' the effective weight is 0.01 g and when on position 'd' the effective weight is 0.0045 g on the pan. The distance between two small divisions represents a weight of 0.0001 g.

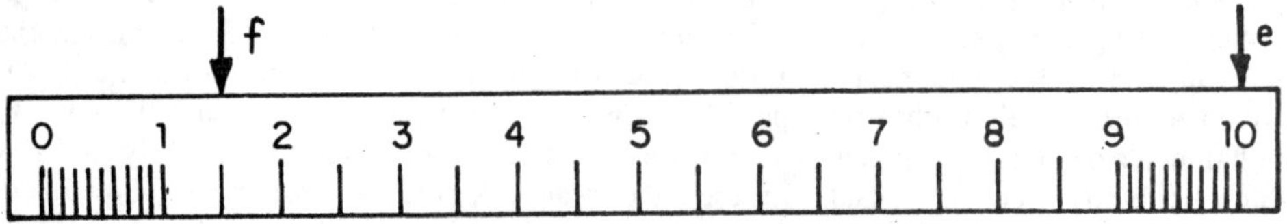

Fig. 1.10c. Graduated beam of a two pan balance

A third type of graduated beam is shown in Fig. 1.10c. In this case the scale divisions cover only half the effective length of the beam and a 10 mg rider is used. Here the zero position of the rider is at the zero division on the beam & effective weight of the rider is on the right-hand pan. If the rider is placed at position "e" i.e. the effective weight on the pan is 0.01 g and if at position 'f' it represents an effective weight of 0.0028g. The scale is subdivided in fifths and each small division is equal to 0.0002g.

(b) *Single-pan Analytical Balance* : The single-pan balance has the advantage of convenience as well as saving a lot of time on weighings. Different manufacturers have put up their own designs of single-pan balances but they have common features and operational procedures (Fig 1.11c).

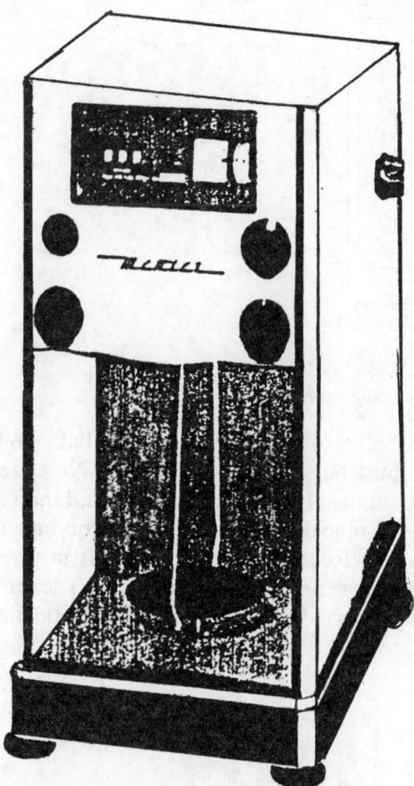

Fig. 1.11(a) Single-pan, constant-load analytical balance

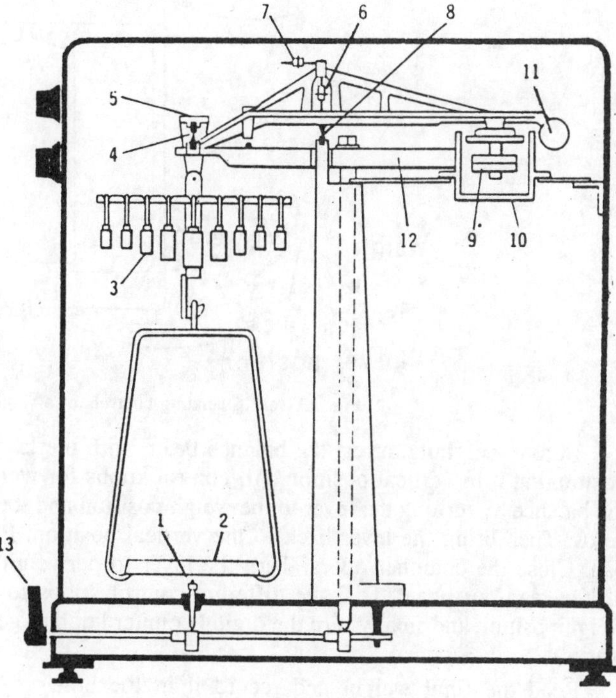

Fig. 1.11(b) single-pan, constant-load balance. 1, pan brake; 2, pan; 3, set of weights; 4, sapphire knife edge; 5, stirrup for hangers and weights; 6, movable weight for adjustment of sensitivity; 7, movable weight for initial adjustment of zero point; 8, main knife edge (sapphire); 9, counterweight; 10, air damper; 11, engraved optical scale; 12, lifting device; 13, arrest lever.

The balance consists essentially of a single pan which together with a set of concealed weights is suspended from a concealed beam. This combination is counter-poised by a fixed weight. The object to be weighed is placed on the pan and equilibrium is reached by removing from the pan end of the beam weights totaling the weight of the object. The beam is thus under a constant load regardless of the weight of the object and therefore the sensitivity of the balance is constant. There are no weight to be handled manually but they are removed by means of control knobs on the front panel of the balance and the figures corresponding to these weights appear on a direct reading scale. The weights less than 0.1 is indicated by the final beam deflection and is registered optically and automatically on an illuminated scale.

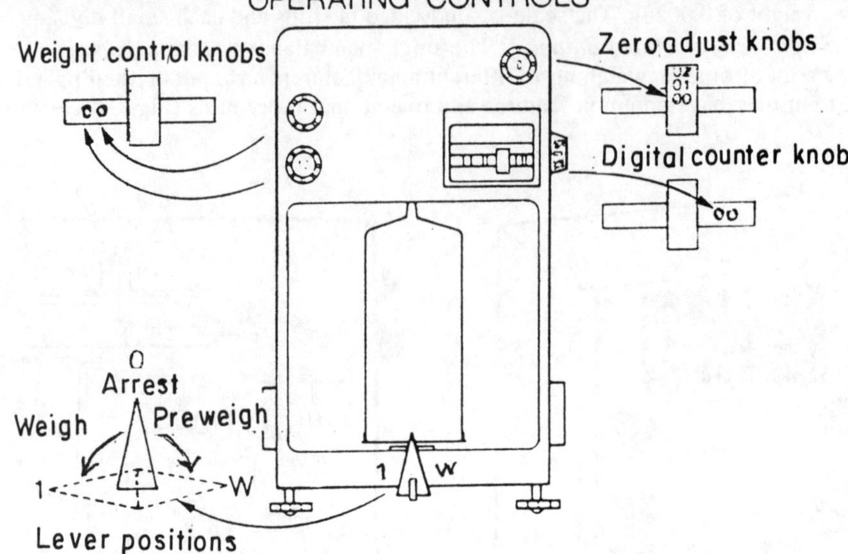

Fig. 1.11(c). Operating controls of a single-pan analytical balance.

Before weighing, arrest the balance beam with the lever at the bottom and centre of the balance by positioning it in vertical position. All control knobs for weights must be set to zero positions. Now, zero the balance by turning the lever to the weigh position and the readout panel or optical scale should indicate zeros. Then bring the lever back to the vertical position. Place the object to be weighed on the balance pan. Close the chamber doors. Turn the lever to perweigh position. Read the preweigh result in grams on the read out panel. Dial the different control knobs to preweigh result systematically. turn lever to weigh position and finally turn the digital counter knob to get the last two digits (weigh up to four decimal places).

Read the final weight and record it in the note book. After recording the weights, arrest the balance and remove the object from the balance pan. Return all knobs to zero positions and clean the balance and the surrounding.

The above procedure of operating a single-pan balance is common for most of them with minor variations. It is advisable to consult operating manuals or learn the operations from the instructor incharge.

(c) *Digital Electronic Balances*: Indian made or imported digital electronic balances are available but they are still expensive. They are easy to use and are direct reading. They are manufactured in various models but their features and operations are common.

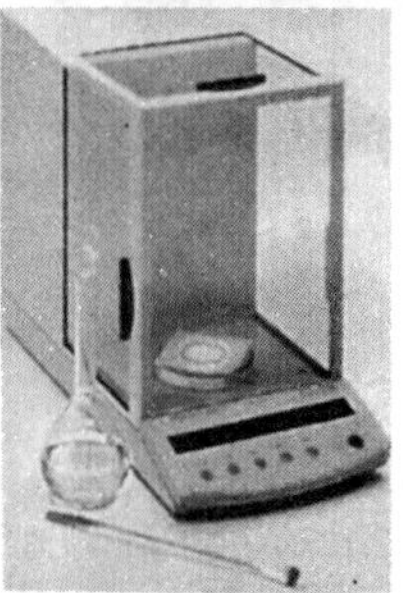

Fig. 1.12 An Electronic Balance

1.6 Methods of Weighing

The samples for analysis work can be weighed by two types of weighing procedures namely; (a) weighing by difference and (b) weighing by addition.

(a) *Weighing by difference*: Weigh accurately the weighing bottle. Place more than the specified amount of sample in the weighing bottle. Weigh the bottle and the contents accurately. Tip out the contents of the bottle into the receiving vessel. When most of the sample has been transferred, replace the stopper carefully to prevent the sample from being blown out of the bottle. Reweigh the bottle and contents. The difference between the two Weighings gives the weight of the sample. If the sample is hygroscopic in nature, exposure to atmosphere should be minimised.

(b) *Weighing by Addition*: In case of a solid sample, weigh the empty watch glass or weighing bottle or the vessel accurately and introduce the sample in small amounts until the correct weight has been added. Weigh the vessel along with the material accurately. Transfer the contents into a receiver slowly and wash the weighing vessel thoroughly with a jet of distilled water, collecting all the washings.

For a water-miscible liquid sample a similar procedure as described above is followed. The liquid sample is added into the weighing vessel by means of a test pipette without touching the rim of the vessel. After correct weight is added the sample is poured gently down into a receiving vessel in the above manner. Weighing vessel is washed down with a jet of distilled water.

In case of a water immiscible liquid sample, the liquid may be weighed directly into the vessel after the vessel is weighed empty. Care is taken that the liquid does not touch the rim of the vessel.

For volumetric work in general, the sample weighings should be within ± 0.0001 g and for gravimetric work, all weighings should be within ± 0.0002 g.

Care of the Balance: the Following rules should be observed in the handling of the analytical balances:

1. Test the adjustment of the balance before weighing and call an instructor if it requires an adjustment.
2. Brush the pan and surroundings of the balance before starting to weigh any substances.
3. No sample should be ever placed directly upon the balance pan.
4. Hot objects must never be placed inside the balance case.
5. After completion of a weighing the balance pan and surroundings should be cleaned.
6. All levers and knobs should be turned carefully and slowly.
7. Personal responsibility for the condition of the balance should be adopted.

1.7 Various Methods Of Drug Analysis

Every analytical determination is based on the measurement of some physical or structural property which is related directly or indirectly to the amount of the desired constituent present in the sample. Consequently various analytical methods available for drug analysis can be classified on the type of physical quantity which is measured. Thus we can identify four major common procedures namely; (a) volumetric (b) gravimetric (c) electrical (d) optical

The volumetric methods involves the measurement of volume. The various categories of volumetric procedures used for analysis are acid-base methods, oxidation — reduction methods, complexo-metric methods etc.

The gravimetric methods involves the measurement of weight. The method consists in the separation of the desired constituent in a form that is of known percentage composition and which can be weighed accurately. The various categories of gravimetric methods are precipitation methods, electrodeposition methods and volatilisation methods depending upon how the desired constituent is separated into a weighable form before its measurement.

The electrical methods of analysis incorporate all those methods in which the primary measurement deals with electrical quantity like voltage, resistance, current etc.

The optical methods of analysis are based on the interaction of radiant energy with matter and thus can be subdivided as absorption methods, diffraction methods etc.

In addition to the above described major procedures of analysis there are other properties which are made use of for analytical determinations e.g. various categories of chromatographic procedures, radiochemical methods, differential thermal analysis, particle size determination etc.

The important criteria for selectivity of a particular method are sensitivity, precision, accuracy and speed. The titrimetric and gravimetric methods are generally precise and give accuracy within one or two parts per thousand, while other methods do not reach this accuracy.

1.8 General Instructions for Analytical Work

In order to be a good successful analyst there are some general points which one should always keep in mind. These are described below:

(a) *Economy in Time*: An analyst whether working in an industry or a university should be consious that the analysis time is properly followed. He should study and plan his work but there should be no speed or callousness in quantitative work. He should understand the principles and procedures involved in our experiment. He should keep at least two operations at a time e.g. while cooling something he can make a weighing etc. or utilize time in between an operation by writting the experiment or making calculations. There should be no hold ups or wastage of time.

(b) *Cleanliness and tidyness:* The laboratory bench top and all glass apparatus should be very clean free from any grease, dust or impurities. All glassware should be cleaned with a cleaning solution or a detergent and then rinsed with distilled water. The bench-top should be dusted off and if possible shinned with wax. The apparatus should be neatly arranged on the bench-top or in the cup-board. All reagent bottles must be returned to their original shelves immediately after use and should not hang around.

(c) *Labelling*: On any quantitative work, all solution, filtrates, precipitates should be labelled as a matter of habit either by means of a glass marking pencil or on gummed labels.

(d) *Reagents*: In general all reagents meant for quantitative work should be pure. For drug analysis, they should meet the requirements as specified in the pharmacopoeias. Technical grade reagents are not pure and are not generally used in analytical work. Reagent grade materials can serve the purpose since the labels on the containers give the analysis and usually are highly purified. A chemical which is of very high purity and can be weighed directly and used. Laboratory instructor should make sure that adequate supplies of materials and reagents are available for a class.

(e) *Duplicate Estimations*: It is advisable to perform estimations in duplicate so that agreement on results can be established with confidence. The two results from a determination can be averaged if they are within 0.4%.

2

Drug Analysis and Quality Control

2.1 Drug Analysis

Drug analysis consists in the estimation of the purity and quality of drugs and fine chemicals which are used in pharmaceutical preparations. It also involves in the analysis of medicinal agents and their metabolites found in animals or human body. The scope of the pharmaceutical analysis can be extended by incorporating the analysis of the chemical constituents found in the human body whose altered concentrations during disease states serves as a diagnostic aid in the practice of medicine. However, the last named aspect can also be placed under clinical or analytical bio-chemistry and thus will not be touched upon as such in this text book.

2.2 Quality Control

A quality control programme for drug and cosmetic industry involves with batch-to-batch uniformity of a product insuring that the final product possesses desired characteristics of identity, purity, potency, uniformity, safety, efficacy and stability within established levels which meet all the legal, professional and company standards. In addition to the above stated requirements the quality control includes packing and storing in a manner that will retain the properties of the product, labelling that adequately describes the product, and expiry date and lastly the distribution in a manner that retains its potency.

The laws and standards for drug quality are laid down by state and central government agencies. These laws are applicable to (i) good manufacturing practices and also for (ii) new drug applications.

If a drug product is suspected to be defective or spurious the following information is collected on it: (a) trade name, dosage form and strength, (b) lot number or batch number, (c) date of purchase, (d) source of purchase, (e) name and address of manufacturer, (f) defect noted and suspected, (g) reporting pharmacists name. the above steps are then followed to determine if the product is indeed defective. This is achieved by (i) sending a portion of the sample to a laboratory for analysis (ii) calling and advising the drug manufacturing company of the defect involved in the product.

2.3 Sources of Impurities in Drug Products

In general, the various types of impurities that may be present in pharmaceutical substances can come from the following four sources: (a) the raw materials used, (b) the method of manufacture adopted, (c) due to the instability of the product and (d) from the atmospheric contaminants.

(a) Raw Materials: The impurities already present in the starting material may be carried through during the various stages of manufacturing process and thus contaminate, the final compound or the active ingredient.

(b) Method of Manufacture: During the manufacturing process, in addition to the impurity that is already present in the starting material new impurities may enter the active ingredient. This can be through (i) reagents (ii) solvents and (iii) reaction vessels.

(i) *Reagents*: There are many ways by which reagents can contaminate a final product, e.g. sodium carbonate contains soluble alkali and its traces are liable to remain if it is not properly washed during a process. Another example is use of hydrogen peroxide which contains traces of barium. Presence of sulphate can be due to use of sulphuric acid in a process.

(ii) *Solvents*: Water in general is commonly used for washings etc in a manufacturing process and thus can commonly give rise to traces of impurities like Na^+, Ca^{2+}, Mg^{2+}, CO_3^{2-}, Cl^- and SO_4^{2-} . However these impurities will not arise if distilled water is used which is prohibitive on a large scale from the point of view of its cost.

(iii) *Reaction Vessels*: These are constructed from various types of metals like Copper, iron, galvanized iron, lead and stainless steel. The solvents when not fully removed may cause corrosion through their action and in this manner traces of metals may pass into solutions and eventually contaminate the final product. If reactor vessels made of glass are used, may give traces of alkali to the solvents.

(c) *Chemical Instability*: It is observed that many drug products undergo chemical decomposition when not stored under proper conditions. The decomposition is facilitated by factors like light, traces of acid, alkali and even air. Therefore , in such cases preservatives and antioxidants are added to prevent any decompositions.

(d) *Atmosphere Contamination*: The drug produces can also pick up impurities from atmosphere and these are likely to come from dust, SO_2, H_2S, CO_2, water vapour and possibly soot, sulpher, silica etc.

2.4 Limit Tests For Inorganic Substances :

These tests have been designed to control the amount of impurities likely to be present in the drug substances and they may come from any of the sources stated above. The limit tests can identify and estimate small quantities of various inorganic impurities. They are usually selective in which case they react with trace amounts of the impurity. Various types of limit tests as prescribed by pharmacopoeias are described below:

(i) Limits of Moisture and Volatile Matter: Some of the drug products are hygroscopic and have tendency to absorb moisture on storage. Such substances when dried may undergo a loss in weight. The amount of heat to which the substance is submitted will vary according to the nature of the substance. The temperatures used are such that decomposition of the material does not occur and substances are dried under specific conditions so that official limits on the weight loss are not crossed. For example ethisterone is heated at 105° for constant weight for several hours whereas mercuric oxide is heated at 105° for 1 hour only. Hyoscine hydrobromide is dried slowly from 20° to 105°C for 30 minutes & then at 105°C for constant weight. For many drug products, drying under vacuum can be applied e.g. Isoprenaline sulphate etc. and then official assay performed. The amount of water present in the hydrated salt is estimated by Karl Fisher method and official limits can be observed. e.g. procain penicillin. In a similar manner when assay procedures are performed for inorganic salt hydrates the official moisture limits should be observed and accordingly weighd, e.g. sodium chloride, sodium sulphate, sodium benzoate, sodium salicylate etc.

(ii) Limits of Soluble Matter: This requirement is applied with the aim to put a limit on the soluble impurities in drugs. The drug itself is completely insoluble in a particular solvent and thus a specific impurity can be detected. For example the amount of barium salts soluble in water can be excluded from Barium sulphate used for X-ray work on patients, the amount of tartaric acid in Potassium Acid Tartrate can be controlled by treatment with 90% ethanol. Other examples are presence of soluble matter is Kaolin which can be removed by and amount of treatment with acid mercuric chloride in mercurous Chloride which can be removed with water.

(iii) Limit of Insoluble matter: The pharmacopoeial monographs specify on the limits of insoluble matter present in the official substances. For example Phenobarbitone contains phenylbarbituric acid which can be removed by boiling with 90% ethanol. Similarly sodium chloride as an inpurity present in chloramine can be removed by treatment with cold dehydrated alcohol. The contamination of Lead acetate with basic acetates can be detected by their solubility in water.

(iv) Limits of Non-volatile Matter: The limits for the presence of non-volatile matter can me applied to both inorganic and organic substance which are readily volatile. However, in case of inorganic substances they are applied in order to control contamination with dirt and other salts. Some of the official substances which can be examined for presence of non-volatile matter are camphor, menthol, anaesthetic ether, chloroform, hydrogen peroxide solution, ammonia solution etc.

(v) Limits of Residue on Ignition: Such limits are imposed on two types of compounds: (a) those which are completely ignited when ignited and (b) those which undergo decomposition leaving a residue of definite composition. The example of the latter type are substances like heavy and light magnesium carbonate. These decompose giving off CO_2 & Water and leaving a residue of oxide. The example for the former group can be yellow mercuric oxide.

(vi) Loss on Ignition: This kind of test is applicable to substances which contain thermolabile impurities. The examples of such substances are light and heavy magnesium oxides containing corresponding carbonates as impurities. Another example is lead monoxide which contains carbonate and moisture and can be submitted to this test or limit.

Method: Heat a clean crucible on a pipeclay triangle in a hot Bunsen burner for 10 minutes. Cool in a desiccator for about 20 minutes and weight. Repeat until constant weight is attained. Introduce about 1 g of sample into the Crucible, reweigh and then heat strongly for about 1 hour. Cool in a desiccator and reweigh. Repeat the heating for further 30 minutes, cool and reweigh. Repeat the heating and cooling until constant weight is obtained.

(vii) Ash Values: In the crude drugs, the amount of ash which is left after incinerations represents the inorganic residue. This residue gives us the drug plus the inorganic matter that may have come from the external source. Thus official limits have been set for ash values in the case of powdered drugs. The determination of these values have following uses:

(i) to establish that undue amount of external inorganic matter such as sand, floor sweepings, earth etc. has not been accidently introduced during collection and subsequent treatments.

(ii) to essure that other components of plant do not get mixed up e.g. cardamom fruit etc.

(iii) to eliminate adulteration with stone cells, starch etc which can change the values.

(iv) to eliminate adulteration or mix up with the exhausted drug material e.g. Ginger etc.

In general four different types of ash values are notified in the pharmacopoeias; namely: (a) total ash (b) acid-insoluble ash (c) Water insoluble ash and (d) sulphated ash.

EXERCISE 1. Determination of total ash in Ginger.

Method: Ignite a silica dish to a constant weight under low uniform temperature over an Argand burner. Weigh about 2 to 3 g of powdered drug and spread it evenly on the bottom of the dish. Ignite again at low temperature until vapours have ceased to evolve and then increase the temperature till just red hot to burn off carbon. Cool in a desiccator and weigh. Repeat the process of heating and cooling until constant weight is obtained. In case Carbon-free ash is not formed, extract the residue with hot water, filter through ashless filter paper, incinerate the residue & filter paper in the silica dish until all carbon is removed using a higher temperature if necessary. Add filtrate to the dish, evaporate to dryness and ignite again to a constant weight. Calculate the percentage of ash with reference to air-dried drug.

EXERCISE 2. Determination of acid-soluble ash in Rhubarb.

Method: Transfer the total ash obtained from above into a beaker using 25 ml dilute HCl. Boil for 5 minutes. Transfer the insoluble residue to a previously prepared, ignited and weighed Gooch crucible. Wash well with hot water, filter under suction to remove water and place it in another crucible. Ignite it to a dull read heat, cool in a desiclator and weigh. Calculate the percentage of acid-insoluble ash with reference to air dried drug.

EXERCISE 3. Determination of water-soluble ash in Ginger.

Method: The procedure is similar to that used for acid-soluble ash except 25 ml of water is used in place of 25 ml acid. The weight of the insoluble residue is subtracted from the weight of the total ash, the difference being the weight of the water-soluble ash. Calculate the percentage of the water-soluble ash with reference to air-dried drug.

EXERCISE 4. Determination of sulphated ash in Acetylsalicylic acid(Aspirin).

Method: Ignite a silica crucible until constant weight is attained. Introduce about 5 g of sample, reweigh, moisten with H_2SO_4 and heat gently at first and then strongly till volatile matter is removed. Ignite more strongly to remove the carbon , cool, remoisten with H_2SO_4 and then reignite until constant weight is attained. Calculate the percentage of sulphated ash. The test can be applied to colchicine, lignocaine HCl, benzyl benzoate, to unorganised drugs like colophony, podophyllum resin, wool alcohols as well as to citric acid.

(viii) Precipitation Methods: This test is applied to detect small amounts of impurities like iron, aluminium, silica etc in potassium hydroxide. The method consists is taking a sample of about 5 g and boiling it with excess of dil HCl. It is then made alkaline on treatment with NH_3. Any metallic hydroxide formed is collected, dried and ignited. The limit for Fe, Al etc. is 0.005 g.

2.5 General Limit Test For Chlorides :

This test is used to limit the amount of chloride as an impurity in inorganic substances. The procedure consists in the precipitation of the chloride from the sample with $AgNO_3$ in the presence of dilute HNO_3. The opalescent solution obtained from the sample is compared with a standard opalescence obtained from a known amount of chloride ions. The two opalescent solutions are compared by placing them in an identical pair of Nessler glasses.

EXERCISE 5. Determination of chloride in sodium sulphate.

Method: As pointed out in above two solutions involved are sample solution and standard solution which are prepared as described below.

Standard Solution : Place 1 ml of 0.01 N HCl in a test tube, add 10 ml of dil HNO_3 and dilute to 50 ml with water. Add 1 ml of 5% $AgNO_3$ solution and stir.

Sample Solution : Weigh the sample as per stated in a monograph and dissolve in water. Add 10 ml of dilute HNO_3 and dilute to 50 ml with water. Add 1 ml of 5% $AgNo_3$ solution and stir. compare the opalescence of two solution after five minutes. The opalescence of test solutions should not be greater than that of standard.

2.6 General Limit Test for Sulphates :

The aim of the test is to control the impurity due to sulphate in inorganic substances. The test is based on the precipitation of SO_4^{2-} ,with barium chloride in the presence of hydrochloric acid and traces of barium sulphate. The opalescent solution so obtained is compared with a standard turbidity containing a known amount of SO_4^{2-} ion.

EXERCISE 6. Determination of sulphate in lactic Acid.

Method : The test is carried out as explained above and following solutions are required.

Barium Sulphate reagent : Prepare M/2 barium chloride solution and dilute 15 ml with 20 ml sulphate free alcohol (95%) and 55 ml water. Add 5 ml of potassium sulphate solution (0.0181% W/V) and dilute to 100 ml with water.

Sample Solution: Weigh the sample as per monograph and dissolve in water. Add 2 ml of dilute HCl and dilute to 45 ml with water. Add 5 ml of freshly prepared $BaSO_4$ reagent and stir.

Standard solution: Pipette 1.25 ml of N/100 H_2SO_4 into a beaker. Add 2 ml of dilute HCl and dilute to 45 ml with water. Add 5 ml of freshly prepared $BaSO_4$ reagent and stir.

The two solutions are transferred into identical pair of Nessler glasses and their turbidity compared after 5 minutes.

2.7 General Limit Test for Iron

The test depends on the formation of a purple colour by reaction of the iron with thioglycollic acid in a solution buffered with ammonium citrate and comparison of the colour produced with a standard colour containing a known amount (0.04 mg) of iron. The purple colour obtained is due to formation a coordination compound ferrous thioglycollate while ferric iron is reduced to ferrous state by the reagent as shown by the following reactions.

$$2Fe^{3+} + 2CH_2\ SHCOOH \longrightarrow 2Fe^{2+} + COOHCH_2\ S.S.CH_2\ COOH + 2H^+$$

$$Fe^{2+} + 2CH_2\ SH\ COOH \longrightarrow \begin{matrix} CH_2\ .SH & & O.CO \\ | & Fe & \\ COO & & HS.CH_2 \end{matrix} \quad +2H$$

EXERCISE 7. Determination of iron in Sodium Chloride.

Method : The test has been explained as in above and following solutions are required.

Standard Iron Solution FeT : This solution is prepared from ferric ammonium sulfate (0.173 g) and 5 ml dilute HCl. The mixture is further diluted to 1000 ml. Each ml of solution now contains 0.02 mg of iron.

Sample Solution: Weigh the specific amount of sample as per monograph. Dissolve in 35 ml of water. Add 2 ml of 20% W/V aqueous citric acid, FeT and then 2 drops of thioglycollic acid. Make the solution alkaline with dilute NH_3 solution, FeT and then dilute to 50 ml with water.

Standard Solution: Dilute 2 ml of standard iron solution FeT with 40 ml of water. Add 2 ml of 20% W/V aqueous citric acid FeT and then add 2 drops of thioglycollic acid. Make the solution alkaline with dilute NH_3 solution FeT and dilute to 50 ml water.

The colour of the two solutions is compared after 5 minutes. The colour of the test solution should not be more intense than the standard solution.

2.8 TEST FOR LEAD

This test is based on principle that traces of lead salts if present are converted to lead sulphide by the addition of Na_2S to a slightly alkaline solution buffered by a high concentration of ammonium acetate. The brown colour obtained due to the presence of colloidal PbS in the sample solution is compared with that obtained from a known amount of lead. The contamination due to lead varies greatly with the substance and depends on the source and the method of manufacture.

Method: The following solutions are required for its determination.

Dilute lead solution PbT: It is a solution of lead nitrate (0,016g) containing nitric acid (0.5 ml) diluted to 1 litre with water. Thus each ml of solution will contain equivalent of 0.01 mg of lead.

Primary Solution: Dissolve X g or as specified in monograph of the sample in hot water containing specific volume of acetic acid. Boil the solution to remove any CO_2 present. Add dilute ammonia PbT until solution becomes alkaline and then 1 ml of Potassium cyanide solution PbT (10%).

(The purpose of addition of KCN is to convert Cu & Fe if present to cyanides so that they do not precipitate as sulphides). Filter the solution. Dilute the solution to 50 ml with water. Add 2 drops of sodium sulphide solution PbT and stir.

Auxillary solution: Dissolve y g or as specified in the monograph of sample in hot water containing specific volume of acetic acid. Boil the solution to remove CO_2 if any. Add specified amount of dilute lead solution PbT. The rest of the steps are as indicated in the preparation of primary solution.

Finally, the colour of the two solutions are compared, the colour of the primary solution should not be darker than that of the auxillary. It should be remembered that the acetic acid required in the test should not contain more than 1 PPM lead and is not needed if the substance is acidic in nature. Further the method requires modification depending upon he nature of the substance.

2.9 Test For Arsenic

The test for arsenic is based on the procedure in which all arsenic if present is converted into arsine (AsH_3) by reduction with zinc and hydrochloric acid. The reaction of the issuing gases with mercuric chloride paper producers a yellow stain which can be compared with that produced from a known amount of arsenic. The presence of a small amount of stannous chloride in HCl ensures a quick reaction between zinc and acid with the evolution of hydrogen. Pure zinc is not reactive towards HCl and thus the presence of a small quantity of tin increases the rate of reaction. The hydrogen formed reduces any arsenic present to arsine, AsH_3 which passes out and reacts with mercuric chloride as shown by the reaction: $2AsH_3 + HgCl_2 \longrightarrow Hg(AsH_2)_2 + 2HCl$. Other arsenic salts like $AsH(HgCl)_2$, As (HgCl) and As_2Hg_3 may also be formed. These products on reaction with mercuric chloride paper produce a yellow spot. The test is applied at the same time on two solutions, one containing the sample and the other containing a known amount of arsenic. The stains produced on the mercuric chloride paper are compared, the depth of the colour produced is proportional to the amount of arsenic present.

Specific methods in pharmacopoeias may be consulted on individual substances for the determination of arsenic.

EXERCISE 8. Determination of arsenic in calcium lactate.

Method: The following solutions are required for its determination.

Dilute arsenic solution As T: It is prepared from 0.0132 g of arsenic trioxide to which is added 5 ml HCl and diluted to 1000 ml with water. Each ml of the solution contains 0.01 mg of As. This solution serves as a standard solution.

Sample Solution: Dissolve 5 g of sample in 50 ml of and 12 ml of stannated HCl and transfer to a bottle. Add 1 gm of KI to the solution which produces HI to convert Pentavalent arsenic to trivalent state and during which arsine is also formed through reduction. Add 10 g of granulated zinc AsT to the solution and fix a delivery tube to which is attached a mercuric chloride paper. Allow the reaction to proceed at room temperature for 40 minutes and warm to 40° if needed.

Standard Solution: Dilute the arsenic solution AsT between 0.2 and 1 ml. Add 10 ml of standard HCl AsT and then dilute with 50 ml water The rest of the procedure is same as in the sample solution.

After 40 minutes compare the yellow stain from the sample and the standard. The colour of the sample should not be darker than that of the standard stain.

Calcium lactate should not contain more than 2 PPM of As.

The colours prduced by a 5 g sample and 1 ml of dilute arsenic solution AsT are compared. If the colours from the two are equal we have :

5 g of sample contains 1×10^{-5} of As

$$\therefore \quad " \quad " \quad " \quad " \quad " \quad " \quad \frac{1 \times 10^{-5}\, g}{5g}$$

$$\therefore \quad 1{,}000{,}000 \text{ g sample contains } \frac{1 \times 1000{,}000 \text{ g}}{100000 \times 5 \text{ g}}$$

$$= 2.0 \text{ g of As}$$

2.10 Tests For Heavy Impurities

In general, metallic type of impurities are detected by standard procedures of inorganic qualitalive analysis which involve colour and precipitation reaction. The procedures are briefly outlined below.

(i) Heavy Metals: For heavy metals setting aside alkali and alkaline earths the two reagents used are hydrogen sulphide or sodium and ammonia. Addition of an excess of NH_3 to the sample may or may not produce a colour or precipitate and conclusions may be drawn accordingly as shown in table below.

Insoluble in excess NH_4OH	Soluble in excess NH_4OH		Precipitation prevented by adding NH_4 salts	Precipitated in the presence of phosphate
Hg^+ , Hg^{2+} , Pb,	Cu	Blue Solution	Co, Ni, Mn,	Mg, Ca, Sr, Ba
Bi, Sn, Al,	Ni		Zn, Mg,	
Fe(Co)(Mg)	Ag		Fe^{2+}	
(Mn)	Cd	Colourless Solution		
	Zn			
	Cr	Pale violet solution		

In a similar manner the heavy metal impurities precipitated as sulphides by the addition of H_2S or Na_2S are shown in the table below. Conclusions are accordingly drawn.

Precipited in the presence of mineral acid	Precipited in the presence of a weak acid	Precipited by NH_3 and H_2 S	
		KCN absent	KCN present
Ag,Hg,Pb, Bi,Cu,As, Sb,Sn,(Cd)	Zn,Ni,Co	All the metals in the preceding Columns,	A large group of Metals form complex salts with KCN from except AS, which they are not Sb(Sn) PPtd. as sulphides by H_2S. The following give ppts with KCN. Pb(black), Zn(white), Cd(Yellow).

(ii) Alkaline Earth Metals : As barium salts are usually used in the removal of large amounts of sulphate ions, they become a common impurity. They are tested by the addition of dilute H_2SO_4. Calcium sulphate does not get precipitated unless present in large quantity because it is soluble. Strontium is not generally found as impurity but will precipitate along with Ba if present. Calcium can be precipited with ammonium oxalate in presence of NH_3. Magnesium is precipited along with calcium as phosphate in the presence of NH_3.

(iii) Alkali Metals: Although no specific tests are applied but the common method to limit them is to boil the sample with water, filter, evaporate the filtrate to dryness and weighed.

(iv) Acid radical Impurities: Simple procedures are available to detect and limit the presence of nitrate, oxalate, phosphate, fluoride, and silicate. Pharmacopoeias should be consulted for their specific tests.

2.11 Impurities In Organic Medicinal Substances :

So far we have discussed the contamination among the inorganic substances and how to control them by limit tests. It is to be understood that organic medicinal substances get contaminated in exactly the same manner during their manufacturing processes.

Since the organic drug substances belong to a very wide range of chemical groups and at the same time the contaminating impurities being of varied nature the task of detecting impurities becomes a difficult job. Therefore, the contaminating impurities for organic medicinal compounds can be classified into (a) inorganic impurities (b) organic impurities and (c) contamination by chemical intermediates.

(a) Inorganic Impurities: The control of inorganic impurities has already been dealt upon in some detail. However for organic medicinals there are some special specific test to detect ammonium salts, heavy metals, acid radicals as well as free halogen and halide ions. These tests can be found in pharmacopoeias.

(b) Organic Impurities : One of the most common method of limiting the organic impurity is the determination of melting points for active ingredients. In some of the medicinals a melting point range is allowed e.g. phenobarbitone (m.p. 174-77°) atropine (m.p. 115-18°) etc. to give an allowance for storage effect. Along with melting point other physical constants like refractive index, optical rotation and weight/ml etc. wherever applicable can also be measured as a criteria for purity.

In addition to the above stated physical constants specific organic impurities can be controlled by performing functional group tests to determine contamination by say e.g. sugars, ketones, aldehydes and unsaturated substances etc.

Anaesthetic ether, ethyl oleate etc. can be submitted for peroxide contamination since peroxides are toxic.

Ethyl alcohol used for galenicals etc. can be tested for contamination due to methanol.

(c) Contamination by chemical Intermediates: The organic synthetic drug products can get contaminated by trace amounts of intermediates used in their manufacture. Tests are given in official monographs to detect and control their presence.

2.12 Quality Control for Alkaloids

It is a well known fact that the plant materials do not contain alkaloids as single constituents but rather in the form of a mixture of constituents or in combination with other chemical substances. Separation of alkaloids is very tedious and contamination from other alkaloids cannot be avoided. However, a provision for exclusion of such impurities is necessary and such tests are given in official monographs.

2.13 Quality Control for Fixed Oils and Fats

An impression has been created among people that some unscrupulous manufacturers have tendency to adulterate fixed oils and fats by sophisticated means or their storage facilities are not good and thus they become rancid. The adulteration in the edible oils and fats can be established by determining acid value, saponification value, iodine value and ester value etc.

2.14 WATER CONTENT

Many official drugs contain varying amounts of water either in the form of water of crystallisation i.e. hydrates or in absorbed form. Therefore it is important to specify limits of water content in order to maintain some sort to uniformity in these drugs. It is necessary to determine accurately the water or moisture content in crude drugs and other substances so that when they are sold their active constituents conform to the official specifications of the assay.

Water content can be determined by any one of the following procedures: (a) gravimetric, for drugs containing no constituents other than water volatile at 105°C; (b) gravimetric, for drugs containing ether-soluble constituents volatile at 105°C; (c) Azeotropic; (d) Karl Fisher (Titrimetric); (e) dew point; (f) hygrometric.

For the procedure (a) about 10 g of drug is accurately weighed and dried in an oven at 105°C for 5 hrs. After 5 hrs. the sample is weighed and again dried at 1 hr intervals until weight loss is not more than 0.25% in 1 hr of drying. The weight loss of the drug represents the moisture present in the drug sample.

The method (C) is also known as ''xylene method'' or ''toluene distillation method'' and requires a small apparatus for collection of water. The method has disadvantage that large amount of drug about 50-100 g are required for the estimation.

EXERCISE 9. Determination of the Moisure content of Digitalis by Azeotropic precedure.

Method: Place in a dry 500 ml round bottom flask 50 g of accurately weighed substance. Introduce a few capillary melting point tubes, sealed at the upper end to prevent any bumping. Place about 200 ml of toluene in the flask, connect the Liebig condenser and the moisture-tube receiver as shown in the Fig. 2.1

Heat the flask gently for 15 minutes, when the toluene begins to boil, distil at the rate of 2 drops per second until most of wate has passed over, then increase the rate of distillation to about 4 drops per second.

When the water has distilled over, rinse the inside of the condenser tube with toluene and brush it down the tube. Continue the distillation for 5 mins, then remove the heat and allow the apparatus to cool to room temperature. Force down any water droplets which adhere to the walls of the moisture receiver tube either by rotating or by tapping the tube. When water and toluene layers have separated completely, read the volume of water and calculate its percentage in the substance.

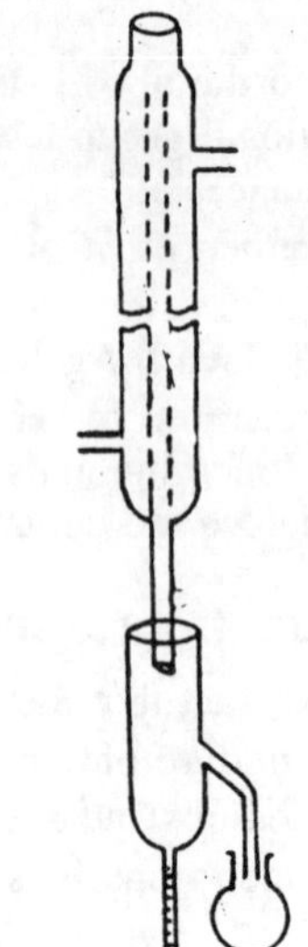

Fig. 2.1 Dean stark distillation appartus

Electrometric Determination of Water: The most important method of determination of water content is the Karl Fisher electrometric titration method. It is widely applied for moisture determination of drug substances because it is very rapid, specific and requires very small amounts of sample.

The method consists of titration of sample in methanol in Karl Fisher reagent which incorporates iodine, sulpher dioxide, pyridine and methanol. The reactions involved are shown as:

$$I_2 + SO_2 + H_2O \longrightarrow 2HI + SO_3$$

$$SO_3 + C_5H_5N \longrightarrow C_5H_5N.SO_3 \text{ (Pyridine—sulfur-trioxide)}$$

$$HI + C_5H_5N \longrightarrow C_5H_5N.HI$$

$$C_5H_5N.SO_3 + CH_3OH \longrightarrow C_5H_5N.\ HSO_4CH_3$$

It is clearly seen that 1 mol of water is equivalent to 1 mol of iodine. Pyridine reacts with SO_3 forming a complex which neutralises HI thereby prevents its oxidation to I_2. Methanol reacts with pyridine—sulpher-trioxide. In the absence of methanol water reacts with the complex, and 2 moles of water is then equivalent to 1 mol of iodine.

$$C_5\ H_5N.SO_3 + H_2O \longrightarrow C_5H_5N.\ H_2SO_4$$

Karl Fisher titration apparatus is commercially available and consists of one or two automatic buretts, a tightly covered tiration vessel fitted with electrodes and a magnetic stirrer. The air in the systems kept dry with P_2O_5, anhydrous $CaCl_2$ or silica gel.

The procedure consists in setting of a movable contact of a potentiometer to the position which gives a current of 5 to 10 mA through the circuit with the platinum electrodes immersed in the solution to be titrated. Before the titrant is added the resistance of the cell is high and most current coming from the battery flows in the upper leg of the circuit, thereby causing an increase to be shown by the microammeter. The end point is taken when the current flow increase to between 50 & 100 mA for 30 seconds or longer depending on the solution being titrated.

EXERCISE 10. Standardistion of Karl Fisher reagent.

Method: Place 36 ml of methanol in the titration vessel and add sufficient amount of Karl Fisher reagent to give the characteristic end point. Weigh accurately 150-350 mg of sodium tartrate ($Na_2C_2H_4O_6.2H_2O$) and transfer it to the titration vessel and titrate to the end point.

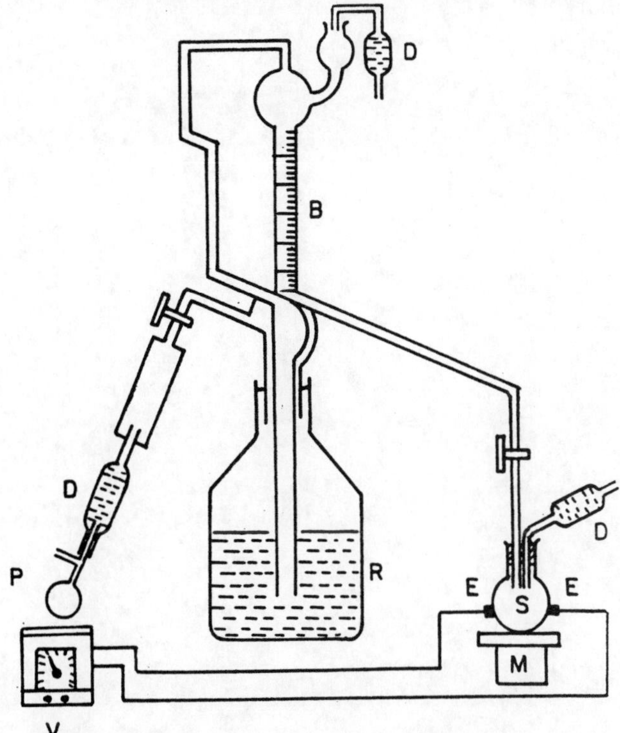

Fig. 2.2a. Karl Fisher titration apparatus
B = burrete, D = desicant, E = Platinum electrodes, M = magnetic stirrer, P = pressure bulb, R = reservoir for solution, S = stirring bar, V = Polarizer indicator.

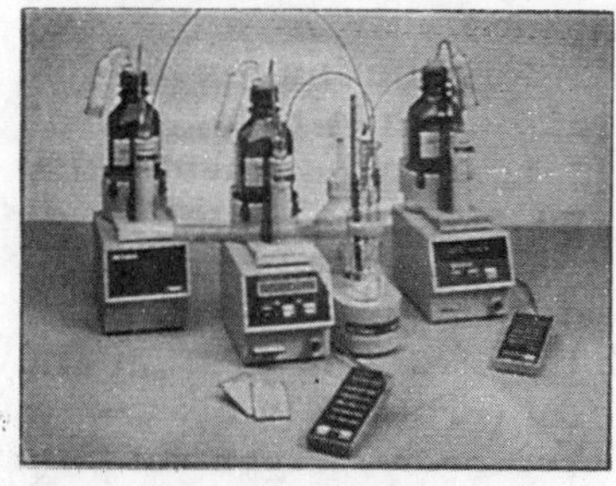

Fig. 2.2b. A modern Karl Fisher titration apparatus
(Courtesy of Metrohm Ltd.)

The water equivalence factor F, in mgs of H_2O per ml of reagent is calculated according to the formula $0.1566 \times \frac{W}{V}$, where W is the weight in mgs of sodium tartrate and V is the volume in ml of the reagent.

Each mg of sodium tartrate is equivalent to :

$$\frac{2H_2O}{Na_2C_4H_4O_6.2H_2O} = \frac{36.04}{230.08} = 0.1566 \text{ mg of } H_2O$$

Therefore, if V ml of Karl Fisher is required in titration of W mg of sodium tartrate, each ml of reagent is equivalent to $0.1566 \times \frac{W}{V}$ mg of H_2O. As the titration progresses the colour changes to brownish yellow which becomes amber colour at the end point when a slight excess of reagent has been added.

SECTION-B
CHEMICAL OR CLASSICAL METHOD OF ANALYSIS

3

Acidimetric And Alkalimetric Methods

3.1 General

The definitions for acids and bases have been put forward by Lowry and Bronsted and also G.N. Lewis. According to Bronsted and Lowry an acid is a substance which when dissolved in water undergoes dissociation with the formation of hydrogen ions, e.g. nitric acid and hydrochloric acid dissociate as follows :

$$HNO_3 \rightleftharpoons H^+ + NO_3$$

$$HCl \rightleftharpoons H^+ + Cl^-$$

A base is defined as a substance which when dissolved in water undergoes dissociation with the formation of hydroxyl ions e.g. sodium hydroxide and potassium hydroxide dissociate as :

$$Na\,OH \rightleftharpoons Na^+ + OH$$

$$KOH \rightleftharpoons K^+ + OH$$

On the basis of Lewis definition an acid is a substance that can accept an electron pair from a base and a base is a substance that can donate a pair of electrons to an acid. In other words a Lewis acid has an incomplete electron shell so that it can accept an electron pair from a Lewis base to complete that electron shell. Another consequence of these definitions is that the loss of proton by a Bronsted - Lowey acid gives rise to the formation of corresponding Bronsted - Lowry base which is called the ''conjugate base''of the parent acid.

In the same way, the addition of a proton to any Bronsted-Lowry base leads to the formation of ''conjugate acid'' of the parent base, e.g.

$$H_2O \rightleftharpoons HO^- + H^+$$

$$H_3O^+ \rightleftharpoons H_2O + H^+$$

$$NH_4^+ \rightleftharpoons NH_3 + H^+$$

$$HCO_3^- \rightleftharpoons CO_3^{2-} + H^+$$

It is to be remembered that the hydrogen ions do not exist by itself in the solution, but combine with one or more molecules of water to form hydronium ions.

$$H^+ + H_2O \rightleftharpoons H_3O^+$$

Further, one should realise that the inherent tendency in an acid to lose its proton is very much related to the affinity of the solvent for proton and therefore will determine the "strength" of an acid. For example, hydrochloric acid in water will behave as a stong acid and the reaction will proceed to the right because water acting as a base has much stronger affinity for a proton than does the chloride ion.

$$HCl + H_2O \rightleftharpoons Cl^- + H_2O$$

On the contrary, hydrochloric acid behaves as a weak acid in methanol because methanol molecules do not attract protons as readily as do water molecules, i.e. this reaction does not proceed to the right.

$$HCl + CH_3OH \rightleftharpoons Cl^- + CH_3OH_2^+$$

By the same explaination, an aqueous solution of ammonia acts as a weak base because tendency for ammonia to accept a proton from water is much greater than tendency for $\overline{O}H$ ion to accept a proton from N^+H_4 ion.

Thus a "strong acid" or a 'base" is one in which solute acid or base reacts fully, with the solvent, whereas a "weak acid" or 'base' solution is one in which only partial or insignificant reaction with solvent occurs. One can also relate the strength of acid or base with the extent of "ionization". For example, hydrochloric acid is a strong acid in water because it is completely ionized whereas acetic acid is a weak acid in water because it is slightly ionized.

So, it can be pointed out that the strength of an acid is related to the concentration of H^+ ions that are produced on ionisation and at any given concentration will depend upon the value of degree of dissociation α . The acid dissociation constant K_a gives a relationship between α and the concentration and hence is a measure of acid strength. In the same way the strength of the base is related to its dissociation constant.

The relationship between the dissociation constants of an acid (HA) and its conjugate base (A^-) can be obtained from the equilibrium reactions involved as :

$$HA \rightleftharpoons H^+ + A^-$$

$$A^- + H_2O \rightleftharpoons HA + \overline{O}H$$

$$\text{But} \quad k_a = \frac{[H^+]\,[A^-]}{HA}$$

$$\text{and} \quad k_b = \frac{[HA]\,[\overline{O}H]}{[A^-]}$$

$$\therefore \quad k_a \cdot k_b = \frac{[H^+]\,\cancel{[A^-]}}{\cancel{[HA]}} \; \frac{\cancel{[HA]}\,[\overline{O}H]}{\cancel{[A^-]}}$$

$\therefore \quad k_a \cdot k_b = [H^+] \cdot [\bar{O}H]$

$\therefore \quad k_a \cdot k_b = k_w$

From the above it can be implied that the stronger the acid the weaker is its conugate base and vice-versa.

Since the dissociation constant of weak acids and weak bases are numerically small, therefore logarithmic notation is used.

The dissociation constant exponent, pk is obtained from the dissociation constant in a manner similar to the derivation of pH from hydrogen ion concentration, i.e.

$$pk_a = -\log_{10} k_a$$

Thus higher the value of k_a, the smaller will be the value of pk_a which means that stronger the acid the smaller the pk_a value.

3.2 Autoprotolysis of Water

It is well known that pure water is slightly ionized because it is capable of accepting a proton from a second molecule of water as shown by the reaction.

$$H_2O + H_2O \rightleftharpoons H_3O^+ + \bar{O}H$$

The above described equilibrium reaction is called "autoprotolysis". This equilibrium expression can be written in terms of "activities" or effective concentrations, as :

$$K = \frac{(H_3O^+)\,(\bar{O}H)}{(H_2O)^2} \quad \text{or } K = \frac{a_{H_3O^+} - a_{\bar{O}H}}{a^2 H_2O}$$

However, the expression is simplified by following the thermodynamic convention that pure liquid has unit activity and this convention is assumed to be also applicable for relatively dilute solutions. Hence, the activity for each species equals the actual equilibrium concentration. Accordingly, we can rewrite the above equation by the ion-product expression by water :

$$K_w = [H^+]\,[\bar{O}H]$$

The term $[H_2O]^2$ remains constant since it is present in large excess and the term $[H^+]$ is written instead of $[H_3O^+]$. The constant K_w is called "dissociation Constant" or ion-product constant or ionization constant of water. Its value is temperature dependent, ranging from 1.14×10^{-15} at 0°C through 1.01×10^{-14} at 25° and 5.47×10^{-14} at 50°C to 5.4×10^{-13} at 100°C. The value at 22°C is 1.00×10^{-14} which is used in all calculations involving K_w.

The main purpose of acid and base titrations is the determination of acid which is required to exactly neutralize a given amount of a base. The point at which this is obtained is known as the "end point" or equivalence point or "stoichiometric point". Thus neutralization involves reaction between acid and alkali such that at the end point the solution consists of salt and water only. However, the correct end point is characterised by a definite value of the hydrogen ion concentration of the solution.

3.3 pH

The concept of hydrogen ion concentration (pH) has a great importance in pharmaceutical analysis because many analytical methods require optimum pH condition for reactions to complete. Also, in the neutralisation reactions the pH of the solution at the equivalence point determines what types of indicators can be used for the estimations. One should also note that the pH values below or above certain limits can cause physicochemical changes in pharmaceutical or drug substances.

The acidity, basicity or neutrality of a solution can be indicated in terms of molar concentrations of hydrogen ions or by means of pH.

The simplest definition of pH is expressed as the negative logrithm (base ten or decimal) or of the molar concentration of hydrogen ions, i.e.

$$pH = - \log [H^+] \qquad \text{-----(1)}$$

It is also defined as the logarithm of the reciprocal of the molar concentration of hydrogen ions.

$$pH = \log \frac{1}{[H^+]} = -[\log H^+]$$

However, pH can also be defined as the logarithm of reciprocal of hydrogen ion activity.

$$pH = \log \frac{1}{aH^+} = \log (1) - \log a_{H^+}$$
$$= \log a_{H^+}$$

One can utilise the ion product constant expression of water and rewrite :

$$K_w = [H^+] = 1.00 \times 10^{-14}$$

Taking the negative logrithm for each term, one can write the equation as:

$$-\log k_w = -\log [H^+] - \log [\overline{O}H] = 1.0 \times 10^{-14}$$

$$\text{or } pk_w = pH + pOH = 14 \qquad \text{-----(2)}$$

The above equation is used for the calculation of p OH or pH of solutions. The first definition is generally used for solving problems on acid-base titrations, for selection of end-point indicators or designing of new titration methods etc.

3.4 Methods for pH Calculations for Solutions of Acids and Bases

The main aim of this portion of the capter is to illustrate methods for calculation of pH of acids & bases and of aqueous solutions of medicinal substances containing an acid, a base, a salt or a mixture containing any of these components. It is to be remembered that in all these calculations, the solution temperature is 25°c and that the ion-product of water is taken as 1.00×10^{-14} for the sake of convenience. Further, molar concentrations are used instead of "activity" and Debye-Huckel correction factor is used for non-ideality of solutions.

3.4.1 Strong Acid Solutions

Before proceeding with any such calculations on medicinal agents one should inspect the structural formula of these substances and establish if a medicinal agent is acidic, basic and neutral in character.

PROBLEM 1 : 1 Calculate the pH of (a) 0.00140M HCl and (b) 1.00 litre of solution containing 0.080 gm of HCl.

(a) $[H^+] = 0.00140 = 1.40 \times 10^{-3}M$

$pH = - \log [H^+] = 2.85$

(b) Number of moles of HCl = 0.080 gm

$$= 0.08 \text{ gm} \times \frac{1 \text{ mole}}{36.46 \text{ gm}}$$
$$= 2.194 \times 10^{-3} \text{ mole}$$

Concentration of HCl = 2.194×10^{-3} mole/litre

$$[H^+] = 2.194 \times 10^{-3} \text{ M}$$

$$pH = -\log H^+ = 2.65$$

3.4.2 Strong Base Solution

In this case, it should be noted that the hydroxide concentration is directly related to the original concentration of the base. Therefore, the pH can be calculated from the hydroxide concentration and the ion product constant for water.

PROBLEM 2: Calculate the pH of a 0.0024 M barium hydroxide solution. Since two hydroxide ions are involved in the ionization of Ba $(OH)_2$ hence,

$$[\bar{O}H] = 0.004 \text{ M} = 4.8 \times 10^{-3} \text{ M}$$

$$p\,OH = -\log [OH^-]$$
$$= 2.35$$

$$pH = 14.00 - pOH$$
$$= 11.65$$

3.4.3 Weak Acid Solutions

It was explained above that in general a weak acid or a weak base is incompletely ionized in an aqueous solution. As a consequence the hydrogen ion concentration or the hydroxide ion concentration is always less than the original concentration of the weak acid or weak base respectively.

A few examples of weak acids consisting in the form as uncharged chemical species are acetic acid, penicillin G, nicotinic acid etc.

The following quadratic formula

$$[H_3O^+] = \frac{-k_a + \sqrt{k_a^2 + 4k_a c}}{2} \qquad .....(3)$$

Can be used for all calculations involving the hydronium ion concentration of weak monoprotic acids. However an approximation formula

i.e. $$[H_3O^+] = \sqrt{k_a C} \qquad .....(4)$$

gives values with 5% of those obtained by quadratic formula and thus can also be used in such calculations. The term C in equation 4 is analytical concentration which is equal to the total number of moles of solute, both ionized and unionized.

PROBLEM 3: Calculate the pH of a 0.100 M acetic acid solution.

The dissociation of acetic acid and ionization of water can be explained by the following equations::

$$CH_3COOH \rightleftharpoons CH_3\,COO^- \; ; \; k_a = 1.75 \times 10^{-5}$$

$$H_2O \rightleftharpoons H^+ + OH \; ; \; k_2 = 1.00 \times 10^{-14}$$

It should be noted that since acetic acid is a stronger acid and also, hydrogen ion will suppress dissociation of water the contribution from the ionization of acetic acid can only be taken into account :

$$\frac{[\,H^+]\,[\,CH_3COO^-\,]}{[\,CH_3COOH\,]} = k_a = 1.75 \times 10^{-5}$$

But each molecule of acetic acid which undergoes ionization produces one molecule of H^+ ion & one molecule of acetate ion, Thus we have :

$$[H^+] = [CH_3\,COO^-]$$

Further at equilibrium the concentration of acetic acid is equal to initial concentration (0.1.00 F) minus the amount ionized which can either be concentration of H^+ ion or concentration of acetate ion i.e.

$$[CH_3COOH] = 0.100 - [H^+]$$

By Substution above in the original equilibrium expression, we have

$$\frac{[\,H^+\,]}{0.100 - [\,H^+\,]} = 1.75 \times 10^{-5}$$

The above expression is solved by quadratic formula* for $[H^+]$ ion concentration i.e.

$$[\,H^+\,] = \frac{1.75 \times 10^{-5} \pm \sqrt{(1.75 \times 10^{-5})^2 - 4(1)\,(1.75 \times 10^{-5}}}{2} = 1.32 \times 10^{-2}\ M$$

or pH = 2.88

PROBLEM 4: Calculate the pH of a 10^{-3}M Phenoxymethyl penicillin solution, $k_a = 1.79 \times 10^{-3}$. Penicillin V has two amide and a carboxyl groups. The two amide groups are neutral in nature. As the value of k_a is less than 1, therefore it is a weak monoprotic acid.

We use quadratic formula to calculate H_3O^+ concentration:

$$[H_3O^+] = \frac{-0.00179 + \sqrt{(0.00179)^2 + (4)\,(0.00179)\,(10^{-3})}}{2}$$

$$[H_3O^+] = 7.147 \times 10^{-4}$$

3.4.4 Salts of Weak Bases and Strong Acids

A few examples of medicinal compounds in this class are ephledrine hydrochloride, procaine hydrochloride, chlorpromazine and sulfate salts of organic bases. The derivation of equation to calculate the H^+ ion concentration and pH for above category of compounds (i.e. $R_3N^+HCl^-$) comprises of the following equilibrium reactions.

$$2H_2O \rightleftharpoons \bar{O}H,\ K_w = [H_3O^{+\,\prime}]\,.\,[\bar{O}\,H] \qquad (1)$$

$$R_3NH^+ + H_2O \rightleftharpoons H_3O+ + R_3\,N,\ K_a = \frac{[H_3O^+\,]\,[R_3N\,]}{[R_3NH^+\,]} \qquad (2)$$

* The following is the quadratic formula, $\{x = -b \pm \frac{\sqrt{b^2 + 4ac}}{2a}$ and is derived from $ax^2 + bx + c = 0$

$$R_3N + H_2O \rightleftharpoons R_3NH^+ + \bar{O}H, K_b = \frac{[R_3NH][OH^-]}{[R_3N]} \quad (3)$$

It should be noted that the anions of these salts do not react much with H_2O and thus do not affect the pH of the dilute solutions.

An examination of the equilibrium equation No. 2 shows that each ion of $R_3 N^+H$ which reacts with water produces one molecule of conjugate base R_3 NH and one hydronium ion. Further that the contribution of water is negligible and for equation 3 the equilibrium position stay towards the left, i.e.

We can write:

$$[H_3O^+] .= [R_3N]$$

we can write equation 3 as

$$k = \frac{[H_3O^+]^2}{R_3N^+H}$$

or $[H_3O^+] = \sqrt{k_a [R_3NH^+]}$ (4)

Let C be the analytical concentration of the salt, then

$$C = [R_3N^+H] = [R_3N]$$

Since $[H_3O^+] = [R_3N]$

$\therefore \quad C = [R_3N^+H] + [H_3O^+]$ and $[R_3NH] = C - [H_3O^+]$

substitute the values into eq. (4)

$\therefore \quad [H_3O^+] = \sqrt{k_a(C - [H_3O^+])}$ (5)

If $[H_3O^+]$ is very small than C, we can say

$$[H_3O^+] = \sqrt{K_aC} \quad (6)$$

PROBLEM 5 : Calculate the pH of a 6.52×10^{-2}M procaine HCl solution having k_b of being 6.9×10^{-6}.

To begin with, one should know that procaine HCl is a salt of a weak base and a strong acid and that the protonated tertiary amino group behaves as a weak monoprotic acid in an aqueous solution. It also should be noted that the arylamine component will behave as a weak base and will not affect the pH of the solution and is not be involved in the calculations.

The value of k_a for the hydrochloride salt is obtained from k_b value i.e. from procaine.

$$k_a = \frac{K_W}{k_b}$$

$$= \frac{1 \times 10^{-14}}{6.9 \times 10^{-6}} = 1.45 \times 10^{-9}$$

As the value of k_a is less than 1, the cation is a weak acid. The approximation formula can be used for calculation of H^+ ion concentration for salts of strong acids and weak bases.

$$[H_3O^+] = \sqrt{K_aC_A} = \sqrt{1.45 \times 10^{-9} \times 6.52 \times 10^{-2}} = \sqrt{9.45 \times 10^{-11}}$$

$$pH = -\log(9.7232 \times 10^{-6}) = 5.012$$

The hydronium-ion concentration can also be obtained by an alternate procedure as shown below:

Since $k_a = \frac{k_W}{k_b}$ the same can be substituted into eq. (6)

We have :

$$[H_3O^+] = \sqrt{\frac{K_W C_A}{k_b}} = \left(\frac{K_W C_A}{k_b}\right)^{1/2}$$

which can be rewritten in the form of logs as

$- \log [H_3O^+] = 1/2 (-\log k_w - \log k_b - \log C_A)$

$pH = 1/2 \ (pk_w - pk_b - \log C_A)$

or $pH = 1/2 \ (pk_w - \langle pk_b - \langle \log C_a (7)$

By using the given values in above eq. (7) we have

$$pH = 1/2 \ (14 - 5.012 + 1.185)$$

$$pH = 5.0865$$

3.4.5 Weak Base Solution

As already explained weak bases produce small amount of $\bar{O}H$ ion concentration because their ionization in water does not reach to completion, medicinal agents with weak base character are, morphine, atropine, chlorpromazine, or sulphonamide anion, penicillin ion, barbiturate ion, as well as anionic ions of salts of weak acids and strong bases ($Na^+ A^-$). Ammonia and acetate ion also fit in this category.

PROBLEM 6: Calculate the pH of a solution of 0.0100 ammonia ($pk_b = 1.80 \times 10^{-5}$).

The following method will be adopted :

Since ammonia is much stronger a base than water, we may consider ammonia as the only source of $\bar{O}H$ ions and ignore the ionization of water. Thus we can equate the concentration of $N^+ H_4$ ion and $\bar{O}H$ ion from the ionization of ammonia as :

$$[N^+H_4] = [\bar{O}H]$$

At equilibrium the concentration of NH_3 is given by

$$[NH_3] = 0.0100 - [\bar{O} H]$$

The equilibrium between ionized and unionized species in an aqueous solution of ammonia is as follows :

$$NH_4OH \rightleftharpoons N^+ H_4 = \bar{O}H$$

But less than 30% of the dessolved ammonia exists as ....while the predominant species is NH_3 so the equilibrium in reality can be written as:

$$NH_3 + H_2O \rightleftharpoons N^-H_4 + O^-H.$$

However, it is difficult to differenciate between NH_3 and NH_4OH so the ionization reaction can be represented by:

$$\frac{[N^+H_4][O^-H]}{[NH_3]}] = k_b = 1.80 \times 10^{-5}$$

By substiting the values into the above expression we have

$$\frac{[O^-H]^2}{0.100 - [O^-H]} = 1.80 \times 10^{-5}$$

or by successive approximations we have

$$[O^-H]^2 = 1.80 \times 10^{-7} \text{ or } [O^-H] = 4.24 \times 10^{-4} M$$

$$pOH^- = -\log [OH^-] = 3.37$$

$$pH = 14.00 - pOH = 10.63$$

3.4.6 Weak Bases, Uncharged Chemical Species

The equations which are used for the calculation of the hydronium ion concentration and pH of a weak base comprising of an uncharged chemical species involves the reactions given below :

$$2H_2O \rightleftharpoons H_3O^+ + \bar{O}H$$

$$k_w = [H_3O^+]\ \bar{O}H \qquad (1)$$

$$R_3N + H_2O \rightleftharpoons R_3\ N^+H + O^-H$$

$$K[H_2O] = k_b = \frac{[R_3N^+H]\ [\bar{O}H]}{[R_3N]} \qquad (2)$$

Where k = equilibrium constant

k_w = ionization constant of weak base.

R_3N = molar concentration of unionized base

$R_3\ N^+H$ = molar concentration of conized species/conjugate base

The following approximation formula can be utilized for the calculation of hydronium ion concentration of a weak base:

$$[\bar{O}H] = \sqrt{kbc}$$

A quadratic formula can also be used for the calculation of hydronium ion concentration for weak bases.

$$[O^-H] = \frac{-k_b + \sqrt{k_b^2 + 4k_b c}}{2}$$

The values obtained with approximation formula has errors within 5% of that obtained by quadratic formula and are allowed.

PROBLEM 7. Calculate the pH of 10^{-3}M ephedrine solution, ($k_b = 2.28 \times 10^{-5}$).

As per the value of k_b and structural formula for epheridine, it is a weak monoprotic organic base. The quadratic formula can be used to determine the $\bar{O}H$ ion concentration as indicated below :

$$[\bar{O}H] = \frac{-0.0000228 + \sqrt{(0.0000228)^2 + (4)(0.0000228)(20^{-3}}}{1}$$

$$[OH\} = 3.03 \times 10^{-4}$$

$$pOH = -\log \bar{O}H = -\log 3.03 \times 10^{-4}$$

$$= -(0.48 - 4.00) = 3.52$$

$$\text{But } pH = pk_w - pOH$$

$$pH = 14.00 - 3.52$$

$$= 10.48$$

3.4.7 Salts of Strong Bases and Weak Acids

The examples of such types of bases are salts like sodium acetate, sodium pentobarbital, potassium pencillin G, sodium sulphadiazine etc.

The following approximation formula can be used for the calculation of $[\bar{O}H]$ .concentration :

$$[O^-H] = \sqrt{kbc}$$

PROBLEM 8: Calculate the pH of a solution which is 0.100 M in sodium acetate ($pk_a = 1.75 \times 10^{-5}$).

The equations involved in this process will be following:

$$H_2O \rightleftharpoons H^+ + \bar{O}H$$

$$H^+ + CH_3COO^- \rightleftharpoons CH_3COOH$$

It is observed that one H^+ & one $\bar{O}H$ are formed for each molecule of H_2O on ionization and one molecule of acetic acid is formed on consumption of one H^+. Thus at equilibrium we have

$$[H^+] = [\bar{O}H] - [CH_3COOH]$$

$$\text{or} \quad [CH_3COOH] = [\bar{O}H] - [H^+]$$

Since the solution is basic, the concentration of H^+ will be small and can be ignored so

$$[CH_3\ COOH] = [\bar{O}H]$$

The above can also be obtained by considering the equation

$$CH_3\ COO^- + H_2O \rightleftharpoons CH_3COOH + \bar{O}H$$

Thus the equilibrium reaction will be as:

$$k_{eq} = \frac{[CH_3COOH]\ [\bar{O}H]}{[CH_3COOH^-]}$$

Multiply the numerater and denominator of the right side of above equation by $[H^+]$

$$k_{eq} = \frac{[CH_3COOH]\ [\bar{O}H]\ [H^+]}{[CH_3COO^-]\ [H^+]}$$

But $[H^+]\ [\bar{O}H] = k_w$ and

$$\frac{[H^+]\ [CH_3COO^-]}{[CH_3COOH]} = k_a$$

So we can right:

$$\frac{[CH_3COOH]\ [\bar{O}H]}{[CH_3cOOH-]} = k_{eq} = \frac{k_w}{k_a} = \frac{1.00 \times 10^{-14}}{1.75 \times 10^{\ 5}}$$

We have already established that

$$[CH_3\ COH] = [\bar{O}H]$$

The equilibrium concentration of acetate ion is equal to the original acetate concentration (0.100 M) minus that which is converted to acetic acid.

$$[CH_3COO^-] = 0.0100 - [\bar{O}H]$$

Since the initial acetate concentration is large, while k_{eq} is very small, the equilibrium concentration of acetate ion can be assumed to be just 0.100M then

$$\frac{[CH_3COOH]\ [\bar{O}H]}{[CH_3COO^-]} = \frac{[\bar{O}H][\bar{O}H]}{0.10} = 5.71 \times 10^{-10}$$

$$\text{or} \quad [\bar{O}H]^2 = 5.71 \times 10^{-11}$$

$$[O^-H] = 7.56 \times 10^{-6}$$

$$pOH = 5.12$$

$$pH = 14 - 5.12 = 8.88$$

PROBLEM 9. To calculate the pH of a 10^{-4}M phenobarbital sodium, $pk_a = 3.8 \times 10^{-8}$.

It should be noted that phenobarbital sodium is a salt of a strong base. It can be written in enol form in which state it acts as a weak monoprotic base and the imide hydrogen has no effect on the pH of the solution..

Consider the following two equilibrium equation that are involved.

$$A^- + H_2O \rightleftharpoons HA + \bar{O}H, \quad k_b = \frac{[HA]\ [\bar{O}H]}{[HA]} \qquad (1)$$

$$HA + H_2O \rightleftharpoons H_3O^+ + A^-, \quad k_a = \frac{[H_3\bar{O}]\ [A^-]}{[HA]} \qquad (2)$$

Multiply the reaction (1) and (2) above

$$k_b \,.\, k_a = \frac{\cancel{[HA]}\ [O^-H]}{\cancel{[HA]}} \times \frac{[H_3O^+]\cancel{[A^-]}}{\cancel{[HA]}} = [H_3O^+]\ [O^-H] = k_w$$

$$\therefore \quad k_b \,.\, k_a = k_w$$

$$k_b = \frac{k_w}{k_a} = \frac{1 \times 10{-}14}{3.8 \times 10^{-8}} = 2.6 \times 10^{-7}$$

Since the value of k_b is less than 1, this anion is a weak base and therefore the approximation formula may be used for calculation of hydronium-ion concentration.

$$[\bar{O}H] = \sqrt{K_bC} = \sqrt{2.6 \times 10^{-7} \times 10^{-4}} = 5.1 \times 10^{-6}$$

$$pOH = -\log(5 \times 10^{-6}) = 5.29$$

$$pH = pk_w - pOH$$

$$= 14.00 - 5.29 = 8.71$$

We can also make use of the following equation and substitute the values.

$$\log\ [H_3O^+] = \frac{1}{2}\ \log\ k_w + \frac{1}{2}\ \log\ k_a\ \frac{1}{2}\ \log c$$

$$-\log\ [H_3O^+] = -\frac{1}{2}\ \log\ k_w - \frac{1}{2}\ \log\ k_a - \frac{1}{2}\ \log C$$

$$pH = \frac{1}{2}\ pk_w = \frac{1}{2}\ pK_a + \frac{1}{2}\ \log c$$

$$= \frac{1}{2}\ (14.00 + 7.42 - 4.00)$$

$$= \frac{1}{2} \times 17.42 = 8.71$$

3.5 Salts

A salt is defined as a chemical substance other than water which is produced by the neutralization of an equivalent amount of (i) a strong acid and a strong base (ii) a weak base and a strong acid, (iii) a strong base and a weak acid and (iv) a weak acid and a weak base. Further it should be noted that (a) the pH of a salt solution obtained by the dissolution of the crystalline form of a salt is the same as that obtained during the neutralization reaction of chemically equivalent quantities of acid and base and (b) that salts exist in solution as ions.

3.5.1 Salt Solution of a Strong Acid and a Strong Base

In salt solutions of this type the equilibrium reaction of water is not seriously affected and the pH will remain constant as that of water i.e. 7.00.

The examples of these salts are sodium chloride, sodium nitrite, potassium sulphate.

3.5.2 Salt Solution of a Weak Base and a Strong Acid

In salt solution of this kind the cationic portion is considered the weak acid and reacts with water to produce hydronium ions. The pH equation is represented by $pH = (pk_w - pk_b - \log c)$. The examples of these salts are ammonium chloride, ephedrine sulphate, atropine hydrochloride, chlorpromazine hydrochloride.

3.5.3 Salt Solution of Weak Acid and a Strong Base

In salts of this nature, the anionic portion is considered the weak base and reacts with water to produce hydroxyl ions. The derivation of the pH equation is $pH = (pk_w + pk_a + \log c)$

3.5.4 Salt Solution of a Weak Acid and a Weak Base

Ammonium acetate may be considered such a case and it undergoes hydrobysis in aqueous solution as shown belows:

$$N^+H_4 \rightleftharpoons H^+ + NH_3$$

$$CH_3COO^- + H_2O \rightleftharpoons CH_3COOH + \bar{O}H$$

$$N^+H_4 + CH_3COO^- + H_2O \rightleftharpoons NH_3 + CH_3COOH + H^+ + OH$$

Since H^+ and $\bar{O}H$ ions are produced in equal amounts they can be removed from the total expression so we have

$$NH_4 + CH_3COO^- \rightleftharpoons NH_3 + CH_3COOH$$

The hydronium ion concentration can by given by:

$$[H_3O^+] = \sqrt{\frac{K_w\, k_a}{k_b}}$$

taking logarithms we have :

$$\log[H_3O^+] = \frac{1}{2}\log k_w + \frac{1}{2}\log k_a - \frac{1}{2}\log k_b$$

$$\therefore \quad pH = \frac{1}{2} pk_w + \frac{1}{2} pk_a - \frac{1}{2} pk_b$$

3.6 Buffer Solutions

A buffer solution is a solution that has an ability to resist a change in the hydrogen ion concentration (pH) upon addition of a small amount of acid or alkali. A buffer solution can be obtained from a mixture of a weak acid or a base and its salt, for example from acetic acid and solid acetate or ammonia and ammonium chloride. The buffer action in a solution obtained from a weak acid & its salt is explained in terms of that hydrogen ions are removed by the anions of a weak acid to form unionized molecules as:

$$H^+ + A^- \rightarrow HA$$

The hydroxyl ions are also removed by neutralization as per equation

$$\bar{O}H + HA \rightleftharpoons H_2O + A^-$$

The concentration of H^+ ion in such a buffer solution will be determined by the dissociation constant of acid according to the following equation :

$$k_a = \frac{[H^+]\,[A^-]}{HA}$$

$$\therefore \quad \log k_a = \log [H^+] + \log \frac{[A^-]}{[HA]}$$

$$\therefore \quad -\log k_a = \log [H^+] + \log \frac{[A^-]}{[HA]}$$

$$\therefore \quad pk_a = pH - \log \frac{[A^-]}{[HA]}$$

$$\therefore \quad pH = pk_a + \log \frac{[A^-]}{[HA]}$$

In the above HA is weak acid and partially ionized which would imply that HA will be numerically equal to the initial concentration of acid and $[A^-]$ will be equal to initial concentration of salt.

$$pH = pk_a + \log \frac{[salt]}{[Acid]}$$

The above is known as Henderson Equation,

If [Salt] = [Acid] we have

$$pH = pk_a + \log 1$$

or $pH = pk_a$

The resistance of buffer solution to a pH change is a measure of *buffer capacity*.

The buffer action of a solution of a weak base and its salt is explained by the fact that hydroxyl ions are removed by the salt cations (BH^+) to form unionized molecules:

$$\bar{O}H + BH^+ \rightleftharpoons B + H_2O$$

Hydrogen ions are removed by neutralization

$$H^+ + B \rightleftharpoons BH$$

The concentration of the weak base and its salt with respect to $\bar{O}H$ ions in the solution will be determined by the dissociation constant of the base as indicated below:

$$k = \frac{[BH^+]\,[\bar{O}H]}{[B]}$$

$$\therefore \log k_b = \log [\bar{O}H] + \log \frac{[BH^+]}{[B]}$$

$$-\log k_b = -\log [\bar{O}H] - \log \frac{[BH^+]}{[B]}$$

$$\therefore pk_b = pOH - \log \frac{[BH^+]}{[B]}$$

But $pOH = pk_w - pH$

$$\therefore pk_w - pH - \log \frac{[BH^+]}{[B]}$$

$$pH = pk_w - pk_b - \log \frac{[BH^+]}{[B]}$$

It is to be observed that the base is weak and slightly ionized. Its ionization is suppressed by the large concentration of cations BH^+ from the fully dissociated salt. Also [B] is numerically equal to the initial concentration of base and [BH^+] is numerically equal to the initial concentration of salt.

$$\therefore pH = pk_w - pk_b - \log \frac{[\text{salt}]}{[\text{Base}]}$$

$pk_w - pk_b = pk_a$ can be substituted in the above equation so we have,

$$pH = pk_a - \log \frac{[\text{acid}]}{[\text{salt}]}$$

$$\text{and } pH = pk_a + \log \frac{[\text{salt}]}{[\text{Acid}]}$$

This is due to the fact that [BH^+] is the conjugate acid of base B, and it can be equated to the initial concentration of the salt.

PROBLEM 10. Calculate the pH of a solution which contains 2.50×10^{-3} mole of sodium acetate and 3.0×10^{-4} mole of acetic acid in 1 litre of solution ($pk_a = 4.74$).

Using the following equation and substitute the known values :

$$pH = pk_a + \log \frac{[\text{Conj. base}]}{[\text{acid}]}$$

$$= 4.74 + \log 2.5 \times 10^{-3} - \log 3.0 \times 10^{-4}$$

$$= 4.74 + [-2.6 + 3.5]$$

$$= 5.74$$

PROBLEM 11. Calculate the pH of 200 ml of a solution containing 0.20 M of ammonium chloride and 0.20 M of ammonia.

The following equations are involved :

$$NH_3 + H_2O \rightleftharpoons N^{+}H_4 + \bar{O}H$$

The equilibrium expression is

$$\frac{[N^{+}H_4][\bar{O}H]}{[NH_3]} = 1.80 \times 10^{-5}$$

Further, $[N^{+}H_4] = 0.200 + [\bar{O}H]$

and $[NH_3] = 0.200 - [\bar{O}H]$

$$\therefore \quad \frac{(0.200)[\bar{O}H]}{0.20} = 1.80 \times 10^{-5}$$

$$[\bar{O}H] = 1.80 \times 10^{-5} \text{ M}$$

$$p\,OH = 4.74$$

$$pH = 9.26$$

3.7 Solutions of Polyprotic Acids and Their Salts

So far in this chapter we have studied only those acids, bases, and salts which are capable of single proton transfer reactions. In addition to these, there is another group of important acids, called polyprotic acids. They possess two or more ionizable hydrogen ions and include such acids as sulphuric (H_2SO_4), oxalic ($H_2C_2O_4$), carbonic (H_2CO_3) and phosphoric acids (H_3PO_4). In the same manner salts of these acids will exist, that will behave like bases and accept two or more protons, e.g. sodium carbonate can accept up to three protons to produce phosphoric acid. Thus phosphoric acid can undergo ionization in three separate steps as shown below:

$$H_3PO_4 \rightleftharpoons H^+ + H_2PO_4^- ; \; k_1 = 7.5 \times 10^{-3}$$

$$H_2PO_4^- \rightleftharpoons H^+ + HPO_4^{-1} ; \; k_2 = 6.2 \times 10^{-8}$$

$$HPO_4^{--} \rightleftharpoons H^+ + PO_4^{-3} ; \; k_3 = 4.8 \times 10^{-13}$$

3.8 Acid Base Indicators

Theoritically speaking the *equivalence point* in a titration is defined as that point at which the quantity of titrant added is stoichiometrically equivalent to the substance being determined. Whereas *end point* is an experimental phenomenon which indicates that the equivalence point has been reached. The end point does not always coincide with the equivalence point although in a titration the difference between these two points must be very small.

In an acid base titration the end point can be determined by the following two common procedures: (a) the course of titration can be followed with a glass electrode pH meter and the full titration curve is recorded. The inflection point or maximal slope of the titration curve is then located as the end point, (b) the second method| *involves* the use of acid-base indicators which are simply organic dye substances. An acid-base indicator has the ability to serve as a pH indicator because of the fact that it exists in two states; the acid form has one colour which by loss of proton changes into a base form having different colour. This equilibrium between the acid and the base form can be represented as:

$$In_A \rightleftharpoons H^+ + In_B \quad \text{OR} \quad HIn \quad H^+ + \quad In^-$$

Colour A   Colour B   Unionized Colour   Ionized Colour

Where In_A is the acid form of the indicator with colour A and In_B is the base form of the same indicator with a different colour B. Most of the indicators are very intensely coloured and can be used in dilute solution in very small quantities so much so that the acid base equilibrium which is under examination is not disturbed by the addition of the indicator. Being weak acids or bases they are able to reach instantaneous equilibrium with the system and the colour of the solution will range between the extreme colours of the two forms as the proportion of the acidic and basic forms automatically adjusts itself to the pH of the solution.

In acid solution, the excess of H^+ ions will suppress the ionization of the indicator. The concentration of In will be small, and that of HIn large so the colour will be that of unionized form. On the other hand the alkali will bring up the removal of hydrogen ions from the system with an increase in the concentration of ionized form (In^-) consequently the colour of the solution will have ionized colour.

$$k_{In_a} = \frac{[H^+]\,[In^-]}{[HIn]}$$

$$[H^+] = KIn_a \frac{[HIn]}{[In^-]}$$

$$\therefore \quad -\log [H^+] = -\log kIn_a - \log \frac{[HIn]}{[In^-]}$$

$$\therefore \quad pH = pk_{In_a} + \log \frac{[In^-]}{[HIn^-]}$$

Similarly derivation for an indicator functioning as a weak base can be derived as shown below:

$$In + H_2O \rightleftharpoons In\,H^+ + O^-H$$

Unionized colour   Ionized colour

$$k_{In_b} = \frac{[InH^+]\ [O^-H]}{[In^-]}$$

$$pH = pk_w - pk_{In_b} - \log \frac{[InH^+]}{[In]}$$

3.8.1 Tautomeric Indicators

The behaviour of some of the indicators is difficult to explain, the colour changes are brought about by tautomeric changes in the structure of the molecule. e.g. the action of phenolphthalein can be explained in terms of quinonoid structure

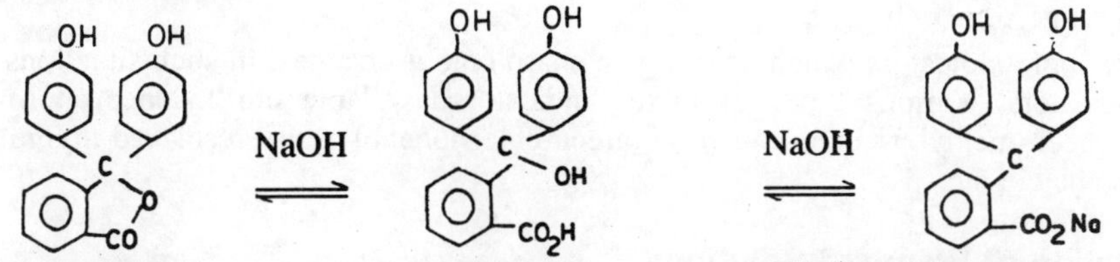

NaOH ⇌ NaOH ⇌

Acid solution colourless HIn — Colourless pH 7-8 HIn — Alkaline solution pH 8-10 red colour

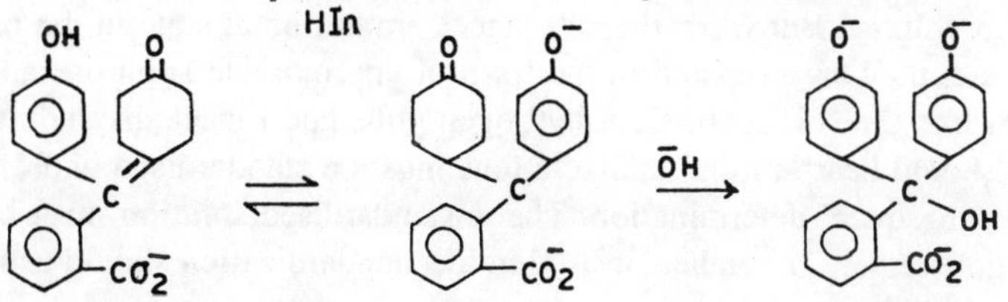

$\bar{O}H$ →

Coloured (In^-) — colourless pH 12

That observed colour of a two-colour indicators is determined by the ratio of the concentrations of ionized and unionized forms. The average colour-change interval or range of an indicator is supposed to be about two pH units. The observed colour changes within the indicator range occur in the form of a gradual change of tint or shade from one extreme colour to the other. The shade of colour is independent of the quantity of indicator present, but too much indicator should not be used because, then slight changes will become difficult to be detected.

In case of a single colour indicator like phenolphthalein, the intensity of the colour is important and not shade difference, therefore the concentration of the indicator should be properly controlled.

It is good to have a wide variety of indicators available to cover the complete pH scale.

3.8.2 Selection of Indicators

The following criteria should be kept in mind while making decisions concerning the proper selection of end point indicators.

(a) Three drops of indicator test solution should be used unless otherwise directed.

(b) In a titration between a strong acid with a strong alkali or vice-versa methyl orange, methyl red or phenolphthalein should be used.

(c) When a weak acid is titrated against a strong acid, phenolphthaleine should be used as an indicator.

(d) In a titration between a weak alkali and a strong acid, methyl orange can be used as the indicator.

(e) A weak acid and a weak alkali should not be titrated against each other since no indicator will give a sharp end point.

(f) In a titration, it is advisable to titrate wherever possible to the appearance of colour rather than to disappearance.

3.8.3 Mixed Indicators

The most important criteria for a good indicator should be a sharp difference between the two colours which it exhibits in the acid and alkaline conditions and that this colour change should take place over a very small range of pH changes.

There are some indicators which do not give sharp colour changes. In such situations one can resort to mixed indicators. Various types of mixed indicators available are xylenecyanol-methyl orange, bromocresol green-methyl red, bromocresol green-chlorophenol red, cresol red-thymol blue, thymol blue-Phenolphthalein etc.

3.9 Preparation of Standard Solutions

When the reagents are available in a pure state, the exact quantity is weighed, dissolved in water and then made up to volume. But when the substances are not obtainable in the pure state e.g. mineral acids, caustic alkalis etc. they are prepared in the form of approximate solutions and then standardised against a pure standard like the A.R. potassium hydrogen phthalate for alkalis and anhydrons sodium carbonate for acids. One should bear in mind that solutions must be standardised under the same conditions as will be used in the subsequent determination. The unstandardised solution must be placed in the burette and not in the titration vessel. The indicator used in the standardization should usually be the same to be used in the subsequent determination.

The concentrations of standard solutions can be indicated by means of "normality" i.e. the number of equivalents of solute per litre of solution (milliequivalents per millilitre) or in terms of "molarity" i.e. number of moles of solute per litre of solution. While in some cases "molality" i.e. number of moles of solute per 100 gm of solvent is used.

A normal solution (N/1), is thus a solution which contains one gram equivalent of a substance per litre of solution. Solutions which are not normal but have different strengths can be accordingly represented like:

2 N = Twice normal

N/2, 0.5N = half normal

N/10 or 0.IN = Deci normal

N/100 or 0.0IN = Centi-normal

The equivalent weight of an acid or base is that weight of it which contains 1.008 g of replaceable hydrogen or its equivalent like the hydroxyl group. In case of oxidation-reduction titrations the equivalent weight is that weight which yields or combines with 1.008 gm of available hydrogen or 8.00 g of available oxygen for use in oxidation or reduction during a reaction. In a similar manner in precipitation reaction i.e. in argentimetry equivalent weight of a substances contains or combines with 1g atom of a univalent atom. In a way equivalent weight is determined from the actual that may occur in a particular situation.

Calculation of Equivalent weight:

Hydrochloric acid:

$$HCl \equiv H$$

$$\therefore \quad 36.47g\ HCl \equiv 1000\ ml\ N/1$$

Sulphuric Acid:

$$H_2SO_4 \equiv 2H$$

$$98.08\ g\ H_2SO_4 \equiv 2H \equiv 2000\ ml\ N/1$$

$$\frac{98.08}{2}\ g\ H_2SO_4 \equiv 1000\ ml\ N/1 \text{ since 98.08 is 2 equiv.}$$

$$49.04\ g\ H_2SO_4 \equiv 1000\ ml\ N/1$$

Sodium carbonate :

$$Na_2\ CO_3 + 2\ HCl = 2\ NaCl + H_2O + CO_2$$

$$Na_2\ CO_3 \equiv 2HCl \equiv 2H$$

$$\therefore \quad 106\ g\ Ns_2CO_3 \equiv 2000\ ml\ N/1$$

$$\therefore \quad 53\ g\ Na_2\ CO_3 \equiv 1000\ ml\ N/1$$

Sodium Oxalate :

(a) As an acid : $NaHC_2O_4 + Na\ OH = Na_2C_2O_4 + H_2O$

$$\therefore \quad NaHC_2O_4 \equiv Na\ OH = H$$

$$\therefore \quad 112g\ NaHC_2O_4 \equiv 1000\ ml\ N/1$$

(b) As a reducing agent:

$$NaHC_2O_4 + O = Na\ OH + 2\ CO_2$$

$$\therefore \quad NaHC_2O_4 \equiv O \equiv 2\ H$$

$$\therefore \quad 112\ g\ NaHC_2H_4 \equiv 2000\ N/1\ ml\ N/1$$

$$\therefore \quad 56\ g\ NaHC_2H_4 \equiv 1000\ ml\ N/1$$

In the preparation of a standard solutions, of known strengths, it is usually easy to make approximately N/1, N/2 or N/20 etc. The relationship of the exact strength of such a solution to the nominal normality is then shown by means of factor. The factor is defined in terms of number of ml of exact N/1, N/2 etc solution which are equivalent to 1 ml of solution of the same nominal normality. It is the number by which the actual volume of the solution of approximate strength must be multiplied to obtain the equivalent volume of a standard solution of exact normality. Suppose in a standardisation of N/1 (approx) $H_2\ SO_4$ by N/1 $Na_2\ CO_3$ we find that 25 ml of N/1 Na_2CO_3 was neutralized by 24.5 ml. of N/1 (approx) $H_2\ SO_4$

Then

$$24.5\ ml\ N/1\ (approx)\ H_2SO_4 \equiv 25\ ml\ N/1\ Na_2\ CO_3$$

$$\therefore \quad 1\ ml \quad \text{"} \quad \text{"} \quad \text{"} \quad \equiv \frac{25\ ml\ N/1}{24.5} \equiv 1.020\ ml\ N/1$$

Therefore the strength of $H_2 SO_4$ solution is N/1 (1.020). The factor is 1.020 and all volumes of this solution when multiplied by 1.020 will give the equivalent volume of the normal solution i.e. the exact normality of H_2SO_4 is 1.020 N.

In the above equation one should note that the unknown strength is placed on the left hand side.

EXERCISE 1. Standardization of N/1 HCl :

Method: The most commonly method makes use of exsiccated sodium carbonate. Dilute 85 ml of hydrochloric acid to 1000 ml. Weight accurately 1.5 g of A.R. grade anhydrous sodium carbonate (primary standard) that has been previously heated at about 270°C to remove traces of moisture. Dissolve it in 100 ml of water, and 2 drops of methyl red TS. Add the acid slowly from burret with constant stirring until solution becomes faintly pink. Heat the solution to bioling & continue the titration, repeat the same until the faint pink colour is no longer affected by boiling. Calculate the normality of HCl. Each 52.99 mg of anhydrous $Na_2 CO_3$ is equivalent to 1 ml of 1 N HCl.

The following equations may be considered

$$NaHCO_3 \longrightarrow Na_2CO_3 + H_2O + CO_2 \uparrow$$

$$Na_2CO_3 + 2HCl \longrightarrow 2NaCl + H_2O + CO_2$$

Sodium bicontains carbonate small amounts of moisture and on heating the sample at 270°C moisture is removed and $NaHCO_3$ is changed to Na_2CO_3.

Further, the CO_2 generated in the nentralization reaction makes the solution acidic and can introduce error if it is not removed. So, after the first end point is reached the solution is boiled to remove CO_2 and titration is continued to a point where 1 drop of titrant makes a colour change.

Calculations

Concentrated HCl is 36.5% and has specific guavity of 1.18 so 85 ml in 1000 ml will give approximately 1 N HCl i.e. 1 litre of 1 N HCl should contain 36.46 g or 1 g equiv. of HCl. However, this solution contains:

$$85 \times 1.18 \times 0.365 = 36.61\text{g HCl}$$

Say, a pure sample of sodium carbonate weighing 1.5250 g was used and say 30.10 ml of acid was needed in the titration.

Equiv. Wt. of $Na_2 CO_3$ = 105.99/2 = 52.00g

$$\therefore \text{meq of } Na_2 CO_3 = \frac{1.5250}{0.0599}$$

$$\text{ml} \times N = \frac{\text{wt. of } Na_2CO_3}{\text{meq}}$$

$$N = \frac{1.5250 \text{ g}}{30.10 \times 0.5299 \text{ g}} = 0.9511$$

It is also possible to standardise a solution of HCl using a standard solution of NaOH or KOH as a secondary standard. Say, if 25.30 ml of 0.9705 N Na OH is needed in titration of 25.00 ml of a solution of HCl, the normality can be found by the formula : $V_A \times \text{Normality}_A = V_B \times \text{Normality}_B$

$$\text{OR} \quad \text{ml} \times N = \text{ml} \times N$$

$$25.0 \times N = 25.30 \times 0.9705$$

$$N = \frac{25.30 \times 0.9705}{25.00}$$
$$= 0.9821$$

EXERCISE 2. Standardisation of 1 N Sulphuric Acid:

Method : Add 30 ml of sulphuric acid to about 1020 ml of water with stirring and cooling. Determine the normality by titration against sodium carbonate as described previously.

Sulphuric acid (95%) is a diprotic acid having specific gravity of about 1.83 at 25°c, 1000 ml of normal solution will contain 98.08/2 = 49.04g consequently, 30 ml of concentrated acid should contain 30 × 1.83 × 0.95 = 52. 15g of H_2SO_4. The method of calculating the normality is similar to that described for 1 N hydrochloric acid.

EXERCISE 3. Standardisation of IN sodium Hydroxide:

Method: Dissolve 45g of sodium hydroxide in 950 ml of water. Freshly prepared saturated solution of barium hydroxide is thereafter added until no precipitate is formed. The mixture is shaken and left overnight in a stoppered bottle. Decant or filter the solution and standardise it as described below:

About 5 g of potassium biphthalate (primary standard) which has been previously crushed and dried at 120° is accurately weighed. It is dissolved in 75 ml CO_2— free water and drops of phenolphthalein TS are added. The solution is titrated with sodium hydroxide solution to the production of permanent colour. Calculate the normality. Each 204.23 mg of pure dried potassium biphthalate is equivalent to 1 ml of 1 N NaOH.

Calculations :

$$KH\ C_8H_4O_4 + NaOH \longrightarrow KNaC_8H_4O_4 + H_2O$$

204.23 g

1 mol or 204.23 g of pure dried potassium is 1 equiv.

$\therefore$ 1 meq $\equiv$ 0.20423 g.

Say, the exact weight of sample of dried potassium diphthalate is 4.9551g and say 24.25 ml of NaOH were required in the titration the normality of the solution would be as:

$$ml \times N = \frac{\text{wt. of } KHC_8H_4O_4}{0.20423}, \qquad \therefore\ N = \frac{4.9551\ g}{24.25 \times 0.20423\ g} = 1.00$$

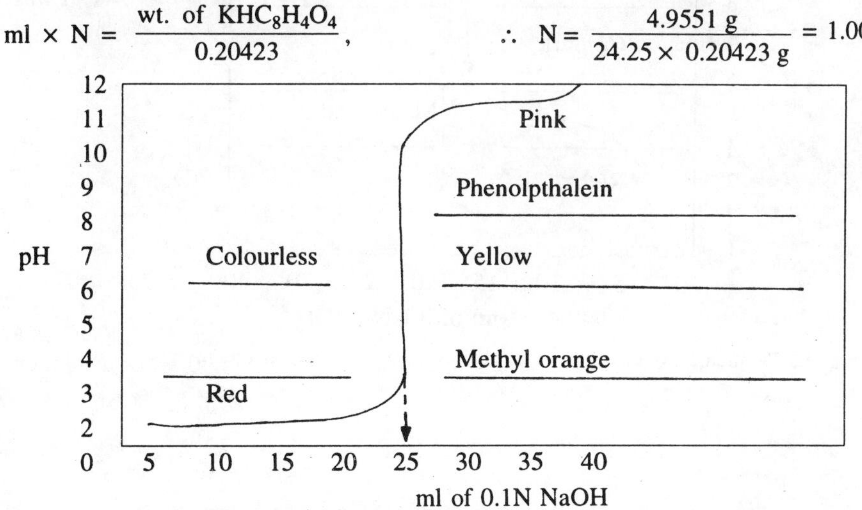

Fig. 3.1 Titration curve of hydrochloric acid (0.1 N) using 0.1 N NaOH as titrant

In the above standardisation example it is to be noted that an excess of (1 equiv = 40.00g) sodium hydroxide is weighed since it is hygroscopic in nature and also the solution is treated with barium hydroxide to precipitate any carbonate that may have been formed due to the action of CO_2. Phenolphthalein is sensitive to CO_2, but methyl orange is insesitive to CO_2.

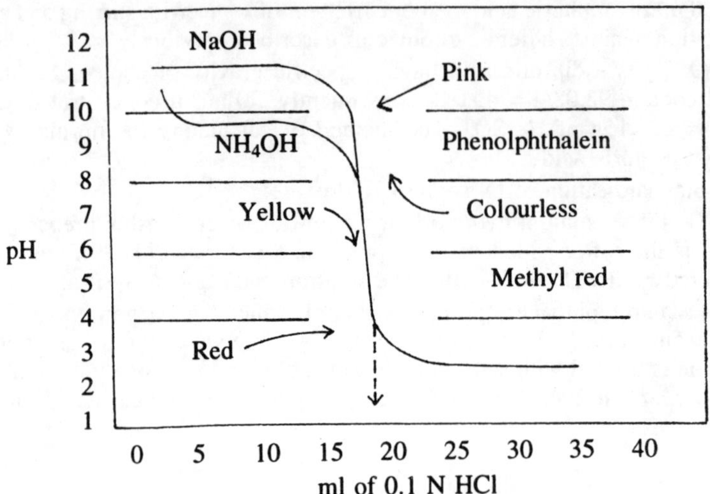

Fig. 3.2 Titration curve of a strong and weak bases (NaOH) with a strong acid Hcl)

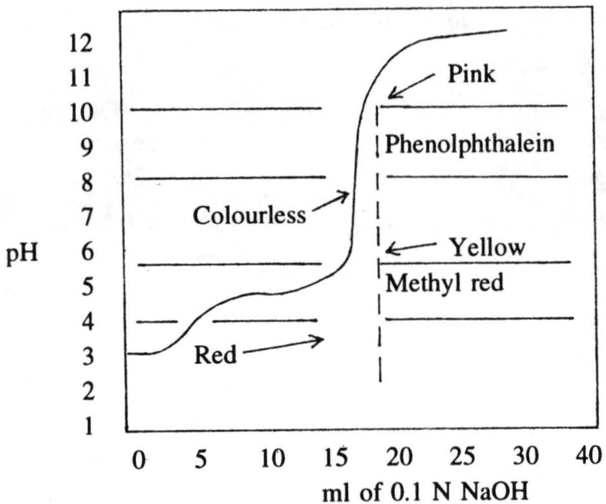

Fig. 3.3 Titration curve of 0.1 N acetic acid using 0.1 N NaOH as titrant.

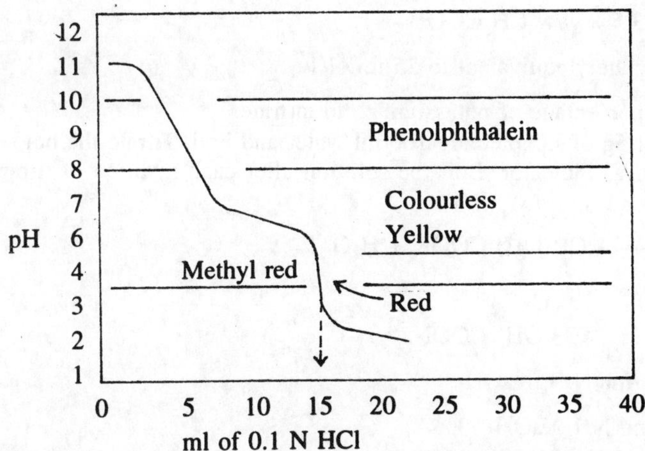

Fig. 3.4 Titration curve of sodium carbonate using HCl as the titrant

3.10 Important Assay Preparations

3.10.1 Direct Titration of strong Acids.

EXERCISE 4. Determination of percentage W/V of HCl

The equations involved are:

$$HCl + NaOH = NaCl + H_2O$$

$$36.46 \text{ g. } HCl \equiv H \equiv 1000 \text{ ml N/1 NaOH}$$

$$0.03646\text{g } HCl \equiv 1 \text{ ml N/1 NaOH}$$

Method: In a stoppered bottle weigh out accurately 4g of sample. Transfer the acid into a stoppered flask containing 40 ml of water. Titrate with N/1 NaOH using methyl orange as indicator taking the first definite orange colour as the end point.

The proportion of HCl in the sample is calculated by the formula:

$$\% \text{ W/W} = \frac{\text{ml base} \times N \times 0.3646 \times 100}{\text{Wt of the Sample}}$$

3.10.2 Direct Titration of Weak Acids

EXERCISE 5. Determination of percentage w/w of Acetic acid:

Method: Accurately weigh about 5g of sample using a stoppered weighing bottle. Transfer the acid into a stoppered flask using 50 ml of water. Titrate with N/1 NaOH using phenolphthalein as indicator. The end point is recorded as the first shade of pink colour.

The stoichiometric reactions involved are:

$$CH_3COOH + NaOH \equiv CH_3COONa + N_2O$$

$$60.05\text{g } CH_3COOH \equiv 1 \text{ ml N/1 NaOH}$$

$$0.0605\text{g } CH_3COOH \equiv 1 \text{ ml N/1 NaOH}$$

Acetic acid (I.P.) contains 32.5–33.5% w/w CH_3COOH

∴ 5 g of sample is approximately equivalent to 25 ml N/1.

EXERSICE 6. Determination of percentage of potassium acid tartrate.

Method: weigh accurately about 1.5g of sample, add 100 ml water and boil. Titrate the hot solution with N/5 NaOH using phenolphthalein as indicator. Boil the solution after each addition of titrant. The reactions involved are indicated below:

$$\begin{array}{l} CH(OH)\,COOK \\ | \\ CH(OH)\,COOH \end{array} + NaOH \longrightarrow \begin{array}{l} CH(OH)\,COOK \\ \\ CH(OH)\,COONa \end{array} + H_2O$$

$C_4H_5O_6K \equiv NaOH \equiv 1000$ ml N/1 NaOH

188.2 g $C_4H_5O_6K \equiv 1000$ ml N/1 NaOH

0.03764g $C_4H_5O_6K \equiv$ 1 ml N/5 NaOH

Similarly substances like p-aminbenzoic acid, citric acid, nicotinic acid, oxalic acid, phosphoric acid, potassium hydrogen phthalate, salicylic acid, sulphanilic acid can be determined.

3.10.3 Direct Titration of Strong Bases

EXERCISE 7. Determination of percentage of sodium carbonate in exsiccated sodium carbonate.

Method: Accurately weigh 1 g of sample into a conical flask containing little water and titrate against N/2 HCl using 1 drop of methyl orange as indicator. The end point is orange colour nearest to yellow. The determination is based on the following equations:

$$Na_2CO_3 + 2\,HCl \longrightarrow 2\,NaCl + CO_2 + H_2O$$

$Na_2\,CO_3 \equiv 2\,HCl = 2H$

106 g $Na_2\,CO_3 \equiv$ 2000 ml N/1 HCl

26.50 g Na_2 CO $\equiv$ 1000 ml N/2 HCl

0.02650g $Na_2CO_3 \equiv$ 1 ml N/2 HCl

EXERCISE 8. Determination of percentage of sodium salicylate.

Method: Accurately weigh about 3 g of sample, dissolve in 50 ml of water and transfer the solution to a separating funnel. Add 50 ml ether and 20 drops of bromophenol blue indicator and titrate with N/2 HCl until full green colour is obtained (yellow in strong acid, green in slight acid & blue in alkali).

During titration the separatory funnel is shaken at intervals. Draw off the aqueous layer into a clean separating funnel rinse the stem with 2ml of water. Wash the ether layer twice with 5 ml of water and add to the aqueous layer in the 2nd separator. Again rinse the stem of the first separator. To this aqueous solution add 20 ml ether and shake well. The salicylic acid still left in the aqueous layer becomes redistributed between ether and aqueous layer and very little salicylic acid remains in the aqueous solution; the aqueous solution thus becomes blue again. Continue the titration with shaking at intervals until green colour is obtained.

The equations involved in the titration are:

$$C_6H_4\,(OH)COO\,Na + HCl = C_6H_4\,(OH)\,COOH + NaCl$$

C6H4 (OH) COONa ≡ H

$$160.1g\ C_6H_4\ (OH)\ COONa \equiv 1ml\ N/1\ HCl$$

$$0.800\ 5g\ C_6H_4\ (OH)\ COONa \equiv 1ml\ N/2\ HCl$$

The percentage purity of sample is calculated by the formula:

$$\% = \frac{ml \times N \times meq}{Sample\ Wt.}$$

Table 3.1
Acidimetric Assays (Direct titration with acid)

Substance	Indicator	Official Requirements, %
Aminophylline	m.o	$C_2H_8N_2$ = 13.5-15
Aminophylline injection	"	" = 20 mg
" Tablets	"	" 97-103
Potassium hydroxide	Phen	KOH = 85 total alkalinity
" "	mo	K_2CO_3 = 3.5
Pyrazinamide	mb	—
Sodium bicarbonate	mo	$Na_2\ CO_3$ = 95-105
" " Injection		
" " Tablets	mo	" "
Sodium carbonate	mo	Na_2CO_3 = 99.5-100.5
Sodium Hydroxide	Phe	NaOH = 95-100.5 Total alkalinity
Ammonia spirit aromatic	mo	$(NH_4)_2\ CO_3$ = 3.5-4.5
Ammonium chloride injection	mr	NH_4Cl = 94-106
Sodium salicylate tablets	bpb	$C_7H_5NaO_3$ = 95-105

mo = methyl orange; mr = methyl red; bpb = bromophenol blue; Phe = Phenolphthalein; mb = methylene blue.

Table 3.2
Acidimetric Assays (Titration of excess acid with base)

Substance	Indicator	Official Requirement %
Alumina and magnesia tablets	bpb	Acid cosuming 10 ml/tablet
calamine	mo	ZnO-98–100.5
Lidocaine	bcg/mr	$C_{14}H_{22}N_2O$ = 99–101
Milk of Magnesia	mr	$Mg\ (OH)_2$ = 7.0–8.5
Magnesium oxide	mo	Mgo = 96–100.5
Magnessium Trisilicate	mo	Mgo = 20
Naphazoline HCl	mr	$C_{14}H_{14}N_2$ HCl = 98–100.5
Zinc oxide	mo	ZnO = 99-100.5
Zinc Undecylenate	mo	$C_{22}H_{38}O_4$ Zn = 98.102
Magnesium citrate solution	Phe	$C_6H_8O_7$ = 7.59g/100 ml.
Potassium sodium tartrate	mr/mb	$C_4H_4kNaO_6$ 99–102
Thiotepa	Phe	$C_6H_{12}N_3PS$ = 97–102

bpb = bromophenol blue; mr = methyl red; mo = methyl orange;
Phe = Phenolphthalein; bcg = bromocresol green

3.10.4 Direct Titration of Weak Bases

EXERCISE 9. Determination of percentage of Ethylenediamine.

The sample is dissolved in water and titrated with N/10 H_2SO_4 to the green colour of bromocresol green.

3.11 Back Titrations

An estimation which involves a back titration requires an addition of an excess of a standard volumetric solution by a pipette to the weighed amount of sample and then determination of excess not required by the sample. Therefore the amount of volumetric solution used by the substance is actually estimated. The method can be applied to substances such as NH_3, $CaCO_3$, lactic acid, formaldehyde etc.

EXERCISE 10. Determination of percentage of Zinc oxide.

Method: Weigh accurately about 1.5 g of freshly ignited zinc oxide and 2.5g of ammonium chloride. Dissolve the above substances in 50 ml of 1 N H_2SO_4 with the aid of gentle heat. When the solution is complete, add methyl orange TS and titrate excess of H_2SO_4 with IN NaOH. Each millilitre of 1 N H_2SO_4 is equivalent to 40.69 mg of ZnO. The equations involved are shown below.

$$ZnO + H_2SO_4 \longrightarrow Zn\ SO_4 + H_2O$$

$$ZnO \equiv H_2SO_4 \equiv 2H \equiv 2000 \text{ ml N/1 } H_2\ SO_4$$

$$\therefore\ 81.38g\ ZnO \equiv 2000 \text{ ml N/1 } H_2\ SO_4$$

$$0.04069g\ ZnO \equiv 1 \text{ ml N/1 } H_2SO_4$$

The percentage of Zinc and zinc oxide in the sample is calculated by the formula:

$$\% = \frac{(ml_a \times N) - (ml_b \times N) \times \text{meq wt} \times 100}{\text{sample wt}}$$

Where $ml_a \times N$ = total amount of $H_2\ SO_4$ used and $ml_b \times N$ = amount neutralized by standard NaOH in back titration.

EXERCISE 11. Determination of percentage of sodium potassium tartrate (Rochelle Salt). ($C_4H_4O_6$ Na K. 4 H_2O).

Method: When alkali metal salts of aliphatic acids are heated strongly the organic portion of the molecule is destroyed and the metals are converted into Na_2CO_3 or $K_2\ CO_3$ which can be determined by titration.

Weigh accurately about 2 g of the salt in a clean, dry tared crucible and ignite gently at first, untill the salt is thoroughly carbonized, protecting the sample from contact with the flame all the time. One may use another crucible to serve as a jacket. It strong heat is applied in the beginning, loss of a portion of the sample may take place due to spattering. It heated strongly or if the flame comes into the contact with the carbonized mass, the alkali carbonate may be converted into the oxide. Cool the crucible, place it in a glass beaker, and break up the carbonised mass with a glass rod. Add 50 ml of water and 50 ml of 0.5 N H_2SO_4 and boil the solution for 30 min. Filter the solution & wash with H_2O untill it is neutral to litmus. Cool the combined filtrate and washings, add methyl red-methylene blue TS, and titrate the excess acid with 0.5N NaOH.

The following equations are involved in this assay.

$$2\ C_4H_4O_6\ NaK.\ 4\ H_2O \xrightarrow{\text{heat}} Na_2CO_3 + K_2CO_3$$

$$2\ C_4H_4O_6\ NaK\ 4\ H_2O \equiv 4H$$

$$564.4\ g\ C_4H_4O_6\ NaK\ 4H_2O \equiv 4000\ ml\ N/1\ H_2SO_4$$

$$0.07056g\ C_4H_4O_6\ Na\ K.\ 4H_2O \equiv 1\ ml\ N/2\ H_2SO_4$$

The percentage of the salt is calculated by the formula given below.

$$\%\ C_4H_4O_6\ NaK = \frac{(ml_a \times N) - (ml_b \times N) \times meq\ \ wt \times 100}{Sample\ \ wt}$$

3.11.1 Back Titrations With Blank Determinations

In any estimation if the volumetric solution is unstable or if its strength alters during the course of analysis a blank determination is performed. Blank determinations are also carried out in assays which involve heating a liquid containing excess of standard alkali, cooling and back titrating the excess. Heating and cooling an alkaline solution causes a change in the strength when certain indicators are used. This may be due to interaction with glass or due absorption of atmospheric CO_2. Therefore the alkali must be standardized, under the conditions to be used in the determination; this is called a blank determination.

EXERCISE 16. Determination of percentage W/W of lactic acid and lactide together as CH_3 CHOH COOH.

Method: Weigh accurately about 3 to 4g of sample in a weighing bottle. Wash out the sample through a funnel into a conical flask, using 50 ml water. With the aid of a pipette add 50 ml of N/1 (approx) NaOH. Boil the solution on a water bath for 5 minutes. Cool the flask to room temperature and titrate the excess of alkali with N/1 HCl using phenolphthalein as the indicator. If the pink colour of the indicator fades immediately add a few more drops. Perform a blank determination without lactic acid using 50 ml of N/1 (approx) Na OH. The volume of N/1 HCl used in the blank titration measures the amount of alkali available to react with the lactic acid and lactide in the sample and the volume of N/1 HCl used, when the sample is present gives the volume of excess alkali.

The assay is based on the fact that lactic acid is composed of lactide and free acid. The purpose of this analysis is to determine both lactide and lactic acid calculated as CH_3 CHOH COOH.

EXERCISE 16. Determination of the percentage acetylsalicylic acid (Aspirin, CH_3COO C_6H_4COOH).

Method: The assay is based on the principle which involves the hydrolysis of aspirin to acetic acid and salicylic acid and immediate formation of their salts. About 1 gm of aspirin is accurately weighed in a weighing bottle and transferred into a conical flask. Add 100 ml of N/2 (approx) Na OH from a pipette. Heat the solution on a boiling water bath for 10 minutes. Cool the flask to the room temperature. Back titrate the excess of alkali with N/2 HCl using phenol red as indicator with yellow colour as the end point. Perform a blank determination without aspirin using 50 ml of N/1 (approx) NaOH in a similar manner. The volume of N/2 HCl used in the blank titration measures the amount of alkali available for hydrolysis of aspirin to acetic acid and salicylic acid and the volume of N/1 HCl used when the sample is present gives the excess of alkali.

The reactions involved in the assay are indicated below.

$$CH_3COOH\ C_6H_4COOH + 2\ NaOH = Na + C_6H_4\ (OH)\ COO\ Na$$

$$H_3COO\ C_6H_4COOH \equiv 2\ NaOH = 2H = 2000\ ml\ N/1$$

$$180.1\ g\ C_9H_8O_4 \equiv 2000\ ml\ N/1$$

$$0.04504\ g\ C_9H_8O_4 \equiv 1\ ml\ N/2\ NaOH$$

Table 3.3
Alkalimetric Assays (Titration of Excess acid with base)

Substance	Indicator	Official Requirement %
Acetycholine	Phe	CH_3CHO = 23.2-24.2
Aspirin	Phe	$C_9H_8O_4$ = 99.5-100.5
Benzyl Benzoate	Phe	$C_{14}H_{12}O_2$ = 99.0-100.5
Chloral hydrate syrup	Phe	$C_2H_3O_2$ = 95-110
Dimenhydrinate syrup	mr	$C_{17}H_{21}NO$ C_7H_7 cl N_4O_2 295-330 mg/100 ml
		HCH = 37
Formaldehyde solution	btb	9 10 3
Methyl salicylate	Phen	$C_8H_8O_3$ = 98
Succinyl choline injection	btb	$C_{14}H_{30}cl_2N_2O_4$ = 93-107
Surose octacetate	Phen	$C_{28}H_{38}O_{19}$ = 98-100.5

btb = bromothymol blue; Phe = phenolphthalein, mr = methyl red.

3.12 Determination of Organically Combined Nitrogen

EXERCISE 14. Determination of percentage of amphetamine sulphate.

Method: Weigh accurately about 0.4g of the sample and dissolve in 120 ml water. Add 2 ml of sodium hydroxide solution and distill the volatile base into excess of N/10 HCl. The distillation is continued untill 5ml liquid is left in the distillation flask. The excess of acid is titrated with N/10 sodium hydroxide using methyl red solution as indicator. The analysis is based on the following reactions:

$$(C_9H_{13}N)_2\ H_2SO_4 + 2\ Na\ OH = 2\ C_9H_{13}\ N + Na_2\ SO_4 + 2H_2O$$

$$(C_9H_{13}N)_2\ H_2SO_4 \equiv 2Na\ OH \equiv 2H \equiv 2000\ ml\ N/1$$

Table 3.4
Alkalimetric Assays (Direct titration with a base)

Substance	Indicator	Official Requirement %
Acetic acid glacial	Phe	$C_2H_4O_2$ = 99.5-100.5
" " irrigation	Phe	$C_2H_4O_2$ = 237.5-262.5 mg
Anticoagulant Citrate	Phe	$C_6H_3O_7$ = 95-105
Phosphate solution	Phe	$C_6H_8O_7$ = 95-105
Benzoic acid	Phe	$C_7H_6O_2$ 99.5-100.5
Benzoic and salicylic acid ointment	Phe	$C_7H_6O_2$ = 90-110
Chlorambucil	Phe	$C_{14}H_{19}cl_2NO_2$ = 98-101
Cholic acid (R)	Phe	$C_{24}H_{40}O_5$ = 98
Citric acid	Phe	$C_8H_8O_7$ = 99.5-100.5
Furosemide	btb	$C_{12}H_{11}$ ClN_2O_5S = 101
Hydrochloric acid	mr	HCl = 35-38
Meprobamate	Phe	$C_9H_{18}N_2O_4$ = 97-100.5
Saccharin	Phe	$C_7H_5NO_3S$ = 98-101
Salicylic acid	"	$C_7H_6O_3$ = 99.5-101.5

(*Contd.*)

Sulfamic acid	"	$HSO_3\ NH_2 = 99.5$
Sulfinpyrazone tablets	"	$C_{23}H_{20}N_2O_3S = 93\text{-}107$
Sulphur, precipitator	"	$S = 99.5\text{-}100$
Tolbutamide	"	$C_{12}H_8N_2O_3S = 98\text{-}101$
Undecylenic acid ointment	"	$C_{11}H_{20}O_2 = 4.5\text{-}5.5$
Benzyl benzoate lotion	"	$_{14}H_{12}O_2 = 26\text{-}30$
Boric acid	Phe	$H_3BO_3 = 99.5\text{-}100.5$
Dehydrocholic acid tablets	"	$C_{24}H_{34}O_5 = 94\text{-}106$
Indomethicin	Phe	$C_{19}H_{16}\ ClNO_4 = 98\text{-}101$
Methylthiouracil	"	$S = 22.2\text{-}22.8$
Niacin	"	$C_6H_5NO_2 = 95\text{-}101$
Oxandrolone	"	$C_{19}H_{30}O_3 = 97\text{-}100.5$
Oxyphenbutazone	btb	$C_{19}H_{20}N_2O_3 = 98\text{-}100.5$
Sorbic acid	Phe	$C_6H_8O_2 = 99\text{-}101$
Tartric acid	"	$C_4H_6O_6 = 99.7\text{-}100.5$

Phe = Phenolphthalein thb = thymol blue; bpb = bromophenol blue; mo = methyl orange; btb = bromothymol blue; mr = methyl red; mb = methylene blue;

EXERCISE 15. Determination of percentage of Nicotinamide.

Method: The analysis of the substance is based on the hydrolysis with sodium hydroxide and distilling the ammonia into 4% W/V solution of boric acid. The distillate is titrated with standard acid using methyl red as indicator. A blank determination without the sample is also performed. The reaction involved is shown below.

$$C_5H_4N\text{-}CONH_2 + NaOH = C_5H_4N\text{-}CO\,Na + NH_3$$

$$\therefore\ C_{10}H_{14}ON_2 \equiv NH_3 \equiv H$$

3.12.1 Nitrogen Determination By Kjeldahl Method

In some cases it so happens that nitrogen is firmly combined and ammonia is not quantitatively liberated from the organic-nitrogen compound by acid or alkaline hydrolysis as described in the previous example. Therefore a much more severe treatment is required before nitrogen is obtained quantitatively as NH_3. The organic portion of the molecule is destroyed and the carbon oxidized untill a clear liquid is obtained. The method involves in the digestion of the substance with concentrated H_2SO_4 using either sodium or potassium sulphate to raise the boiling point of the acid and catalysts such as mercury, selenium and copper to hasten the reaction. This method is not applicable when nitrogen is present as nitro, azo, cyano or hydrazo; etc groups.

EXERCISE 16. Determination of percentage of urethane ($C_3H_7O_2N$).

Method: Weigh accurately about 0.2 g of the sample and transfer into a kjeldal flask (long-necked flask). Add anhdrous $Na_2\ SO_4$ (3g), nitrogen free HgO (0.3g) and nitrogen free H_2SO_4 (6.7 ml). Shake the contents of the mixture. The flask is covered with a funnel then inclined at about 60° on a stand and mixture heated untill all frothing ceases. The solution is further heated untill the mixture refluxes in the flask and becomes clear. Finally it is boiled for 2 more hours. The mixture is cooled, diluted with 75 ml water. Add a few pieces of grannulated zinc (to prevent bumping), a solution of NaOH (10g) & $Na_2S_2O_6$

(2 g in 15 ml water). The flask is now set up for distillation and the liberated NH_3 passed into 4% boric acid (W/V in 20 ml H_2O). The distilate is titrated with N/10 H_2SO_4 using methyl red as indicator. A blank titration without the sample is also performed. The difference between the two titrations gives the amount of NH_3 liberated. The equation involved in the analysis are given below.

$$NH_2\ COO\ C_2\ H_5\ \equiv\ N\ \equiv\ NH_3\ \equiv\ H$$

$$89.00\ g\ NH_2\ COOC_2\ H_5\ \equiv\ 1000\ ml\ N/1$$

$$0.08909\ g\ NH_2\ COO\ C_2\ H_5\ \equiv\ 1\ ml\ N/1$$

∴ 0.2 g of the sample is approximately

equivalent to 20 ml of N/10 $H_2\ S_4$.

Table 3.5
Acidimetric Assays (Nitrogen Determinations)

Substance	Factor	Official Requirement, %
L-Aspargine (R)	0.140	N = 18.4-18.8
Calcium pantothenate	1.401	N = 5.7-6.0
Casein (R)	1.401	N = 15.2-16.0
Glucagon	0.140	N = 16.0-18.5
Heparin Sodium	0.140	N = 2.5
Insulin injection	0.140	N = 0.70 mg/100 units
Insulin zinc suspension	0.140	N = 0.70
L-Lysine (R)	1.401	N = 15.88-16.44
Peptone dried (R)	1.401	N = 14.2-15.5
Protamine sulfate	0.140	N = 22.5-25.5
Protein hydrolysate injection	0.140	N = 1.4 mg - amino
Pyridoxal HCl (R)	1.401	N = 6.7-7.1
Sodium glycocholate (R)	1.40	N = 2.6-3.2
Thioguanine	1.401	N = 40.6-43.1
Yeast extract	1.401	N = 7.2-9.5

R = reagent

4

Non-Aqueous Titration Methods

4.1 General

With the introduction of many new complex organic medicinal substances many of which were poorly soluble and weakly reactive in water the problem of quality control became difficult. Substances which are either too weakly acidic or too weakly basic do not produce sharp end points in aqueous solution, but they can be titrated in non-aqueous media. With the application of non-aqueous titrations that could not be carried out in aqueous medium because of poor solubility or weak reactivity. The speed, precision and accuracy of non-aqueous methods are close to those of the classical acidimetric and alkalimetric titrations. The apparatus involved is also the same but moisture and CO_2 are to be avoided in nonaqueous methods because H_2O which is a weak base can compete with a weak nitrogen base and the end point would not be sharp at all. It has been observed through experiments that the moisture content in non-aqueous titration should not be more than 0.05%. Further, the temperatures during standardization in nonaqueous titrimetry should not be allowed to vary.

In an aqueous solution, neutralization is understood as a reaction between proton donor and a proton acceptor i.e. an acid and a base. On the contrary, in non-aqueous solvents the neutralization can be considered as a reaction between a weakly protophyllic substance which tends to accept a pair of electrons and a highly protophyllic substance which tends to provide a pair of electrons in the formation of covalent bonds by coordination. The protophyllic solvents are basic in character and react with acids to form solvated protons, while protogenic solvents are acidic substances like H_2SO_4 and exert a levelling effect. The third type, i.e. the amphiprotic solvents have both protophillic and protogenic properties, examples being water, acetic acid and alcohols. They are weakly dissociated. Thus if a very strong acid like $HClO_4$ is dissolved in CH_3COOH, the latter can function as a base and accept protons from $HClO_4$ as indicated in the reactions.

$$HClO_4 \rightleftharpoons H^+ + ClO_4^-$$

$$CH_3COOH + H^+ \rightleftharpoons CH_3COOH_2^+$$

The onium ion i.e. $CH_3COOH_2^+$ can readily donate its proton to a base which means that $HClO_4$ in glacial acetic acid functions as a strong acid. For example, pyridine which is a weak base when dissolved in acetic acid, the latter exerts its levelling effect and enhances the basic properties of pyridine. Therefore, one can titrate a solution of a weak base in acetic acid with $HClO_4$ in acetic acid and obtain a sharp end point which otherwise cannot be attained in an aqueous solution.

$$HClO_4 + CH_3COOH \rightleftharpoons CH_3COOH_2^+ + ClO_4^-$$

$$C_5H_5N + CH_3COOH \rightleftharpoons C_5H_5N^+H + CH_3COO^-$$

$$CH_3COOH_2 + CH_3COO^- \rightleftharpoons 2CH_3COOH$$

Add

$$HClO_4 + C_5H_5N \rightleftharpoons C_5H_5N^+H + ClO_4^-$$

The above titration can not be carried out in presence of H_2O because water being a weak base will compete with pyridine as shown by the equations:

$$H_2O + HClO_4 \rightleftharpoons H_3O^+ = ClO_4^-$$

$$C_5H_5N + HClO_4 \rightleftharpoons C_5H_5N^+H + ClO_4^-$$

The equivalence point in non-aqueous titrations is ascertained potentiometrically or by an indicator which will give the sharpest colour change near the end point.

4.2 Acidimetry in Non-Aqueous Solvents

Theory: As already explained above water is amphiprotic in nature i.e. it can act either as an acid or a base depending upon experimental conditions and will compete with the basic species in solution. Therefore the solvent must be altered to eliminate this competing reaction of water and also to increase the strength of the basic species. Unless the weak bases have pk_b values greater than 10^{-6} they cannot be satisfactorily titrated in water. The nonaqueous method involves titration of the weak bases in glacial acetic acid against $HClO_4$ as the titrant. Some of the examples of weak bases come from amines, amine salts, heterocyclic nitrogen compounds, alkali salts of organic acids, alkali salts of weak inorganic acid and amino acids etc. The solvents selected for acidimetry should be either neutral or acidic in nature. The neutral solvents are acetonitrile, alcohols, chloroform, benzene, dioxane, ethyl acetate because they do not enhance dissociation to a great degree. The acidic solvents are formic acid, acetic acid, propionic acid, acetic anhydride, sulphonyl chloride because they are protogenic in nature and can be utilised for weak bases. The reactions involved with a weak base are indicated below:

$$B + CH_3COOH \rightleftharpoons BH^+ + CH_3COO^-$$

$$HClO_4 + CH_3COOH \rightleftharpoons CH_3COOH_2^+ + ClO_4^-$$

$$CH_3COO^- + CH_3COOH_2 \rightleftharpoons 2CH_3COOH$$

Overall reaction is as $B + HClO_4 \longrightarrow BH^+ + ClO^-_4$

It is thus possible to perform analysis of a mixture of two bases of different strengths with the use of two solvents.

The most widely used titrant for weak bases is perchloric acid in glacial acetic acid or in the neutral solvent dioxane. It is the strongest of the known common acids and gives very good results with all the known weak bases. Hydrogen bromide and certain organic sulphuric acids can also be used.

The indicators which can be used in the titration of weak bases and their salts comprise crystal violet, methybrosaniline chloride, quinaldine red, x-naphtholbenzein, malachite green etc.

EXERCISE 1. Preparation and standardization of 0.1 N Perchloric Acid.

Method : Mix slowly 8.5 ml of 70–720% (sp. gr. 1.6) of perchloric acid with 500 ml glacial acetic acid and 30 ml of acetic anhydride, cool the solution and add glacial acetic acid to make the total volume 1000 ml. Allow the solution to stand for 24 hours (Perchloric acid undergoes a spontaneous decomposition and should be handled with care). Meanwhile weigh accurately 500 mg of previously dried (at 120° for 2 hrs) potassium hydrogen phthalate in a 100 ml conical flask. Attach a reflux condenser fitted with a drying tube and add 25 ml of glacial acetic acid. Warm the solution until the salt has dissolved and cool. Add 2 drops of 0.5% W/V acetous crystal violet test solution and titrate with N/10 $HClO_4$ unitl violet colour changes to emarald green.

The equations involved in the titration are:

$$C_6H_4(COOK)_2 + HClO_4 \longrightarrow C_6H_4(COOH)_2 + KClO_4$$

$\therefore$ 204.14 g $C_8H_4O_4K \equiv HClO_4 \equiv H \equiv$ 1000 ml N/1

$\therefore$ 0.204.14 g $C_8H_5O_4K \equiv$ 1 ml N/1

$\therefore$ 0.020414 g $C_8H_5O_4K \equiv$ 1 ml N/10 $HClO_4$

EXERCISE 2. Determination of percentage of adrenaline ($C_9H_{13}O_3N$).

Method : Accurately weigh about 0.3 g of the substance into a 250 ml conical flask. Dissolve in 50 ml glacial acetic acid with warming if necessary. Cool and titrate with N10 acetous $HClO_4$ using crystal violet as an indicator.

The equations involved in the assay are:

$$(HO)_2C_6H_3-CH(OH)CH_2NH.CH_3 + HClO_4 \rightarrow (HO)_2C_6H_3-CH(OH)-CH-CH-NH-CH.ClO_4^-$$

183.2 g $C_9H_{13}NO_3 \equiv HClO_4 \equiv H \equiv$ 1000 ml N/1

0.01832 g $C_9H_{13}NO_3 \equiv$ 1 ml N/10 $HClO_4$

EXERCISE 3. TITRATION OF HALOGEN ACID SALTS OF BASES

For assay of halogen acid salts of bases it is to be noted that halide ions chloride, bromide and iodide are too weakly basic to react quantitatively with acetous $HClO_4$. Mercuric acetate is added to the halide salt to replace halide ion by acetate ion which is a strong base in acetic acid as indicated in the equations below :

$$2\,RNH_2.HCl \rightleftharpoons 2RN^+H_3 + 2Cl^-$$

$$(CH_3COO)_2Hg\text{ (undissociated)} + 2Cl^- = HgCl_2\text{ (undissociated)} + 2CH_3COO^-$$

$$2CH_3COOH_2^+ + 2CH_3COO^- \rightleftharpoons 4CH_3COOH$$

The general procedure involves weighing of the drug sample and dissolving it in warm glacial acetic acid. Mercuric acetate in glacial acetic acid (5% W/V) is then added and the solution is titrated with N/10 acetous $HClO_4$ using 0.2 ml of crystal violet (0.5% in acetic acid) as indicator.

4.3 Alkalimetry in Non Aqueous Solvents

The weakly acidic medicinal compounds can be titrated in an appropriate nonaqueous solvent with a sharp end point just like the weak bases as explained earlier. The different types of weak organic acidic substances comprise acid halides, anhydrides, acids, amino acids, enols like barbiturates, xanthines, imides, phenols, pyrroles, sulphonamides and organic salts of inorganic acids.

The basic solvent like ethylenediamine can enhance the acidic strength of the weakly acidic compounds such as phenols so that they can be titrated with a standard solution of lithium or sodium methoxide. The important characteristics for choosing a basic solvent are : (a)solubility of the substance for analysis, (b) the relative base strength of the solvent, (c) the sharpness of the end-point change and (d) the non-reactivity of the solution. The strong base solvents which can be used for weak acids like enols are ethylenediamine, n-butylamine & morpholine. The somewhat weaker base solvents which can be used for titration of medium-strength acidic substances are DMF & pyridine. For example with the proper selection of basic solvents it is possible to titrate selectively simple mixtures of sulphonamides e.g. sulfanilamide & sulphathiazole.

Sodium methoxide and lithium methoxide are the bases which are used as titrants in the titration of weak acids. Potassium methoxide produces gelatinous reaction products and is not commonly used. Other base titrants like sodium aminomethoxide & sodium triphenylmethane can be used for compounds like phenols and pyrroles.

The equivalence or the end point in a non-aqueous titration of a weakly acidic substance is commonly determined with a potentiometer, i.e. the mid-point of the inflection part of the curve in which ml of titrant is titrated against mV produced in the reaction. It has been observed that azoviolet is the indicator of choice in the titration of acids of weak or intermediate strength in butylamine as the solvent while thymol blue is the indicator of choice for the determination of intermediate to strong acids in DMF as the solvent. In metal alcoholate titration azoviolet will change colour before thymol blue. O-nitro-aniline is the indicator used for titration of very weak acids. Other indicators are thymolphthalein and p-hydroxyazohenzene.

EXERCISE 4. Preparation and standardization of 0.1 N sodium methoxide.

Method : Place in a 1000 ml volumetric flask 150 ml MeOH and Cool in ice. Add in small portions 2.5 g of fresh cut prices of sodium metal. When the metal has dissolved, add sufficient benzene to make 1000 ml and mix. Store in the reservoir of an automatic delivery burette protected from CO_2 and H_2O.

Weigh accurately 400 mg of benzoic acid (Primary standard) in a flask and dissolve in 80 ml of DMF. Titrate with sodium methoxide using 3 drops of thymol blue (1 in 100 ml DMF) as indicator until the end point is blue. Correct for the volume of $NaOCH_3$ solution consumed by 80 ml of DMF and calculate the normality. Each 12.21 mg of C_6H_5COOH is equivalent to 1 ml of 0.I N $NaOCH_3$. The reaction involved with Na & methanol is :

$$Na + CH_3OH \longrightarrow CH_3O^-Na^+ + 1/2\ H_2$$

Carbon dioxide and moisture should be kept away from sodium methoxide because of the following:

$$H_2O + CH_3O^-Na^+ \longrightarrow CH_3OH + NaOH$$

$$H_2CO_3 + 2CH_3O^-Na^+ \longrightarrow 2CH_3OH + Na_2CO_3.$$

The other reactions involved are :

$$C_6H_5COOH + HCON(CH_3) \rightleftharpoons HCO\overset{H}{N}_+ - (CH_3)_2 + C_6H_5COO^-$$

$$CH_3ONa \rightleftharpoons CH_3O^- + Na^+$$

$$HCO\overset{H}{N}_+(CH_3)_2 + CH_3O^- \longrightarrow HCON(CH_3)_2 + CH_3OH$$

$$C_6H_5COOH + CH_3\bar{O}Na^+ \longrightarrow C_6H_5CO\bar{O}Na^+ + CH_3OH$$

The correction for volume of $CH_3\bar{O}Na^+$ consumed by DMF is in effect a blank determination to account for the interaction between water in the solvent and the titrant.

1.0 g atomic wt. of Na (22.99 g) ≡ 1.0 g mol. Wt of $CH_3\bar{O}Na^+$ (54.029)
0.1 N solution contains 1/10 equiv/lit.
2.5 g . Na will produce 5.4 g. or 1/10 of $Na^+O^-CH_3$.
1 meq weight of C_6H_5COOH ≡ 0.12212 g
0. 400 g of C_6H_5COOH ≡ 3 meq of $Na^+O^-CH_3$ for standardization.

The preparation and standardization of N/10 lithium methoxide and N/10 potassium methoxide is done in a similar manner.

EXERCISE 5. Determination of percentage of Phenobarbitone ($C_{12}H_{12}N_2O_3$).

Method : Transfer 40 ml of DMF into a titration flask. Add 3 drops of quinaldine red solution (0.1% W/V in ethanol) and neutralise by titrating with N/10 lithium methoxide. Accurately weigh about 0.2 g of the drug sample in the flask. Titrate with N/10 lithium methoxide using quinaldine red as indicator avoiding any contamination of lithium methoxide with H_2O and CO_2. The end-point will be when the colour changes from pink to colourless.

As an alternative method this titration can also be carried out with N/10 tetrabutylammonium hydroxide in benzene-methanol using thymol blue as an indicator (2 drops; 0.5% in methanol).

The titration is based on the following equation :

$$O = C\begin{matrix} \diagup NH - CO \diagdown \\ \diagdown NH - CO \diagup \end{matrix}C\begin{matrix} \diagup C_2H_5 \\ \diagdown C_6H_5 \end{matrix} + LiOMe = C{=}O\begin{matrix} \diagup N = C - OLi \\ \diagdown N - C \diagup \end{matrix}\!\!\!\diagdown C \text{———} C_2H_5 + CH_3OH \quad (C_6H_5 \text{ on } C)$$

$$\therefore\ 232.2 \text{ g } C_{12}H_{12}N_2O_3 \equiv \overset{+}{Li}\overset{-}{O}CH_3 \equiv H \equiv 1000 \text{ ml N/1}$$

$$\therefore\ 0.02322 \text{ g } C_{12}H_{12}N_2O_3 \equiv 1 \text{ ml N/10 } \overset{-}{Li}\overset{+}{O}CH_3$$

Table 4.1
Non-aqueous titrations with perchloric Acid

Drug Substance	Indicator	Official Requirement %.
Amitryptyline	crv	$C_{20}H_{23}N.Hcl$ = 99-100.5
Benzotropine HCl	mr	$C_{21}H_{25}NO.CH_4O_3S$ = 98-100.5
Carbachol	crv	$C_6H_{15}COB_2O_2$ = 99-101
Chlordiazepoxide HCl	crv	$C_6H_{14}ClN_3O.Hcl$ = 99-101
Chorpheniramine maleate	crv	$C_{16}H_{19}ClN_2.C_4H_4O_4$ = 98-100.5
Chlorpromazine	crv	$C_{17}H_{19}ClN_2S$ = 98-101
Diazepam	nb	$C_{16}H_{13}ClN_3O$ = 98.5-101
Diethylcarbamazine citrate	crv	$C_{10}H_{21}N_3O.C_6H_8O_7$ = 98-100.5
Diphenhydramine	crv	$C_{17}H_{21}NO.Hcl$ = 98-1000.5
Propantheline Bromide	crv	$C_{23}H_{30}Br\,NO_3$= 98-102
Propanolol	Pnb	$C_{16}H_{21}NO.Hcl$ = 98-101
Propoxyphene HCl	crv	$C_{22}H_{29}NO_2.Hcl$ = 98-101
Pyridoxine HCl	crv	$C_8H_{11}NO_3.Hcl$ = 98-100.5
Thiabendazole	crv	$C_{10}H_7N_3S$ = 98-101
Trihexyphenidyl HCl	crv	$C_{20}H_{31}NO.Hcl$ = 98-100.5

crv = Crystal Violet; mr = methyl red; Pnb = p-naptholbenzein; nb = nile blue

Table 4.2
Non-aqueous titration with Lithium or Sodium Methoxide

Drug Substance	Indicator	Official Requirement %
Chorothiazide	thb	$C_7H_6ClN_3O_4S_2$ = 98-100.5
Dichlorphenamide	thph	$C_6H_6Cl_2N_2O_4S_2$
Dicumarol	azv	$C_{19}H_{12}O_6$ = 98-100.5
Ethosuximide	azv	$C_7H_{11}NO_2$ = 98-101
Idoxuridine	thb	$C_9H_{11}N_2O_5$ = 98-101
Mercaptopurine	thb	C_5H_4S = 97-102
Pentobarbital	thb	$C_{11}H_{16}N_2O_3$ = 98.5-101
Phention	azv	$C_{16}H_{12}N_2O_2$ = 98.5-100.5
Sodium aminosalicylate	thb	$C_7H_6N\,NaO_3$ = 98-101
Sulphisoxazole	thb	$C_{11}H_{13}N_3O_3S$ = 99-101

thb = thymol blue; azv = azoviolet; thph = thymolphthalein;

In addition to above given short list, many more drug substances can be assayed by nonaqueous titration method.

5

Oxidation-Reduction Methods

5.1 General

The analytical proceduces which are based on neutralization and precipitation involve chemical reactions that take place without any change in the valence of the reacting substances. On the other hand oxidation-reduction methods of analysis involve a change in valence.

Oxidation can be defined to involve any of the following :

(i) addition of oxygen, such as $SO_2 + O = SO_3$

(ii) removal of hydrogen e.g. $H_2S + O = H_2O + S$

or (iii) increase in the ratio of the molecule, e.g.

$$Sn^{2+} + 2Cl^- + 2HgCl_2 = Sn^{4+} + 4Cl^- + Hg_2Cl_2$$

$$2Fe^{2+} + 4Cl^- + Cl_2 = 2Fe^{3+} + 6Cl^-$$

The reduction can be defined to involve any of the following :

(i) addition of hydrogen e.g. $CH \equiv CH + 2H = CH_2 = CH_2$.

(ii) removal of oxygen, e.g. $CuO + 2H = Cu + H_2O$

or (iii) increase in the ratio of electropositive to electronegative portion of the molecule.

The other simple examples of oxidation-reduction reactions are (i) combination of oxygen gas with hydrogen gas to form water ($O_2 + 2H_2 = 2H_2O$) in which oxygen is reduced and hydrogen is oxidized, (ii) Carbon is burnt in presence of oxygen to produce carbon dioxide ($C + O_2 \longrightarrow CO_2$) in which case carbon is oxidized and oxygen is reduce and (iii) when carbon reacts with sulphur to produces carbon disulphide ($C + 2S \longrightarrow CS_2$) in which case carbon is oxidized and sulphur is reduced.

Oxidation and reduction occur at the same time i.e. when one substance is oxidized the other substance is reduced and vice versa.

A reactant which loses electrons in an oxidation-reduction reaction is called the *reducing agent.* It can be identified in a chemical reaction as the reactant in which constituent atom or atoms are converted to a higher state of oxidation, e.g.

$$Fe^{2+} \longrightarrow Fe^{3+} + e$$

$$2I^- \longrightarrow I_2 + 2e$$

The electrons lost by the reducing agent are gained by the Oxidizing agent, i.e., the reactant in which the constituent atom or atoms are converted to a lower state of oxidation, e.g.

$$Ce^{4+} + e \longrightarrow Ce^{3+}$$

$$Fe^{4+} + e \longrightarrow Fe^{3+}$$

Therefore, a combination of oxidizing and reducing agents forms a chemical reaction that can be used for determination of one the reactants, e.g. (i) reaction of ferrous sulphate with ceric sulphate can be utilized to assay ferrous sulphate as indicated by the reactions :

$$Fe^{2+} \rightleftharpoons Fe^{3+} + e$$

$$Ce^{4+} + e \rightleftharpoons Ce^{3+}$$

Add

$$Fe^{2+} + Ce^{4+} \longrightarrow Fe^{3+} + Ce^{3+}$$

and similarly (ii) reaction of ferric chloride and potassium iodide can be used for the assay of ferric chloride as shown by the reactions :

$$2I^- \longrightarrow I_2 + 2e$$

$$2Fe^{3+} + 2e \longrightarrow 2Fe^{2+}$$

Add

$$2I^- + 2Fe^{3+} \longrightarrow I_2 + 2Fe^{2+}$$

The amount of the oxidizing agent or reducing agent is determined by measuring chemically equivalent amount of the reducing or oxidizing agent respectively. In the above reaction between ferrous sulphate and ceric sulphate, each molecule of ferrous sulphate loses one electron on oxidation i.e. one mole of ferrous sulphate loses 6.02×10^{23} electrons which is equivalent to faraday or 96,500 C. This amount of electricity is identical with that required to reduce 1 mole of cerric sulphate. Hence, one mole of ferrous sulphate and 1 mole of cerric sulphate are chemical equivalents.

An *equivalent weight* of an *oxidizing agent* is that weight which gains electrons equivalent to 1 faraday (96,500 C). It is calculated by dividing the gram molecular weight by the number of electrons gained by each molecule, e.g. in case of cerric sulphate $Ce^{4+} + e \longrightarrow Ce^{3+}$ the equivalent weight is same as 1 grammolecular weight, 332.24 g while in case of potassium permanganate, $MnO_4^- + 5e \longrightarrow Mn^{2+}$ equivalent weight is 1/5 of gram molecular weight or 31.61 g.

Similarly, the equivalent weight of a reducing agent is that weight which loses electrons equivalent to 96,500 C. It is calculated by dividing the gram-molecular weight by the number of electrons lost by each molecule e.g. the equivalent weight of ferrous sulphate which oxidizes to ferric sulphate ($Fe^{2+} \longrightarrow Fe^{3+}$) is 151.91 g which is the same as its 1 gram molecular weight. It should be noted that in some cases the number of electrons gained by an oxidizing agent depends on conditions particularly pH under which the reaction is carried out, e.g. in case of nitric acid, no uniform reaction occurs so it cannot be used as a standard oxidizing agent.

The chief oxidizing agents used in volumetric analysis are potassium permanganate, potassium dichromate, ferric ammonium sulphate, potassium bromate, potassium iodate, potassium ferricyanide, cerric sulphate, iodine and bromine while the important reducing agents used are oxalic acid, potassium arsenite, ferrous ammonium sulphate, titanium chloride and sodium thiosulphate.

5.2 Titrations Involving Potassium Permanganate

EXERCISE 1. Preparation and standardization of N/10 Potassium Permanganate solution :

When potassium permanganate is used as an oxidizing agent under acid condition the following equations are involved :

$$2KMnO_4 + 3H_2SO_4 = K_2SO_4 + 2Mn\ SO_4 + 3H_2O + 5\ O$$

$$2KMnO_4 \equiv 50 \equiv 10\ H \equiv 10{,}000 \text{ ml N/1}$$

$$2 \times 158.0g\ KMnO_4 \equiv 10{,}000 \text{ ml N/1}$$

$$3.160 \text{ g } KMnO_4 \equiv 1000 \text{ ml N/10}$$

Method : Weigh approximately 3.2 g of $KMnO_4$ on a watch glass. Transfer he sample into a breaker and dissolve in small amount of cold water. Stir the solution throughly and add more water in small portions untill the crystals are completely dissolved Filter the solution through a glass wool and add water untill the volume reaches 1 litre.

In the mean time weigh accurately 6.3 g of pure oxalic acid and transfer it to a 1 litre graduated flask. Dissolve it in water and make up to 1 litre. Pipette out 20 ml of this solution, add about 5 ml of concentrated $H_2\ SO_4$ and warm to 70°C. Titrate his solution against $KMnO_4$ which is added from a burette. The first few drops result in a pink colour which persists for 20 secs. Wait untill colour disappears and continue the titration normally. The end point is obtained when a faint pink colour persists for about 30 seconds after shaking the flask.

Oxalic acid deteriorates on standing and must be restandardized from time to time. The Preparation of a standard solution from pure oxalic acid involves the following equations :

$$\begin{matrix} COOH \\ | \\ COOH \end{matrix}\quad 2H_2O + O = 2CO_2 + 3H_2O$$

$$\therefore C_2H_2O_4 \equiv O \equiv 2H$$

$$\therefore 6.302 \text{ g } C_2H_2O_4.\ 2H_2O \equiv 1000 \text{ ml N/100}$$

EXERCISE 2. Determination of percentage of Ferrous Sulphate (Fe SO_4. $7H_2O$).

Method : Weigh accurately about 1 g of the sample in a conical flask. Add 20 ml of dilute concentrated $H_2\ SO_4$ and titrated with N/10 $KMnO_4$ untill one drop gives a permanent pink colour.

The equations involved are stated below:

$$2Fe\ SO_4 + H_2SO_4 + O = Fe_2\ (SO_4)_3 + H_2O$$

$$\therefore 278.0 \text{ g Fe } SO_4,\ 7H_2O \equiv H \equiv 10{,}000 \text{ N/10 } KMnO_4.$$

$$\therefore 0.02780 \text{ g fe } SO_4.\ 7H_2O \equiv 1 \text{ ml N/10 } KMnO_4.$$

EXERCISE 3. Determination of percentage of sodium Nitrite (Na NO_2).

Method : Weigh about 0.6-0.7 g of the sample in a 250 ml graduated flask. Dissolve it in recently boiled and cooled water and make up the volume to get approximately N/10 solution.

Place this solution in a burrette.

Pipette 25 ml of N/10 $KMnO_4$ into a conical flask and add 30 ml of water. Now add 4-5 ml of concentrated H_2SO_4 while rotating the flask and note the rise in temperature which should not be more than 40°C. Titrate this solution against sodium nitrite while maintaining the temperature of 40°. The flask should be rotated during titration because HNO_2 reacts slowly with $KMnO_4$ at 40ºC or otherwise it will be lost as oxides of nitrogen. The higher temperature will decompose $KMnO_4$. When the colour of the titrated solution becomes pale pink, raise the temperature and continue the addition of $NaNO_2$ dropwise. Towards the end of the titration the solution should be boiling.

If $KMnO_4$ solution turns brown or decomposes during titration, repeat the experiment. Sodium nitrite solution cannot be placed in a flask because HNO_2 produced reacts slowly with $KMnO_4$ and can be lost therefore it is placed in the burette.

The equations involved in the determination of sodium nitrite are following :

$$2NaNO_2 + H_2SO_4 = 2HNO_2 + Na_2SO_4$$

$$HNO_2 + O = HNO_3$$

$$NaNO_2 \equiv HNO_2 \equiv O \equiv 2H$$

$$\therefore 69.0 \text{ g } NaNO_2 \equiv 2000 \text{ ml N/1}$$

$$\therefore 0.003450 \text{ g} \equiv 1 \text{ ml N/10 } KMnO_4$$

The overall reaction between sodium nitrite and $KMnO_4$ is stated as :

$$10NaNO_2 + 4KMnO_4 + 11H_2SO_4 \longrightarrow 10HNO_3 + 4MnSO_4 + 2K_2SO_4 + 5Na_2SO_4 + 6H_2O$$

Each molecule of $NaNO_2$ loses two electrons and the equivalent weight of $NaNO_2$ is 34.50 or 1/2 gram molecular weight. Therefore each millilitre of 0.1NK MnO_4 is equivalent to $0.1 \times 0.0345 = 0.00345$ g or 0.1 meq of $NaNO_2$.

5.3 Titrations Involving Ceric Sulphate

Theory : Ceric sulphate in presence of dilute sulphuric acid (1.8 N) is a powerful oxidizing agent. The acid must be present in sufficient amount to prevent the hydrolysis and precipitation of basic salts. While in Case of $KMnO_4$ there are several oxidation states, ceric has only one oxidation state as.

$$Ce^{4+} + e. \rightleftharpoons Ce^{3+}$$

Ceric sulphate is bright yellow in colour both in solid state and in solution and the cerous salt formed on reduction is colourless. As a practical oxidizing agent ceric sulphate has many advantages over permanganate and dichromate, e.g. (i) the solutions are stable even on boiling and do not need protection from light. (ii) reacts quantitatively with oxalate, arsenite, so sodium oxalate or arsenic trioxide can be used as a primary standard, (iii) the cerous ion is colourless and does not interfere with the indicator, (iv) no intermediates products are formed in the reduction of ceric-cerium. The indicator used in the titrations with Ceric sulphate is ferrous Phenanthroline ion also known as ferroin. The reactions involved are shown as :

$$\underset{\text{Colourless}}{C_{12}H_8N_2} + Fe^{2+} \longrightarrow \underset{\substack{\text{Ferrous complex}\\ \text{(red)}}}{Fe(C_{12}H_8N_2)_3^{2+}} \rightleftharpoons \underset{\substack{\text{Ferric Complex}\\ \text{(Blue)}}}{Fe(C_{12}H_8N_2)_3^{3+}} + e^-$$

The indicator solution is obtained by dissolving 150 mg of orthophenanthroline in 10 ml of a solution of ferrous sulphate which is prepared from 1.48 g of pure ferrous sulphate in 100 ml of water. Strong oxidizing agents change ferrous to ferric complex which is light blue in colour. This blue form is very stable and is not affected further by oxidizing agents. The change in colour from red to blue is reversed by reducing agents.

EXERCISE 4. Preparation and Standardization of N/20 Ceric Ammonium sulphate.

Method : Weigh accurately about 31.63 g of ceric ammonium sulphate Ce $(SO_4)_2$. $2(NH_4)_2$ SO_4 $2H_2O$ and dissolve in 2N H_2SO_4 and make up the volume to 1 litre.

In the mean time, prepare N/20 solution of ferrous ammonium sulphate from 19.61 g of A.R. grade reagent in 1 litre water. Now pipette 20 ml of this solution into a conical flask, add 20 ml of N/1 H_2SO_4 and 2 drops of 0-phenanthroline-ferrous indicator. Titrate with N/20 ceric ammonium sulphate until the colour changes to pale blue.

5.4 Titrations involving Iodine

Theory : The iodometric methods of analysis incorporating the use of iodine are based on oxidation - reduction reactions. The reversible reaction $I_2 + 2e \rightleftharpoons 2I^-$ is utilized indirectly in the analysis of oxidizing agents like ferric cupric salts.

The method involves in reducing the oxidizing agent with excess of potassium iodide whereby an equivalent amount of iodine is produced which is titrated with a standard solution of sodium thiosulphate. This procedure is known as iodometry. On the other hand the reversible reaction $2I^- \rightleftharpoons I_2 + 2e$ is utilized in the analysis of reducing agents like thiosulphates and arsenites by direct titration with a standard solution of Iodine. This procedure is called iodimetry. Hence the above two procedures are also known as iodometric and iodiometric methods.

The presence of iodine is detected by the use of starch indicator solution.

The reaction between iodine and sodium thiosulphate as indicated below shows that

$$I_2 + 2Na_2S_2O_3 \longrightarrow 2NaI + Na_2S_4O_6$$

that 1 gram-atomic weight of iodine i.e. 126.9 g and 1 gram-molecular weight i.e. Na_2 S_2O_3 $5H_2O$ (248.17 g) are equivalent

This uniformity of reaction between I_2 with $Na_2S_2O_3$ forms the basis for using standard solution of I_2 in the analysis of $Na_2S_2O_3$ and use of standard solution of Na_2 S_2 O_3 in the analysis of iodine.

In the determination of arsenious acid the reaction involved is as follows,

$H_3AsO_3 + H_2O + I_2 \rightleftharpoons H_3AsO_3 + 2H^+ + 2I^-$ In this reaction arsenious acid is oxidized.

On the other hand in the assay of cupric sulphate, potassium iodide used is oxidized and an equivalent amount of iodine is formed as shown by the equation :

$2CuSO_4 + 4KI \longrightarrow I_2 + 2CuI\downarrow + 2K_2SO_4$

Since iodine does not dissolve freely in water but dissolves in the presence of potassium iodide due to the reaction $I_2 + I^- \longrightarrow I_3^-$ (i.e. triiodide) therefore standard solutions of iodine are essentially solutions of iodine in potassium iodide solution.

The indicator used consists of starch solution in which the presence of 1 part of iodine in several million parts of solution can be detected. The starch solution is prepared by triturating 1 gm of starch in 10 ml of cold water and then dissolving this paste in 200 ml boiling water which is filtered. In hot water starch granules burst out into β-amylose and amylopectin. β-amylose is soluble starch and is separated from amylopection.

The latter is insoluble and is removed by filtration or decantation. Starch solution on intraction with iodine or iodide ion produces an intense blue colour which can be discharged when iodine is reduced with $Na_2S_2O_3$ or any other reducing agent. The colour change is reversible. The indicator is slightly more sensitive in acid media and at temperatures up to 25°C.

EXERCISE 5. Preparation and Standardization of 0.IN Iodine Solution.

Method : The preparation of iodine solution is based on the following reactions :

$$I_2 + H_2O = 2HI + O$$

$I_2 \equiv O \equiv 2H$

$\therefore$ 126.9 $gI_2 \equiv$ 1000 ml N/1

$\therefore$ 12.69 $gI_2 \equiv$ 1000 ml N/10

Weigh approximately 3.2 g of iodine and transfer to a beaker containing 7.5 g of KI and 10 ml of H_2O. Iodine dissolves in this solution which is made up to 250 ml with water. ($KI + I_2 \rightleftharpoons KI_3$) .

In a separate beaker weigh accurately 0.5 g of arsenic trioxide and add 2 ml of 20% NaOH solution. Warm the solution to dissolve AS_2O_3 and make up the volume to 100 ml with water. Withdraw 25 ml, acidify with dilute HCl (test with $NaHCO_3$), add sodium bicarbonate to remove excess acid.

Add 3 ml of starch TS and titrate with N/10 iodine to a permanent pale straw colour.

The reactions involved in the preparation of arsenic trioxide are :

$As_2O_3 + 20 = As_2O_5$

$\therefore$ 197.8 g AS_2O_5 $\equiv$ 4000 ml N/1

$\therefore$ 0.04946 g $As_2O_5 \equiv$ 100 ml N/10

Arsenic trioxide is slowly soluble in water but dissolves readily in NaOH solution to give sodium arsenite.

$$As_2O_3 + 6NaOH \longrightarrow 2Na_3AsO_3 + 3H_2O$$

If iodide is added to this alkaline solution, sodium hypoiodite is formed which does not react with arsenious ion.

$$2NaOH + I_2 \longrightarrow NaIO + NaI + H_2O$$

The overall reaction between As_2O_3 and I_2 is as follows:

$$As_2O_3 + 2I_2 + 2H_2O \rightleftharpoons Asub2O_5 + 2HI$$

The above reaction is made to go to right by removal of HI with Na HCO_3

$$Na_3AsO_4 + I_2 + 2NaHCO_3 \longrightarrow Na_3AsO_4 + 2NaI + 2CO_2 + H_2O$$

Sodium hydroxide and sodium carbonate cannot be used because they react with iodine.

The normality of iodine solution is determined as follows :

$$N = \frac{\text{Wt Of } As_2O_3 \text{ sample}}{\text{ml Iodine} \times 0.04946}$$

EXERCISE 6. Determination of percentage of Ascorbic acid ($C_6H_8O_6$).

Method : Ascorbic acid is a strong reducing agent and is assaged by titration with iodine solution. In the assay, ascorbic acid is oxidized to dehydroascorbic acid while iodine is reduced to iodine. The reaction involved is as :

$$I_2 + C_6H_8O_6 \longrightarrow C_6H_6O_6 + 2HI$$

EXERCISE 7. Preparation of 0.1 N Sodium thiosulphate solution.

Method : weigh accurately 6.25 g of A.R. sodium thiosulphate and transfer to a 250 ml flask. Dissolve in water and adjust the volume. (In case large quantities of sodium thiosulphate are required for storage, the solution should be stabilized by addition of 2 drops of 20% NaOH to prevent hydrolysis). Pipette 25 ml of N/10 iodine into a consical flask and titrate with standard $Na_2S_2O_3$ solution until just colourless.

The reactions involved in the above titration are as follows :

$$2Na_2S_2O_3 + I_2 = Na_2S_4O_6 + 2NaI$$

$$\therefore 2 \times 248.2 \text{ g } Na_2S_2O_3.5H_2O \equiv 2I \equiv 20,000 \text{ ml N/10}$$

$$\therefore 24.82 \text{ g } Na_2S_2O_3.5H_2O \equiv 1000 \text{ ml N/10}$$

EXERCISE 8. Determination of percentage of Sulphur in Sulphur ointment.

Method : The method is based on the conversion of sulphur to sodium thiosulphate by refluxing with excess of sodium sulphite solution :

$$Na_2SO_3 + S = Na_2S_2O_3.$$

The excess of sodium sulphite which will react with iodine is removed by addition of formaldehyde as formaldehyde bisulfite.

$$HCHO + Na_2SO_3 \longrightarrow HCHO.Na_2SO_3$$

Sodium thiosulphate thus formed is then titrated with N/10 iodine.

EXERCISE 9. Determination of Percentage of iron (Fe) in Iron and Ammonium citrate.

Method : Weigh accurately 0.5 g of the sample and dissolve in 15 ml distilled water. Add 1 ml H_2SO_4 and warm gently until yellow to decompose iron and ammonium citrate complex. Cool, and add dropwise N/10 $KMnO_4$ to oxidize Fe^{2+} to Fe^{3+} until pink colour persists for 5 seconds. Add 15 ml of dilute HCl and 2 g of KI and set aside the solution for 3 minutes to allow the liberation of iodine. Titrate with N/10 $Na_2S_2O_3$ till end point is colourless. No indicator is required.

The assay is based on the reactions given below :

$$2FeCl_3 \text{ (sample + HCl)} + 2HI = 2FeCl_2 + 2HCl + I_2$$

$$2Fe \equiv 2FeCl_3 \equiv I_2 \equiv 2H$$

$$2 \times 55.85 \text{ g Fe} \equiv 2000 \text{ ml N/1}$$

$$0.005585 \text{ g Fe} \equiv 1 \text{ ml N/10}$$

5.5 Oxidation-Reduction Methods with Bromine

Theory : In the determinations for substances like phenol, resorcinol, aniline etc. in place of iodine, bromine is used as an oxidizing agent. The reason being that bromine is easily reduced by organic substances producing quantitatively water-insoluble substitution products. The standard solution does not comprise bromine as such but when equivalent amount of potassium bromate and potassium bromide is mixed and acidified bromine is liberated.

EXERCISE 10. Preparation and Standardization of 0.1 N Bromine solution.

Method : Dissolve 3 g of potassium bromate and 15 g of potassium bromide in enough water and make up the volume to 1 litre. Pipette 25 ml of solution into a iodine flask, dilute with 120 ml water. Add 5 ml of HCl, insert the stopper & shake the flask. Add 5 ml of potassium iodide TS, insert the stopper and shake the flask again. Allow the flask to stand for 5 minutes until iodine is liberated and titrate with 0.1 N $Na_2S_2O_3$ using 3 ml of starch solution as the indicator.

The various reactions involved in the above determination are as follows :

$$5kBr + KBrO_3 + 6HCl \longrightarrow 6KCl + 3Br_2 + 3H_2O$$

$$2KI + Br_2 \longrightarrow 2KBr + I_2$$

$$I_2 + 2Na_2S_2O_3 \longrightarrow 2NaI + Na_2S_2O_6$$

The reactions indicate that 1/2 mole of bromine (1 gram-atomic weight) is 1 equivalent. Further, 1/6 mole (27.833 g) of $KBrO_3$ when treated with KI in the presence of HCl is needed to produce 1 equivalent f bromine. Therefore 0.1 × 27.833 = 2.7833 g (0.1 equivalent) of $KBrO_3$ is required to make 1 litre of 0.1 N bromine.

EXERCISE 11. Determination of Percentage of Phenol (C_6H_5OH).

Method : weigh accurately 2 g of sample and dissolve in water and make up the volume up to 1 litre. Pipette 25 ml into a glass-stoppered bottle. Add by means of a Pipette 50 ml of Br. solution and 5 ml of Concentrated HCl. Shake the bottle for 1/2 hour and set aside for 15 mint. By this process bromination of phenol to tribromophenol is complete. Now, add 1 g of KI, shake the solution and titrate the liberated iodine with standard 0.1 N $Na_2S_2O_3$. As soon as the solution turns pale yellow in colour add 10 ml of $CHCl_3$ and 3 drops of starch mucilage and continue titration until the end point is colourless. Perform a blank determination on 50 ml the bromide-bromate solution.

The equation involved in the assay are as follows :

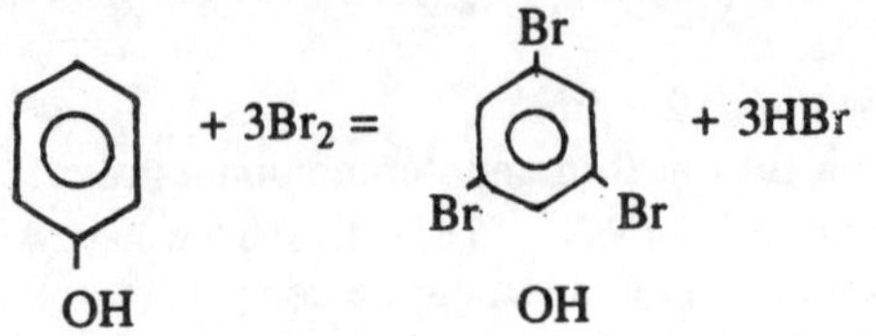

$$C_6H_5OH + 3Br_2 = C_6H_2Br_3OH + 3HBr$$

(Phenol (OH) + $3Br_2$ = 2,4,6-tribromophenol (Br, Br, Br; OH) + 3HBr)

$$\therefore C_6H_5OH + 3Br_2 \equiv 6H$$

$$94.11 \text{ g } C_6H_5OH \equiv 6000 \text{ N/1 Br}$$

$$\therefore 0.001569 \text{ g } C_6H_5OH \equiv 1 \text{ ml N/10 Br}$$

Since the solution of Br_2 is not stable, it is prepared from KBr and $KBrO_3$ as shown :

$$5HBr + HBrO_3 = 3Br_2 + 3H_2O$$

The excess of Br_2 not required for the formation of tribromophenol is estimated by adding KI and titrating the liberated I_2 with $Na_2S_2O_3$.

$$Br_2 + 2HI = 2HBr + I_2$$

5.6 Oxidation-Reduction Methods With Potassium Iodate

Theory : Potassium iodate is available in a high state of purity (99.9%) and a standard solution can be prepared by direct weighing. However, the standardization can be done by any of the following two procedures :

(A) To a definite volume of potassium iodate solution add excess of KI and dilute HCl and titrate the liberated iodine with standard $Na_2S_2O_3$. This method can also be used to standardize $Na_2S_2O_3$.

(B) The standardization can also be done by titration with pure KI solution. Both the above methods are described below.

Method A : Weigh accurately 3.567 g of AR grade potassium iodate and transfer to a 1 litre graduated flask.

Dissolve in water and make up to the volume. Pipette 25 ml of solution into a conical flask, add 2 g of KI and 4 ml of H_2SO_4 and titrate the liberated iodine with N/10 $Na_2S_2O_3$.

The equations involved in standardization are as follows :

$$KIO_3 + 5KI + 3H_2SO_4 = 3K_2SO_4 + 3I_2 + 3H_2O.$$

$$I_2 + 2Na_2S_2O_3 = Na_2S_4O_6 + 2NaI$$

$\therefore$ $KIO_3 \equiv 3I_2 \equiv 6Na_2S_4O_3 \equiv 6H$

$\therefore$ 214.0 g $KIO_3 \equiv$ 6000 ml N/1

$\therefore$ 3.567 g $KIO_3 \equiv$ 1000 ml N/10

Method B : Weigh accurately about 0.5 g of pure sample of potassium iodide. Dissolve in about 50 ml water in a volumetric flask. Add 15 ml of concentrated HCl and 6 ml KCN solution and titrate with M/20 potassium iodate solution.

The various reactions involved in this standardization are explained below.

(a) When the concentration of dilute HCl does not exceed N/1 strength the reaction between KIO3 and KI comes to an end when iodate is reduced to free iodine as :

$$KIO_3 + 5KI + 6HCl = 6KCl + 3I_2 + 3H_2O.$$

(b) When the concentration of HCl, exceeds 4N, iodine formed in the above reaction is further oxidized to ICl as : $KIO_3 + 2I_2 + 6HCl = KCl + 5\ ICl + 3H_2O$. i.e. iodate in exerting its oxidizing action is reduced to I^+ which is present as ICl.

(c) The iodine cation is then stabilized as ICN by the addition of KCN which is less ionized than ICl under these conditions as : $ICl + KCN \rightleftharpoons ICN + KCl$ under these conditions acidity need be only around N/1 i.e. large quantities of HCl will not be required.

(d) When the concentration of HCl exceeds 4N, the reaction between KIO3 and KI is as :

$$KIO_3 + 2KI + 6HCl = 3KCl + 3ICl + 3H_2O$$

If CN^- ions are present the reaction can be written as :

HIO_3 (from KIO_3 & acid) + $2HI + 3HCN \equiv 3ICN + 3H_2O$

$\therefore$ $KI \equiv KIO_3$

$\therefore$ 332.0 g KI $\equiv$ 1000 ml M/1

$\therefore$ 0.01660 g KI $\equiv$ 1 ml M/20

As shown above the iodate solution is expressed in terms of molarity rather than normality. The reason being that KIO_3 is used in the titration of solutions containing both iodide and free iodine and the equivalent of KIO_3 with KI is different from its equivalent when considering its reaction with iodine as:

$2KI \equiv KIO_3 \equiv 2H$ As per reaction a

$2I_2 \equiv KIO_3 \equiv 4H$ As per reaction b

EXERCISE 12. Determination of percentage of Ferrous sulphate tablets ($FeSO_4$).

Method: Weigh accurately 20 tables and dissolve then is 50 ml of 25% W/V Solution of H_2SO_4. Filter if any residue is left, wash with dilute H_2SO_4 and adjust the volume of the filterate to 100 ml. Transfer a measured volume of the solution, equivalent to 0.5 g of exscicated $FeSO_4$ to a stoppered bottle, add 20 ml water, 6 ml of strong solution of iodine monochloride, and 60 ml HCl. Titrate the liberated iodine with M/20 KIO_3. When the solution becomes light brown in colour add 5 ml $CHCl_3$ layer becomes colourless.

The estimation is based on the following equations:

$$4\ Fe^{2+} + 4ICl = 2I_2 + 4Fe^{3+} + 4Cl^-$$

$$2I_2 + KIO_3 + 6HCl = KCl + 5ICl + 3H_2O$$

$\therefore$ $4\ FeSO_4 \equiv 4Fe^{2+} \equiv 2I_2 \equiv KIO_3 \equiv$ 20,000 ml M/20 KIO_3

$\therefore$ 4×151.9 g $FeSO_4 \equiv$ 20,000 ml M/20 KIO_3

$\therefore$ 0.03038 $FeSO_4$ $\equiv$ 1 ml M/20 KIO_3

The procedure involves in dissolving ferrous sulphate tablets in acid & ICl solution is added. Ferrous iron is oxidized to the ferric state and ICl is reduced is to iodine under these conditions. The liberated iodine is estimated with KIO_3 solution.

EXERCISE 13: Determination of percentage of Hydralazine hydrochloride.

Methods: The procedure is similar as can be applied to phenyl hydrazine.

Weigh definite amount of sample (0.2 g) dissolve in water (50 ml) and add concentrated HCl (50 ml). Titrate the solution with M/20 KIO_3 until brown colour produced becomes less intense. Add $CHCl_3$ and continue titration until $CHCl_3$ layer becomes colourless.

The following reaction is involved in the analysis of hydralazine hydrochloride.

$$C_8H_8N_4.HCl + KIO_3 + HCl \longrightarrow ICl + KCl + 3H_2O + N_2\uparrow$$

$$C_8H_8N_4.HCl \equiv HIO_3 \equiv 1000 \text{ ml M/1 } KIO_3$$

$$196.64 \text{ g } 2C_8H_8N_4.HCl \equiv 1000 \text{ ml M/1 } KIO_3$$

$$\therefore 0.00982 \text{ g } 2C_8H_8N_4.HCl \equiv 1 \text{ ml M/20 } KIO_3$$

TABLE 5.1
Assays By Direct Titration with Potassium Permanganate

Drug Substances	Official Requirement, %
Ammonium vanadate	NH_4VO_3 = 98
Hydrogen peroxide solution	H_2O_2 = 2.5—3.5/100 ml
Sodium Ferrocyanide	$Na_4Fe(CN)_6.10.H_2O$ = 98
Dibasic calcium Phosphate	$CaHPO_4$ = 98—100.5
Cherry juice	$C_4H_6O_5$ = 1

TABLE 5.2
Assays By Direct Titration with Ceric Sulphate

Drug Substances	Indicator	official requirement, %
Ferrous sulphate	oPh	$FeSO_4$ = 99.5—104.5
.. .. Tablets	..	$FeSO_4.7H_2O$ = 95—110
Hydroquinone ointment	dPa	$C_8H_8O_2$ = 94—106
Ferrous gluconate	oPh	$C_{12}H_{22}FeO_{14}$ = 95—100.5
.. .. tablets	..	$C_{12}H_{22}FeO_{14}.2H_2O$ = 93—107
Iron soritex injection	..	Fe^{2+} = 8.5 mg/ml
Menadione tablets	..	$C_{11}H_8O_2$ = 96—110

oPh = ortho phenanthroline; dPa = diphenylamine.

TABLE 5.3
Assays By Direct Titration with Iodine

Drug Substances	Official Requirement,%
Antimony & Potassium tartrate	$C_8 H_4 K_2 Sb_2 O_{12}.3H_2O$ = 99—103
Ascorbic acid	$C^6 H_6 O_6$ = 99—100.5
Dimercaprol	$C_3 H_8 OS_2$ = 97
.. .. injection	$C_3 H_8 OS_2$ = 9—11
Sodium thioglycollate	$HSCH_2 COONa$ = 75
Ascorbyl Palmitate	$C_{22} H_{38} O_7$ = 95—100.5
Carbarsone	$C_7 H_9 As N_2 O_4$ = 97.5—101
Stibophen injection	$C_{12} H_4 NaO_{16} S_4 Sb$ = 94—106

TABLE 5.4
Assays By Titrating Liberated Iodine from Potassium Iodide with sodium Thiosulphate

Drug Substances	Official Requirement,%
Diiodohydroxyquin tablets	$C_9 H_5 I_2 NO$ = 99—105
Ethiodized oil	I = 35.2—38.9
Ferrous Fumerate tablets	$C_4 H_2 FeO_4$ = 95—110
Iophendylate injection	$C_{19} H_{29} IO_2$ = 98—102
Levothyroxine tablets	$C_{15} H_{10} I_4 NNaO_4$ = 90—115
Mannitol injection	$C_6 H_4 O_6$ 95—105
Mannitol and sodium chloride injection	$C_6 H_4 O_6$ 95—105
Thyroid tablets	I = 0.17—0.23
Chlorinated lime	Cl = 30
Dextrothyroxine sodium tablets	$C_{15} H_{10} I_4 N NaO_4$ = 90—110
Halazone tablets	$C_7 H_5 Cl_2 NO_4S$ = 90—135

TABLE 5.5
Assays using Bromine solution

Drug Substance	Official Requirements,%
Benzoic & salicylic acid ointment	$C_7 H_6 O_3$ = 90—110
Ethacrynic acid	$C_{13} H_{12} Cl_2 O_4$ = 97—110.2
p-Chlorophenol.	C_6H_5ClO = 99—100.5
Phenol	$C_6 H_6 O$ = 99—100.5
Phenylephrine.HCl	$C_9 H_{13} NO_2.HCl$ = 97.5—102.5
Salicylic acid Plaster	$C_7 H_6 O_3$ = 90—110
Thymol	$C_{10} H_{14} O$ = 99—101

TABLE 5.6
Assays By Direct Titration with Potassium iodate

Drug Substance	Official Requirement, %
Benzalkonium chloride	$[C_6H_5CH_2N(CH_3)_2R]Cl$ = 97—103
Hydralazine HCl injection	$C_8H_8N_4.HCl$ = 95—105
Iodine Tincture	NaI = 2.1—2.6 g/100 ml
Potassium iodide solution	KI = 97.0—103 g/100 ml
Methylbenzethonium chloride	$C_{28}H_{44}ClNO_2$ = 97—103

6

Argentimetric And Complexometric Methods

6.1 Argentimetric Titrations

General:

Argentimetric type of titrations comprise a class of reaction that require the formation of an insoluble precipitate or substance provided that the end point at which precipitation is complete can be determined.

Let us consider a solution of a slightly soluble salt BA in equilibrium with the solid phase BA, i.e.

$$\underset{\text{(solid)}}{BA} \rightleftharpoons \underset{\text{(solution)}}{B^+ + A^-}$$

As per the law of mass action the above equation can be written as :

$$K = \frac{[B^+]\ [A^-]}{[BA]}$$

The concentration of BA in the solution will remain constant in the presence of undissolved BA i.e.

$$K \times \text{constant} = [B^+]\ [A^-] = S_{BA}$$

The term S_{BA} is a constant at constant temperature and is called the *solubility product* of the salt BA.

In any system in which a solid is in equilibrium with its solution, the product of the ion concentrations is determined by the solubility product. Therefore, if an excess of silver ions is added to a saturated solution of silver chloride in water, the solubility product [Ag] [Cl] is exceeded and consequently some silver chloride will be precipitated, equilibrium being reached when the product of silver and chloride ion concentrations become equal to the solubility product. In volumetric procedures, quantitative precipitation can be utilized for estimations provided the end point at which precipitation is complete can be determined. Thus when silver nitrate solution is added to a solution of sodium chloride a precipitate of silver chloride is formed i.e.

$$NaCl + AgNO_3 = NaNO_3 + AgCl \downarrow$$

The end point is the point at which all the silver chloride is precipated. Since the detection of complete precipitation is difficult in actual practice, the use is made of a chemical reaction to produce a coloured precipitate or a coloured solution at the end point.

The various methods of determining the end point in analysis by precipitation methods are following:

(i) Use of internal indicators.

(ii) Cessation of precipitation or appearance of turbidity.

(iii) By potentiometry or amperometry.

The different indicators available for argentimetric titrations are described below :

(a) Ferric ammonium sulphate : It is used in the determination of chlorides, bromides, iodides in acid solution. When excess of standard $AgNO_3$ precipitation of AgCl takes place :

$$Mx + AgNO_3 \longrightarrow MNO_3 + AgX \downarrow$$

The excess of $AgNO_3$ is then back titrated with ammonium thiocyanate :

$$AgNO_3 + NH_4\,SCN \longrightarrow NH_4NO_3 + AgSCN \downarrow$$

At the end point, excess thiocyanate reacts with ferric iron to give the red colour due to formation of ferric ferrithiocyanate :

$$2Fe^{3+} + 6SCN^- \longrightarrow Fe^{3+}\,[Fe(SCN)_6]^{3-}$$

The ferric ammonium TS is prepared by dissolving 8 g of the reagent in 100 ml water.

(b) Potassium chromate : It is used as an indicator in the titration of chloride ions with standard $AgNO_3$ in neutral solution giving a precipitate of red silver chromate at the end point. The end point is reached when Cl^- ions are still present since silver chromate will begin to precipitate as soon as its solubility product is exceeded. The indicator solution is prepared by dissolving 10 g of the reagent in 100 ml water.

(c) Adsorption Indicators : These are acidic or basic dyes which change colour on adsorption on to the precipitate at the end point.

(i) Dichlorofluorescein TS: It is prepared by dissolving 100 mg of the reagent in 60 ml ethanol, 2.5 ml of 0.1 N NaOH is then added and the solution diluted to 100 ml with water.

(ii) Eosin Y TS : This indicator solution is prepared from 50 mg of eosin Y in 10 ml of water.

EXERCISE 1. Preparation and Standardization of 0.1 N silver nitrate.

Method: Weigh accurately 16.989 g of Analar (99.9%) silver nitrate. Dissolve in distilled water and adjust to 1000 ml to obtain an N/10 solution.

In the meantime, dry some Analar sodium chloride at 300°C for 2 hours. Cool in a desiccator and prepare a N/10 solution. Pipette 25 ml of N/10 sodium chloride solution into a conical flask. Add 1 ml of 5% W/V potassium chromate solution until a permanent faint reddish-brown colour is obtained.

The above method is based on the following equations :

$$AgNO_3 + NaCl = NaNO_3 + AgCl \downarrow$$

$$AgNO_3 \equiv NaCl \equiv H$$

$$\therefore\ 169.89\text{ g } AgNO_3 \equiv 58.45\text{ g NaCl} \equiv 1000\text{ ml N/1}$$

$$\therefore\ 0.1699\text{ g } AgNO_3 \equiv 0.005845\text{ g NaCl} \equiv 1\text{ ml N/10}$$

EXERCISE 2. Determination of percentage of carabachol ($C_6\,H_{15}\,O_2\,N_2\,Cl$).

Method : The sample is titrated with N/10 $AgNO_3$ using phenosafranine as an adsorption indicator. The end point is determined when the precipitate in its red form changes to violet. The assay is based on the following reactions :

$$[NH_2\text{—}COOCH_2CH_2\ N^+(CH_3)_3]\,Cl^- = [NH_2COOCH_2\text{—}CH_2\,N^+(CH_3)_3]\,NO_3^- + AgCl \downarrow$$

$\therefore$ 182.7 g $C_6H_{15}O_2N_2Cl$ ≡ $AgNO_3$ ≡ 1000 ml N/1

$\therefore$ 0.01827 g $C_6H_{15}O_2N_2Cl$ ≡ 1 ml N/10 $AgNO_3$

EXERCISE 3. Preparation and standardization of 0.1 N Ammonium thiocyanate (NH_4SCN).

Method: Weigh accurately 8 g of ammonium thiocyanate. Dissolve in distilled water and make up the volume to 1000 ml to obtain N/10 solution. Pipette 25 ml of standard N/10 $AgNO_3$ into a conical flask. Add 5 ml of concentrated. HNO_3 and 3 ml of 10% W/V solution of ferric ammonium sulphate solution. Dilute with 100—150 ml distilled water and titrate with ammonium thiocyanate solution placed in the burette. The end point is the permanent reddish brown colour which does not disappear on shaking.

The reactions involved in the above determination are following :

NH_4 SCN + $AgNO_3$ = NH_4 NO_3 + AgSCN ↓

$\therefore$ NH_4SCN ≡ $AgNO_3$ ≡ H

EXERCISE 4. Determination of percentage of mercuric acetate (C_4 H_6 O_4 Hg).

Method : Weigh accurately about 0.7 g of the sample and dissolve in 40 ml of water. Add 5 ml of dilute HNO_3 and 5 ml of ferric ammonium sulphate indicator. Titrate with N/10 NH_4SCN taking the first permanent brownish-red colour as the end point.

The determination is based on the following equation :

$(CH_3\ CO_2)_2$ Hg + 2NH_4 SCN = $Hg(SCN)_2$ + 2CH_3 CO_2 NH_4 .

$\therefore$ 318.8 g $C_4H_6O_4$ Hg ≡ 2NH_4SCN ≡ 2000 ml N/1

$\therefore$ 0.01594 g $C_4H_6O_4$ Hg ≡ 1 ml N/10 NH_4SCN

EXERCISE 5. Determination of percentage of ammonium chloride (NH_4Cl).

Method : Weigh accurately 0.2 g of the sample and dissolve in 35 ml distilled water. Add 15 ml HNO_3, and 5 ml nitrobenzene and 50 ml N/10 silver nitrate. Shake the mixture vigorously for 1 minute. Add 5 ml of ferric ammonium sulphate indicator and titrate with N/10 NH_4 SCN to the reddish-brown colour as the end point.

The above assay is based on the following reactions:

NH_4Cl + $AgNO_3$ = AgCl ↓ + NH_4 NO_3.

$AgNO_3$ + NH_4 SCN = AgSCN ↓ + NH_4NO_3

$\therefore$ NH_4Cl ≡ $AgNO_3$ ≡ H, $\therefore$ 53.5 NH_4Cl ≡ 1000 ml N/1

$\therefore$ 0.00535 NH_4Cl ≡ 1 ml N/10

Since an aqueous solution of ammonium chloride is slightly acidic, the end point is indistinct when titrated directly with $AgNO_3$ solution. Therefore Volhard method is adopted which is explained as follows: ammonium thiocyanate solution is used alongwith N/10 $AgNO_3$ solution in the estimation of substances which react with $AgNO_3$ but which cannot be determined by direct titration with $AgNO_3$. Excess standard $AgNO_3$ solution is added together with concentrated HNO_3, and the excess $AgNO_3$ titrated with N/10 NH_4 SCN solution.

EXERCISE 6. Determination of percentage of thiourea (CH_4N_2S).

Method: The procedure involves a modification of Volhard method i.e. sulphur contained in thiourea is precipitated as Ag_2S. Thus :

H_2N—CS—NH_2 ≡ Ag_2S ≡ 2H

A solution of the sample is heated with excess N/10 $AgNO_3$ and solution of NH_3 cooled and excess dilute HNO_3 added. This brings about the precipitation of sulpher present as Ag_2S. The precipitate is filtered and washed excess $AgNO_3$ added. The excess $AgNO_3$ in the filtrate and washings are titrated with N/10 NH_4 SCN using ferric ammonium sulphate as indicator.

6.2 Complexometric Titrations

General

The early methods of estimating quantitatively the inorganic pharmaceutical products containing metal ions such as Ca, Mg, Al, Bi and Zn were the gravimetric methods. But these procedures involved a number of steps and were lengthy and time consuming. With the introduction of a new analytical reagent namely — disodium *ethylene diaminetetraacetate* or EDTA a new volumetric method of analysis was developed for the estimation of metal ions. At the same time new metal-ion indicators were also discovered.

When a metal ion combines with a molecule which can donate electrons, the resulting compound is known as a *complex. Thus* a *complexing agent* includes any electron donating system which can form a covalent or a dative bond with a metal ion producing a complex which has different properties from the full metal ion. For example, simple complexing agents are anions in $K^+(BF_4)$, $2K^+(HgI_4)$ in K_3 $Fe(CN)_6$ and $K_4Fe(CN)_6$. The link between the metal and the donor can be covalent involving sharing of two electrons, one form metal and one from the ligand or both from the ligand. But once the complex is formed, there is hybridization and equalization of charges.

O—M = Ionic bond
O—M = Ordinate bond ----
N—M = Coordinate bond.

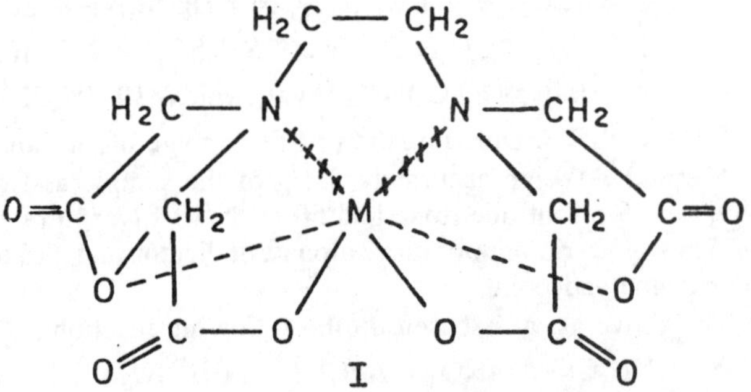

I

In the dative bond, both the electrons are donated by a neutral group such as :NH_3 in the complex $CO(NH_3)_6^{3+}$. These are simple ligands, but there are many organic molecules which possess more than one donating group, neutral or charged and form bi, tri, or polydentate or bi, tri or polyvalent ligands. For example ethylenediamine can form a bidentate ligand while ethylenediamine tetra acetic acid (EDTA) can form a hexdentate ligand (I). In case of polydentate ligands the metal ion is contained in a ring and the ligand is called a *chelating agent.* On the contrary the term *sequestering* agent is used for ligands

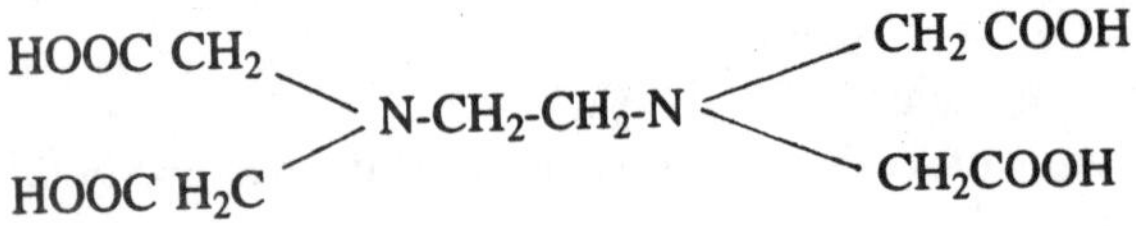

$$(HOOC\,CH_2)(HOOC\,H_2C)N\text{-}CH_2\text{-}CH_2\text{-}N(CH_2\,COOH)(CH_2COOH)$$

II

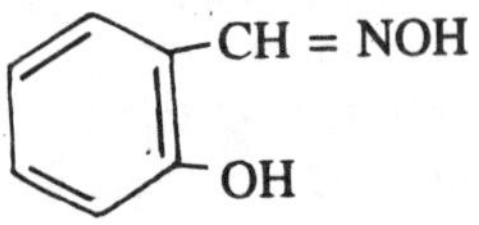

III (benzene ring with —CH = NOH and —OH)

which form water-soluble complexes and differs from the chelating agent in that the metal remains in solution in the chelated condition. A common example of a sequestering agent is EDTA (II) while that of a chelating agent forming an insoluble complex with metals is salicyladoxime (III). Both II and III can form stable complex with copper, that of II is soluble in water while that of III is insoluble but soluble in organic solvents. This is because salicyladoxime does not possess any solubilizing groups like —COOH, SO_3H etc. In all EDTA complextion reaction, the ratio of EDTA to the metal is 1:1. $Y^{4-} + M^{n+} \rightleftharpoons MY^{n-4}$ (where Y^{4-} is the tetraacetylate ion.) It will react with such polyvalent metal ions like Al^{3+}, Bi^{3+}, Ca^{2+}, Cu^{2+}, Hg^{2+}, Zn^{2+}. The dissociation of EDTA can be represented by the following equations :

$$H_4Y \overset{k_1}{\rightleftharpoons} H^+ + H_3Y^-$$

$$H_3Y_{2-} \overset{k_2}{\rightleftharpoons} H^+ + H_2Y^{2-}$$

$$H_2Y_{3-} \overset{k_3}{\rightleftharpoons} H^+ + HY^{3-}$$

$$HY \overset{k_4}{\rightleftharpoons} H^+ + HY^{4-}$$

The predominant form of the dissociated forms of EDTA is dependent upon the pH at which a given complexation reaction is performed.

In a complexometric reaction, the driving force for the reaction is the formation of a stable soluble complex. For example in case of calcium — EDTA complex, on applying the law of mass action the equilibrium constant known as the *stability constant* can be expressed as ;

$$K_s = \frac{[Cay^{2-}]}{[Ca^{2+}] \times [y^{4-}]} = 2.5 \times 10^{11}$$

The stability constant is very large because the complex is slightly ionized and concentration of Ca-EDTA complex is much greater than its constituent ions. Further, since the concentration of Y^{4-} is a function of the pH at which a specific reaction is run, the stability constants are only valid for those pH at which they are determined.

For successful titrations with EDTA, the stability constants of the complex formed must be greater than 8. In case of Li and Na the complex is very weak and cannot be titrated. With anions like Ag and Ba the stability constants are below 8. Metal ions like Fe^{3+} and Cu^{2+} form highly coloured complexes and cannot be titrated visually. The higher the stability constant, the more the pH which complexation titration can be performed. Organic solvents increase the stability of the complex. Neutral salts (Nacl) decrease the stability.

The factors which influence the EDTA reactions are (i) the activity of the metal ion, (ii) the pH at which the titration is run, and (iii) the presence of interfering ions like CN^-, citrate, tartrate and fluoride etc.

The disodium salt is preferred over the free acid in preparing the standard solution of EDTA. It is very stable, much more water soluble and nonhygroscopic, The equivalence point in EDTA titration can be detected visually with an indicator or instrumentally or by electrometric or photometric method and is accompanied by a sharp change in pM which is similar to abrupt change in pH as in acid—base titrations.

The indicators used in EDTA titrations are organic compounds which form coloured complex ions with the metal ion in high dilution. The indicator must possess sharpness of colour change at the end point and also must give up the metal ion to EDTA titrant for complexing and not compete with it.

$$M^{2+} + HIn^{2-} \rightleftharpoons MIn^- + H^+$$

$$\underset{\text{(Red)}}{MIn^-} + H_2Y^{2-} \rightleftharpoons MY^{2-} + \underset{\text{(Blue)}}{HIn^{2-}} + H^+$$

The most commonly used indicator in EDTA titrations is eriochrome black T (IV). It is sensitive to changes in the metal concentrations as well as changes in pH. It forms red complexes with Mg^{2+}, Zn^{2+}, Al^{3+}, Ca^{2+}, Pb^{2+} and Hg^{2+}.

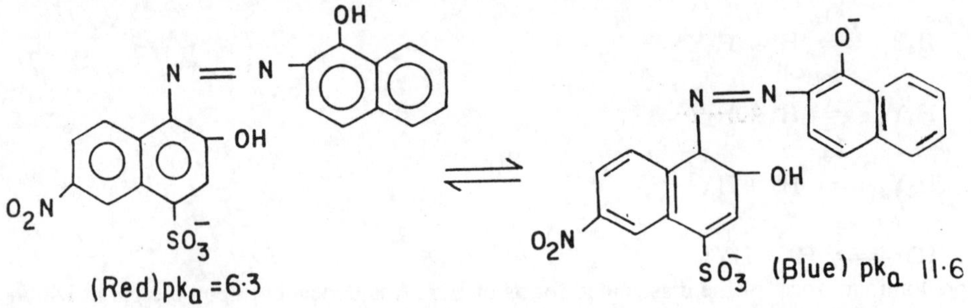

(Red) $pk_a = 6{\cdot}3$ ⇌ (Blue) pk_a 11·6

MASKING

When it is required to titrate a certain cation in a mixture containing other cations which interfere, the latter can be *masked* so that they do not react with the complexing agent or the indicator and therefore are also not included in the titre. This is achieved by adding an auxiliary complexing agent which forms a more stable complex with the interfering ion or ions than does sodium edidate, but does not form a complex with the ion being titrated. Many organic chelating agents can also be used as masking agents in specific cases.

EXERCISE 7. Preparation and standardization of M/100 Sodium edetate.

Theory : It is to be understood that since calcium edetate complex is more stable than the magnesium edetate complex, magnesium ions will liberated in the presence of excess calciums ion. These calcium ions will be completely complexed before magnesium ions as the titration proceeds. At the end point, magnesium, present as a dye-chelate is being titrated and since this has more distinct colour than the calcium dye-chelate, the end point will be sharper.

$$MgY^{2-} + Ca \longrightarrow CaY^{2-} + Mg^{2+}$$

Method: Pipette 20 ml of standard $CaCl_2$ solution into a conical flask, add 1 ml of buffer solution and 3 drops of indicator. Titrate this solution with M/100 sodium edetate solution until the colour changes from wine-red to clear blue. A blank titration is performed without the metal and subtracted from the result. Both, these titrations are repeated for the purpose of reproducibility of result. Standard calcium chloride solution: Weigh accurately 1.001 g of A.R. grade calcium carbonate and dissolve in 25 ml water containing a minimum quantity of dilute HCl. Boil off Co_2, cool and transfer to a 1000 ml flask. Dilute the solution with distilled water to 1000 ml to obtain a final concentration of M/100.

Buffer solution: Dissolve 67.5 g of NH_4Cl in 570 ml of strong NH_4OH solution. Dilute the solution to 900 ml with water. Add a solution of 0.616 g of $MgSO_4$ and 0.93 g of sodium edetate in 50 ml water. Now, add distilled water to make up the final volume to 1 litre.

Indicator : Dissolve 0.5 g of solochrome black WDFA and 4.5 g of hydroxylamine hydroxide in 100 ml ethanol.

TABLE 6.1
Assay by Direct Titration with silver Nitrate

Drug Substance	Indicator	Official requirement %
4-Amino antipyrine HCl.	dcf	$C_{11}H_{13}N_3O.HCl$ = 100.6—108.5
Heparin sòlution	Chrom	NaCl = 0.85—0.95
Diatrizoate meglumine injection	tbph	$C_{18}H_{26}I_3N_3O_9$ = 95—105
Iodipamide	tbph	$C_{20}H_{14}I_6N_2O_6$ = 98—102
Ipodate calcium	eoy	$C_{24}H_{24}CaI_6N_4O_4$ = 97.5—102.5
Mepiridine.HCl	eoy	Cl = 12.2—12.7
Naloxone.HCl	eoy	Cl = 9.54—9.94
Phenylephrine.HCl.	eoy	Cl = 17—17.7
Propantheline bromide	eoy	Cl = 17.5—18.2
Pyridoxine.HCl	eoy	Cl = 16.9—17.6
Succinylcholine chloride	eoy	Cl = 19.3—19.8
Tubocurarine chloride	eoy	Cl = 9.7—10.4
Hydroxy amphetamine.HBr	eoy	Br = 33.6—35.2
Mecamylamine.HCl	eoy	Cl = 17—17.8

dcf = dichlorofuorescein; tbph = tetrabromophenolphthalein; eoy = eosin y.

TABLE 6.2
Assay by Direct Titration with Ammonium Thiocyanate

Drug Substance	Official Requirement, %
Aminophylline Suppositories	$C_{16}H_{24}N_{10}O_4.2H_2O$ = 90—110
Silver Nitrate ophthalmic sol.	$AgNO_3$ = 0.95—1.05
Nitromersol	$C_7H_5HgNO_3$ = 98—100.5
Phenyl mercuric acetate	$C_8H_8HgO_2$ = 98—100.5

TABLE 6.3
Assay by Residual Titration of Silver Nitrate with Ammonium Thiocyanate

Drug Substance	Official Requirement %
Acetylcholine chloride	Cl = 19.3—19.8
Aminophylline injection	$C_{16}H_{24}N_{10}O^4.2H_2O$ = 23.25—26.75
Cyclophosphamide for injection	NaCl = 28.14—31.1
Dextrose and sodium chloride injection	NaCl = 95—105
Dimenhydrinate	$C_7H_7ClN_4O_2$ = 44—47
Mannitol & sodium chloride injection	NaCl = 95—105
Potassium chloride injection	KCl = 95—105
Sodium Chloride injection	NaCl = 0.85—0.95
Theophylline	$C_7H_8N_4O_2$ = 95—101
Trihexphenidyl. HCl	Cl = 10.3—10.7
Ammonium Chloride injection	Cl = 63—70.3
Dibucaine. HCl	Cl = 9.1—9.5
Thiourea	$(NH_4)_2CS$ = 99

TABLE. 6.4
Assay by Direct Titration with EDTA

Drug Substance	Indicator	Official Requirement %
Alumina and magnesia tablets	erio	$Mg(OH)_2$ = 1.7—2.2
Calcium chloride injection	hnb	$CaCl_2.2H_2O$ = 99—100
Calcium gluconate injection	hnb	Ca = 92—102 mg/100 ml
Calcium gluconate tablets	hnb	$C_{12}H_{22}CaO_{14}$ = 95—105
Calcium pantothenate tablets	hnb	Ca = 7.9—9.7
Corticotropin zinc hydroxide	erio	Zn = 0.45—0.55 mg/10 units
Magnesium sulphate injection	erio	$MgSO_4.7.H_2O$ = 93—107.
Zinc oxide ointment	erio	ZnO = 18.5—21.5
Zinc sulphate ophthalmic solution	Pan	$ZnSO_4.7H_2O$ = 95—105
Bismuth subnitrate	XYO	Bi_2O_3 = 79
Calcium stearate	hnb	CaO = 9—10.5

hnb = hydroxynaphthol blue; erio = eriochrome black; XYO = Xylenol orange; Pan = Pyridyl azo naphthol.

7

Gravimetric Methods

7.1 General

Gravimetry consists of isolating and weighing an element or compound in purest form possible. The procedure involves separating a definite weight or volume of the element or compound from the substance under investigation and finally the weight of the constituent is obtained from the weight of the product. The following three different techniques are known : (a) Precipitation from solution (b) Volatilisation or ignition and (c) Solvent extraction.

A few selected examples of gravimetry using above techniques generally performed under pharmaceutical analysis are described below :

7.2 Techniques With Inorganic Substances

7.2.1 Determination Of Aluminium

The procedure is based on the principle that a solution of aluminium salt when treated with ammonium hydroxide in presence of ammonium chloride will precipitate aluminium. This is shown by the reaction as : $Al^{3+} + 3\overset{+}{N}H_4 + 3OH^- = Al(OH)_3 \downarrow + 3NH_4^+$. The fine precipitate obtained is filtered and washed with dilute ammonium nitrate solution. It is converted to the oxide by ignition and finally weighed as Al_2O_3.

EXERCISE 1. Determination of percentage of alum [$KAl(SO_4)_2.12\ H_2O$].

Method : Weigh accurately 1.8 g of sample and dissolve in 200 ml distilled water in a beaker provided with a watch glass and stirring rod. Add 5 g of NH_4Cl and few drops of methyl indicator. (This is to prevent precipitation of Ca^{2+} and Mg_{2+}). Heat the solution to boiling to make the precipitate filterable. Add a strong solution of ammonia and water (1:1) with stirring until the colour of the solution is distinct yellow. Boil the liquid again for 2—3 minutes and then filter through Whatman No. 41 filter paper. Wash the precipitate with a 2% ammonium nitrate which is previously made neutral to methyl red indicator with NH_3. (This prevent the peptisation of precipitate). Repeat the above washing until free from chloride. Cover the mouth of the funnel with a filter paper and place in the oven until most of the moisture has been removed. Transfer the filter paper and the contents to a previously ignited and weighed silica crucible. Heat first gently till the paper is charred and then raise the temperature slowly. Finally the crucible is heated in a muffle furnace at 1200°C for 1 hour. (This produces Al_2O_3). Cool the crucible in a desiccator and weigh. Repeat the heating and cooling until constant weight is obtained. The reaction involved in the method are shown below:

$$2KAl(SO_4)_2.12H_2O \equiv 2Al(OH)_3 \equiv Al_2O_3$$

$$2 \times 474.4 \text{ g } KAl\ (SO_4)_2\ 12H_2O \equiv 102.0 \text{ g } Al_2\ O_3$$

$$9.307 \text{ g } KAl\ (SO_4)_2\ 12H_2O \equiv 1 \text{ g } Al_2\ O_3$$

7.2.2 Determination Of Chloride

The procedure is based on the reaction that when excess of silver nitrate solution is added to the chloride solution containing nitric acid the precipitate of AgCl is obtained which is collected and finally dried at 130—150° to a constant weight.

EXAMPLE 1 : Determination of percentage of Cl in potassium chloride.

Method: Weigh accurately about 0.2—0.3 g of NaCl or KCl and dissolve it in 150 ml water contained in a beaker which is provided with a watch glass and a stirring rod. Add about 0.5 ml of concentrated HNO_3 and place the solution in dark or subdued light. Now, add to the solution N/10 $AgNO_3$ solution slowly with constant stirring until a slight excess is present. ((i) Br^-, I^-, CN^- & sulphide must be absent in the original substance. (ii) AgCl is sensitive to light. (iii) excess of $AgNO_3$ reduces the solubility of AgCl . Allow the precipitate to settle and add a few drops of $AgNO_3$ to check that no further precipitation occurs. Heat the solution to boiling for 2—3 minutes until precipitate coagulates. Add 2 drops of $AgNO_3$ and check again if no further precipitation occurs. Cover the beaker with watch glass and set it aside in the dark for 1—2 hours. Dry a clean No.3 sintered glass crucible to constant weight at 130—150°. Filter the clear cold supernatant solution through the sintered glass crucible under suction. Wash the precipitate in a beaker 2 or 3 times with cold N/100 HNO_3 solution to prevent peptisation of the colloidel precipitate. Transfer all the precipitate to a crucible and wash again with a small amount of N/100 HNO_3 until the last washings collected in a test tube do not give any turbidity with N/10 HCl. (This ensures that all $AgNO_3$ has been removed.) Finally, wash the precipitate with small amounts of water to remove the acid and then small portions of ethanol. Heat the contents of the crucible at 130—150° for 45 minutes, cool in a desiccator and weigh. Repeat the heating and cooling until a constant weight (± 0.0002g) is obtained.

7.2.3 Determination Of Gold

The method is based on the oxidation of organic matter to volatile products on treatment with sulphuric acid. In the process sulphuric acid is reduced to SO_2 and H_2S. Hydrogen sulphide reduces the gold salts to metallic gold which gets precipitated. The subsequent treatment with HNO_3 ensures the complete decomposition of the organic matter as well as oxidation of any sulphur present.

EXERCISE 2. Determination of percentage of gold in sodium auriothiomalate.

Method: Weigh accurately about 0.2 g of the sample into a 100 ml kjeldahl flask. Add 10 ml of concentrated H_2SO_4 and heat gently to boiling under a cupboard. Continue boiling until liquid is clear and pale yellow in colour. cool, add drop wise 1 ml of HNO_3 and boil 1 hour. Cool, dilute with 70 ml water and boil for 5 minutes. Filter the precipitate on a Whatman No. 42 filter paper, wash with hot water, and drain the water. Dry the paper and the precipitate still in the funnel in an oven at 120°. Transfer the paper and the precipitate to an ignited and weighed silica crucible. Heat slowly first to burn off the paper and ignite to a constant weight.

7. 2.4 Determination Of Mercury

The estimation of mercury is based on its conversation to mercuric sulphide which is precipitated as shown by the equation :

$$Hg^{2+} + S^{2-} = HgS \downarrow$$

The mercury contained in a sample is taken in HCl and then treated with H_2S which converts Hg to HgS.

EXERCISE 3. Determination of percentage of mercuric chloride ($HgCl_2$).

Method : Accurately weigh 0.15 g of the sample in a conical flask. Dissolve the sample in H_2O, dilute to 100 ml with H_2O, and add 23 ml dilute HCl. (the presence of group II metals will interfere with this estimation and oxidizing agents must be absent). Place a rubber stopper in the mouth of the flask and pass water-washed H_2S gas through the tube into the flask containing the cold solution of mercuric salt. Gently shake the flask without allowing the liquid to come in contact with tube or the stopper. The precipitate turns completely black as the solution becomes saturated with gas. Allow the precipitate to settle, filter through a Gooch crucible, wash well with cold H_2O, five times with C_2H_5OH, once with CCl_4 and finally with C_2H_5OH. Drain well under suction and finally dry the precipitate at 110—120°.

EXERCISE 4. Determination of Amodiaquine hydrochloride as a free base gravimetrically.

Method : Accurately weigh about 0.3 g of sample in a 100 ml beaker. Dissolve in 50 ml H_2O and add dilute NH_4OH solution with stirring until solution is alkaline. Allow to stand for 30 minutes, and filter through a clean dry No.4 sintered glass crucible. Wash the precipitate with H_2O until washings are free from Cl. Dry the residue to constant weight at 105°.

The method is based on the precipitation of amodiaquine as a free base which is formed when the salt is hydrolysed with dilute ammonia as shown by the reaction below.

$$C_{20}H_{22}ON_3Cl \,.\, 2HCl \,.\, 2H_2O + 2NH_3 = C_{20}H_{22}ON_3Cl \downarrow + 2NH_4Cl + 2H_2O.$$

EXERCISE 5. Determination of weight of Barbitone sodium tablets ($C_8H_{11}O_3N_2Na$) gravimetrically.

Method : Dissolve powder equivalent to 0.3 g of barbitone sodium as complely as possible in dilute NaOH solution. Saturate the solution with NaCl and acidify with HCl. Barbitone is liberated from its salt and NaCl ensures that it is displaced from solution in water. Extract with diethyl ether, dry the residue of barbitone at constant weight.

7.2.5 Determination Of Medicaments In Capsules

The capsules consist of medicament contained in a shell of gelatin which may be either soft or hard. The general method is to weigh the capsules in full and again when all the medicament has been removed. The weight of the contents is calculated by difference. The variation in the weight of the capsules is similar to as occurs in tablet preparations and therefore an average weight or volume per capsule is calculated.

General Method : Weigh 20 capsules and determine the average weight of each capsule. Open the capsules carefully and remove all their contents without any loss. Wash the capsule shells with solvent ether. Allow the shells to dry at room temperature and weigh them. The difference in the weight gives the weight of the contents.

EXERCISE 6. Determination of the average weight of chloramphenicol per capsule.

Method: Weight the contents of five capsules and transfer the material into 60 ml of H_2O placed in a beaker. Extract with four successive volumes of 50 ml of ether. Combine the extracts and evaporate the ether. Collect the residue of chloramphencol, dry at 105° and weigh. Determine the average weight of chloramphenicol per capsule.

TABLE 7.1

Substance	Weighed as	Official Requirements, %
(a) Substances Assayed Gravimetrically		
Magnesium oxide	$CaSO_4$	$CaO \geq 1.5$
Sodium lauryl sulphate	$BaSO_4$	$Na_2 SO_4 \geq 8$
Barium sulfate	$BaCrO_4$	$BaSO_4$ = 97.5—100.5
Aluminium monostearate	$Al_2 O_3$	Al_2O_3 = 14.5—16.0
Magnesium trisilicate	SiO_2	SiO_2 = 45
Undecyclenic acid ointment compound	$C_{18}H_{12}N_2O_2$ Zn	Zn = 1.8—2.2
Aurio thioglucose	Au	$C_6 H_{11} AuO_5S$ = 95—105
Gold sodium thiomalate injection	Au	$C_4 H_3 AuN_2 O_4 S.H_2O$ = 95—105
(b) Substances Assayed Gravimetrically by conversion to Free Acid		
Amobarbital sodium	$C_{11} H_{18} N_2 O_2$	98.5—100.5
Pentobarbital sodium capsules	$C_{11} H_{18} N_2 O_3$	92.5—107.5
Phenytoin sodium capsules	$C_{15} H_{12} N_2 O_2$	93—107
Diethylstilbestrol Dipropinate	$C_{24} H_{28} O_4$	98—100.5
(c) Substances Assay Gravimetrically by conversion to Free Base.		
Papaverine HCl injection	$C_{20} H_{21} NO_4$	95—105
Phenacaine HCl	$C_{18} H_{22} N_2 O_2$	98—102
(d) Substances Assayed Gravimetrically by conversion to Derivatives.		
Choline chloride (R)	Tetraphenylboron	99.5
Piperazine citrate syrup	Dipicrate	93—107
Progesterone injection	Hydrazone	90—110
Benzethonium chloride tincture	Tetraphenyl boron	190—210 mg per 100 ml.
Bethanechol chloride tablets	,,	90—110
Camphor spirit	Hydrazone	$C_{10} H_{10} O$ = 9—11
Dienestrol	Diacetate	98—100.5
Hydroxyamphetamine hydrobromide	Diacetyl	95-105
Phentolamine HCl tablets	Trichloro acetate	93—107

8

Miscellaneous Types Of Analysis

8.1 Sodium Nitrate Titrations

We have already learnt that primary aromatic amines react with sodium nitrite in presence of hydrochloric acid and produce diazonium salts, e.g.

$$NaNO_2 + HCl \rightarrow HNO_2 + NaCl$$

$$C_6\,H_5\,NH_2 + HNO_2 + HCl \rightarrow C_6\,H_5\,N = NCl + 2H_2O$$

Nitrous acid is formed when sodium nitrate solution is added into the acid reaction mixture and reacts with primary amino group forming an unstable nitrite which decomposes with formation of diazonium salt. This product is also unstable and if the reaction mixture is not kept cool, it will decompose. The end point is established by detecting a slight excess of nitrous acid which is present, by using starch-iodide paper as an external indicator :

$$KI + HCl \rightarrow HI + KCl$$

$$2HI + 2HNI_2 \rightarrow I_2 + 2NO \uparrow + 2H_2O$$

The method is applicable to primary arylamino group as in sulpha drugs or local anaesthetics etc. Primary aliphatic amines form an unstable diazonium salt which decomposes to form a primary alcohol.

EXERCISE 1. Determination of percentage of Sulphanilamide powder ($C_6\,H_8\,N_2\,O_2\,S$).

Method : Weigh accurately 500 mg of sulphanilamide powder previously dried at 105°C and transfer to a beaker. Add 50 ml of water and 5 ml of HCl and stir well until dissolved. Cool to 150°C, add 25 g of crushed ice, and titrate slowly with 0.1 M sodium nitrate solution stirring vigorously until a glass rod dipped into titrated solution produces a blue ring when touch to starch-iodide paper. The end point should be reproducible after the mixture has been allowed to stand for 1 minute.

8.2 Fats And Fatty Oils

In the quality control of fats and oils the commonly used procedures of analysis are the determination of a *number* or values known as *constants*. These constants are taken into account along with colour, odour, taste and any special identify tests for establishing the purity and or any adulteration of such substances.

TABLE 8.1
Assays By Direct Titration with Sodium Nitrite

Drug Substance	Official Requirement %
Procainamide HCl injection	$C_{13} H_{21} N_3 O.HCl$ = 95—105
Sulphathiazole	$C_9 H_9 N_3 O_2 S_2$ = 99
Benzocaine	$C_9 H_{11} O_2$ = 98—101
Butacaine sulphate	$(C_{18} H_{30} N_2 O_2)_2 HSO_4$ = 98—101
Propoxycaine HCl	$C_{16} H_{26} N_2 O_3.HCl$ = 98—102
Procaine and tetracaine HCl	$C_{13} H_{20} N_2 O_2.HCl$ = 98—102
Lavarternol injection	$C_{13} H_{20} N_2 O_2.HCl$ = 95—105

8.2.1 Acid Value

The acid value also called acid number is defined as the number of milligrams of potassium hydroxide necessary to neutralize the free acids in 1 g of oil, fat, wax, resin, balsam or such similar organic substances.

The presence of free acids in oils, fats and waxes is mainly due to the hydrolysis of esters contained in them and is caused by bacterial action, by catalytic action of light & heat as well as by chemical action. The freshly prepared fats or oils contain very little or no free acid but upon aging the acid value increases slowly if the substance is not protected from light which if exceeded will indicate that the substances have undergone decomposition on storage.

EXERCISE 2. To determine the acid value of Rosin.

Method : Weigh accurately about 1 g of powdered rosin and dissolve in 50 ml of neutralized alcohol. (Since commercial alcohol is generally acid in reaction, it should be tested before the sample is dissolved. The alcohol can be rendered neutral to phenolphthalein by the addition of standard alkali solution). Add 0.5 ml (1% in 95% ethanol) of phenolphthalein and titrate with N/10 KOH until pink colour persists for 15—30 seconds.

In the titration of fat or oil the sample (about 10 g) is dissolved in mixture of ether (25 ml) and 95% ethanol (25 ml). The mixture is shaken thoroughly after each addition of alkali to ensure complete extraction of the fatty acids from the oily layer.

The analysis is based on the following equations :

$$R\text{—}COOH + KOH = R\text{—}COOK + H_2O$$

$$\therefore \quad KOH \equiv H$$

$$\therefore \quad 56.1 \text{ g KOH} \equiv 10{,}000 \text{ ml N/10}$$

$$\therefore \quad 5.61 \text{ mg KOH} \equiv 1 \text{ ml N/10}$$

$$\therefore \text{ Acid Value} = \frac{\text{Burette reading} \times \text{factor of alkali} \times 5.61}{\text{weight of sample in g}}$$

TABLE 8.2
Acid value limits of Important official substances

Substances	Official Requirement (Acid Value)
Rosin	150—180
White wax	17—24
Carnuba wax	2—7
Oleic acid	196—204
Tolu balsam	112—168

8.2.2 Saponification Value

The saponification value or saponification number is defined as the number of milligrams of potassium hydroxide required to neutralise the free acids and saponify the esters contained in 1 g of fat or volatile oil, wax, resin or other substances of similar origin.

The determination of saponification number is used as an aid in the detection of the presence of glycerides of acids containing less than 16 or more than 18 carbon atoms because the value of this constant is inversely proportional to the mean molecular weight of the acids present. It helps to indicate any adulteration of the sample with unsaponifiable matter like mineral oil.

EXERCISE 3. To Determine the saponification value of cottonseed oil.

Method : Weigh accurately about 2 gms of the sample and place it in a 250 ml conical flask. Pipette 25 ml of N/2 ethanolic KOH into the flask. Attach a reflux condenser and heat the flask on a water-bath for 1 hour. Remove the water-bath and rinse the condenser with 5 ml of neutral ethanol. Remove the condenser and cool the solution. Add 1 ml of phenolphthalein solution and titrate the excess of KOH with N/2 HCl. Perform a blank titration at the same time under similar conditions.

The following equations are involved in the above determination:

$$\text{RCOOR}' + \text{KOH} \equiv \text{R.COOK} + \text{R}'\text{OH}$$

$$\therefore \quad 56.1 \text{ g KOH} \equiv 2000 \text{ ml N/2}$$

$$\therefore \quad 28.05 \text{ g KOH} \equiv 1 \text{ ml N/2}$$

The saponification value is calculated by the formula given below:

$$\text{Saponification Value} = \frac{(b - a) \times (\text{factor}) \times 28.05}{\text{weight of Sampling}}$$

b = Burette reading for blank
a = Burette reading for sample

8.2.3 Ester Value

The ester value is defined as the number of mg of potassium hydroxide required to hydrolyse the esters in 1 g of fatty or volatile oil, fat, wax, balsam, resin or other substances of similar composition.

If the substance does not contain any free acid, the ester number is equal to saponification value. When the free acid is present, the ester value is the difference between the acid and saponification values.

The estimation of ester value is of use in checking any adulteration of rosin, stearic acid and paraffin in yellow and white wax.

TABLE 8.3
Saponification value limits for fatty substance

Substances	Saponification Number
Almond oil	190—200
Cod-—liver oil	180—192
Castor oil	176—182
Corn oil	187—193
Cottonseed oil	190—198
Hydrogenated vegetable oil	188—198
Olive oil	190—195
Peanut oil	185—195
Sesame oil	188—195
Carnuba wax	80—95
Cocoa butter	188—195
Tolu balsam	154—220

Method : Weigh accurately about 2g of the sample and transfer into a 250 ml flask. Add 5 ml of 95% ethanol (previously neutralized) and neutralize the free acid in the solution by titrating with N/10 ethanolic KOH until pink to phenolphthalein (0.2 ml). Add 20 ml ethanolic KOH and reflux in a water bath for 1hour Cool, add 20 ml water and back titrate excess alkali with N/2 HCl using an additional 0.2 ml of phenolphthalein as indicator. Perform a blank determination heating and cooling under same conditions. The difference in the readings gives the amount of alkali required to saponify the ester.

The equations involved in the determination are following:

$$R.COOR' + KOH = R.COOK + R'OH$$

$$\therefore\ R.COOR' \equiv KOH \equiv H \equiv 200 \text{ ml N/2}$$

Ester value gives us the combined acids present in the substance and is obtained by the formula:

$$\text{Ester Value} = \frac{m \times (\text{factor of acid}) \times 28.05}{W}$$

m = Difference in burette readings for sample and blank titrations.

w = weight (in g) of the substance taken

8.2.4. Iodine Value

The iodine value or number is the number of grams of iodine absorbed under specified conditions by 100 g of oil, fat, wax or other similar substances.

The iodine value is a measure of the proportion of unsaturated fatty acids present both free and combined as esters. It is based upon the addition of halogen across carbon-carbon double bond. Iodine itself reacts slowly, therefore iodine monochloride or bromine in pyridine are used as reagents.

The determination of iodine numbers of fats and oils serves to characterise them and also to indicate whether they are pure or admixture. therefore determination of iodine number not only helps to identify the known oil but also to indicate in a definite manner the class to which an unknown oil belongs. Further, when iodine value is considered in conjunction with the saponification number, it not only detects the adulteration but also the nature of adulteration but also the nature of adulterant.

Iodine Monochloride Method : Weigh the required amount of oil (see calculations) and place it in an iodine flask. Add 10 ml of CCl_4 to dissolve the oil. Introduce 20 ml of ICl solution from a burette or a pipette. Insert the stopper previously moistened with KI solution, and set aside in the dark for 30 minutes at a temperature of 25 ± 5°C. Add 15 ml of KI solution and back titrate the excess iodine with N/10 $Na_2 S_2 O_3$ solution using starch mucilage as indicator. Perform a blank determination at the same time with the same quantities of the same reagents and in the same manner, but omitting the sample. Calculate the iodine value from the formula:

$$\text{Iodine Value} = \frac{(b - a) \times 0.01269 \times \text{factor} \times 100}{\text{Weight of the sample in g}}$$

where b = blank reading , a = sample reading.
factor = strength of $Na_2 S_2 O_3$ solution.

The solution of ICl is prepared in the following manner and has the following Composition :

Iodine trichloride	= 8 g.
Iodine	= 9 g
CCl_4	= 300 ml
glacial CH_3COOH	= to 1000 ml

Dissolve 8 g of iodine trichloride in 200 ml glacial acetic acid and dissolve 9 g iodine in 300 ml CCl_4. Mix the two solutions and adjust the volume to 1000 ml with glacial acetic acid.

Calculation of weight of oil required :

Each 20 ml of ICl is equivalent to 40 ml of N/10 $Na_2 S_2 O_3$. Allowing for 100% excess this leaves about 10 ml of ICl (≡ 20 ml of N/10 $Na_2 S_2 O_3$) available for the reaction with the oil.

Sample of oil ≡ 20 ml N/10 $Na_2 S_2 O_3$
≡ 20 × 0.01269 g Iodine
≡ 0.2538 g of iodine.

Let the expected iodine value of sample x.
Then x g of iodine will be absorbed by 100 g of sample

$$\therefore \text{ 0.2 g of iodine will be absorbed by } \frac{100}{x} \times 0.2$$

$$= \frac{20}{x} \text{ g of sample}$$

The weight of oil required for each determination is obtained by dividing the highest expected iodine value into 20.

The analysis is based upon the following reactions :

$$>C=C< \; + \; ICl \longrightarrow \; -\underset{I}{\overset{|}{C}}-\underset{Cl}{\overset{|}{C}}-$$

$$\therefore \; >C=C< \; \equiv \; IOH \equiv ICl \equiv 2I$$

The excess ICl is converted to iodine by the addition of KI and titrated with $Na_2 S_2 O_3$.

$ICl + H_2O = HCl + IOH$
$HCl + KI = HI + KCl$
$HI + IOH = H_2O + I_2$
$ICl = 2I = 20,000$ ml N/10

Pyridine Bromide Method : Weigh the required amount of oil and place it in a stoppered bottle. Add 10 ml of CCl_4 to dissolve the oil. Introduce 25 ml of pyridine bromide solution, stopper and allow to stand in dark for 10 minutes. Add aqueous KI solution and proceed as in iodine monochloride method.

The pyridine bromide reagent is prepared as following and has the composition stated below :

Pyridine	8 g
Sulphuric acid	10 g
Bromine	8 g
Glacial acetic acid to 1,000 ml	

Dissolve 8 g of pyridine and 99 g of H_2SO_4 in 20 ml of glacial acetic acid with cooling. Add 8 g bromine dissolved in 20 ml of glacial acetic acid and dilute to 1 litre with acetic acid.

Calculation of weight of oil required :

Each 25 ml of pyridine bromide solution contains 0.20 g of bromine. Allowing for more than 100% excess, this leaves 0.08 g of bromine (0.125 g I_2) for the reaction with oil.

Let the expected iodine value of sample be x. Then x g of I_2 will be absorbed by 100 g of sample

$$\therefore \quad 0.125 \text{ g of } I_2 \text{ will be absorbed by } \frac{100 \times 0.125}{x} \text{ g of sample}$$

$$= \frac{12.5}{x} \text{ g of sample}$$

Thus the weight of oil (in g) for each estimation is calculated by dividing the highest expected iodine value into 12.5.

TABLE 8.4
Iodine Value limits for fatty substances

Substance	Iodine number (official)
Olive oil	79—88
Peanut oil	84—100
Sesame oil	103—116
Stearic Acid	≤ 4
Stearyl alcohol	≤ 2
Almond oil	95—105
Cod—liver oil	145—180
Oleic acid	85—95
Cetyl Alcohol	≤ 2
Corn oil	102—128
Cottonseed oil	109—116
Hydrogenated vegetable oil	≤ 5
Castor oil	83—88
Cocoa butter	35—43

8.2.5. Acetyl Value

The acetyl value is defined as the number of mg of potassium hydroxide required to neutralise the acetic acid liberated by the hydrolysis of 1 g of acetylated substance.

The acetyl value is found by acetylating hydroxy fatty acids determining the saponification number of product. The acetyl value is calculated from the saponification value of the acetylated fatty acid and the acid value of the original fatty acid.

Method : Acetylated 30 g of the substance with 30 ml of acetic anhydride under reflux for 2 hours. Pour the mixture into 50 ml distilled water and boil gently for 15 min while bubbling CO_2 through the mixture. Remove most of the water and repeat the boiling operation with two successive 500 ml portions of distilled water. Transfer the acetylated oil into a separatory funnel and wash with two 200 ml portions of warm (50°C) distilled water. Remove as much as of water and dry with 5g of anhydrous sodium sulphate (15 min) and filter.

From the acetylated substance weigh approximately 2 g sample and determine its saponification number. Separately, the acid value of the original fatty acid substance is also determined. The acetyl value is calculated from the following formula :

$$A = \frac{S - F}{1 - 0.000755}$$

Where A = acetyl value of free fatty acids

S = saponification value of acetylated fatty acids.

F = acid value of the original fatty acid.

The factor 0.00075 gives the number of gms of acetyl group that corresponds to 1 mg of KOH. The denominator 1-0.00075 Corrects for any discrepancy between the molecular weight of acetylated substance used for the determination of saponification and that of the original fatty acids used for the determination of acid value.

8.2.6 Hydroxyl Value

The hydroxyl value or hydroxyl number, is the number of milligrams of potassium hydroxide equivalent to the hydroxyl content of 1 g of substance.

The hydroxyl value gives an indication of the identity and purity of fatty substances possessing alcoholic hydroxyl groups. It is inversely proportional to the molecular weight. Thus an abnormally low value is indicative of adulteration with higher molecular weight alcohols or with non-alcoholic fatty substances like paraffin, petroleum oil etc.

EXERCISE 4. To determine the hydroxyl value of Cetyl alcohol.

Method : Weigh accurately, 2 g of cetyl alcohol and transfer it into a 250 ml iodine flask. Add 2 ml of pyridine and 10 ml of toluene. To the mixture add 1.5 M acetyl chloride in toluene (1.5 M acetyl chloride is prepared by dissolving 10 ml of acetyl chloride in 90 ml of toluene) and heat in a water bath at 60-65°C for 20 min. Add 25 ml of distilled water, stopper the flask and shake it vigorously for few minute. Allow the mixture to stand for 5 min to decompose the excess acetyl chloride. Titrate the reaction mixture with 1 N NaOH to a pink end point using 1 ml of phenolphthalein TS as an indicator. Perform a blank titration under identical conditions without the substance.

The reaction involved is as follows :

$$CH_3(CH_2)_{14}-CH_2-OH + CH_3COCl \longrightarrow CH_3(CH_2)_{14}\ CH_2-O-\overset{\overset{\displaystyle O}{\|}}{C}-CH_3 + HCl$$

The hydroxyl number is given by the formula :

$$\frac{\text{ml of 1 N NaOH} \times 56.11}{\text{Wt. of Sample}}$$

The hydroxyl value of cetyl alcohol is 218-238 while that of stearyl alcohol is 200-220

EXERCISE 5. Determination of percentage (W/W) of Benzyl Alcohol.

Method : Accurately weigh 1.5 g of the substance and reflux with a mixture of acetic anhydride (1 part by volume) and pyridine (1 part by volume) on a water-bath for 30 min. Cool and dilute the mixture with 25 ml of water. Titrate the excess acetic anhydride and acetic acid with N/1 NaOH to a pink end point using phenolphthalein as an indicator. Perform a blank titration in an identical manner. The difference in titrations is equivalent to the benzyl alcohol.

The above determination is based on the following reactions :

$$C_6H_5CH_2OH + (CH_3\ CO)_2O = C_6H_5\ CH_2O\overset{\overset{O}{\|}}{C}—CH_3 + CH_3\ COOH$$

$$(CH_3CO)_2\ O + 2NaOH = 2CH_3COONa + H_2O$$

$$\therefore \quad C_6\ H_5\ CH_2\ OH \equiv (CH_3\ CO)_2O \equiv CH_3\ COOH \equiv NaOH \equiv H$$

$$(CH_3\ CO)_2O \equiv 2Na\ OH_2 \equiv 2H$$

$$\therefore \quad 108.1\text{ g } C_6\ H_5\ CH_2OH \equiv 1000\text{ ml N/1 NaOH}$$

$$\therefore \quad 0.1081\text{ g } C_6\ H_5\ CH_2OH \equiv 1\text{ ml N/1 NaOH}$$

Benzyl alcohol is heated with acetic anhydride in presence of pyridine to produce benzyl acetate. Each molecule of acetic anhydride reacts with alcohol to produce one molecule of acetic acid which is then titrated with standard alkali using phenolphthalein as an indicator.

8.3 Analysis of Alkaloids

8.3.1 General

Alkaloids are defined as chemical substances which contain organic nitrogen in their structure, are obtained from plant, animal or synthetic sources and generally possess pharmacological activities.

A small number of alkaloidal preparations are used as drugs in therapeutics and many of them have potent actions. When such preparations are administered, it is obvious that a slight deficiency of the alkaloid in a preparation may cause a marked decrease in the physiological effect, while a slight excess may cause toxic effect. Therefore, it is necessary that estimation of such alkaloidal drugs and preparations is performed for the purpose of ensuring their purity standardization, and pharmacolegal aspects as a necessary component of quality control and pharmaceutical analysis. Various types of quantitative methods of analysis have been developed for alkaloidal drugs and these can be classified as (i) volumetric, (ii) gravimetric, (iii) spectrophotometric, (iv) electrochemical as well as (v) physiological.

The different samples of the same drug may show variation in the amount of alkaloid content present in crude drugs. The variation may be due to several factors, namely: (i) the age of the plant when it is collected; (ii) the season of the year when the drug is harvested, (iii) the soil and climate in which the drug is grown; (iv) the conditions under which the drug is collected, dried and stored.

The quantity of the alkaloid present in the galenical preparations is also subject to variation because of different reasons such as: (i) the quality of drug used, (ii) the menstruum used in the extraction of the alkaloid, (iii) the amount of decomposition of the alkaloid during the process of extraction and of storage.

It is to be noted that the rate of deterioration of alkaloidal preparations will depend upon (i) the nature of the alkaloid, (ii) the pH of preparation, (iii) heat and light. Therefore it becomes necessary to restandardise the alkaloidal drugs and preparations. Further, since the content of the alkaloid i s not more than 1 % of the crude drug preparation special care must be used to separate it from the other constituents such as proteins, gums, fatty acids, glycosides, resins, volatile and fatty oil and colouring matter.

In order to understand the principles upon which the various methods of analysis of alkaloids are based, one should also known their peculiar physical and chemical characteristics. These are briefly stated below :

1. Since the nitrogen in the alkaloid may be primary amine, secondary or tertiary amine the formula R3N is used to represent the *free alkaloid.* The amino nitrogen has basic properties and has a free pair of electrons which reactions with H^+ to form *alkaloidal salts* $R_3N^+ HCl^-$ The free alkaloids are sporingly soluble in water but soluble in most organic salts while alkaloidal salts are freely soluble in water and sparingly soluble in organic solvents.
2. They form highly insoluble precipitates with a number of reagent e.g. with salts of heavy metals like Hg, Au and Pt etc.

In general, the methods used in the analysis of dosage forms containing alkaloids and other amine drugs involve two major steps : (i) the separation and collection of the alkaloid from other constituents present in the dosage form and (ii) analysis of the alkaloid itself by a suitable method. The separation of the alkaloid is achieved by liberating the free amine from the alkaloid salt by treatment with sodium hydroxide followed by exhaustive extraction of the aqueous layer with an organic solvent like other. The organic solvent is freed from alkali by washing it with aciduated water.

The analysis of the crude drugs is classified according to the manner in which the percent of extractive is determined. If the percent of the extractive represents the total of a class of the plant principles like alkaloids or glycosides or flavenoids etc the assay is called the *proximate assay.* If, on the other hand, the percent of extractive from a crude drug represents a single chemical species like morphine, strychnine etc, the assay is called an *ultimate assay.*

EXERCISE 1. Assay of Belladona tincture

Method : Measure 100 ml of the sample and reduce it to 10 ml by evaporation at 100°C.

Transfer the concentrated liquid into a separatory funnel containing 25 ml $CHCl_3$. Rinse the container with small portions of dilute ethanol and add them to the separatory funnel. Add 25 ml of water and render the mixture alkaline by the addition of ammonia T.S.

Extract the alkaloids completely with successive quantities of $CHCl_3$. Transfer the extract to a separatory funnel using diethyl ether. Extract with the successive portions of 0.5 N H_2SO_4. Render the combined acid extracts alkaline with NH_3 TS and extract at once the alkaloids with successive portions of $CHCl_3$. Evaporate the combined extracts on a steam bath to dryness and then heat on a water-bath for 15 min. Dissolve the residue in a small volume of $CHCl_3$, again evaporate to dryness and heat on a water bath for 15 min. Dissolve the residue in a few ml of $CHCl_3$, add 15 ml of 0.02 N H_2SO_4, remove $CHCl_3$ by evaporation, cool, add methyl red TS and titrate the excess with 0.02 N NaOH. Each ml of 0.02 N acid is equivalent to 5.788 mg of alkaloids of belladona leaf, calculated as hyoscyamine or atropine.

EXERCISE 2. Determination of the percentage of Morphine calculated as anhydrous Morphine.

Method : Place 8 g of sample in a mortar and triturate with 30 ml water and 2 g of calcium hydroxide. (This liberates morphine and narcotine and converts them into water soluble Ca-salts). Transfer the mixture to a tared flask and make up to 90 g with water. Shake the mixture occasionally and filter through a Buchner funnel. Transfer exactly 52 ml of the filterate into a clean dry conical flask and add 2 g of ammonium chloride, 25 ml ether & 5 ml 90% ethanol. [Ammonium chloride decomposes the ca-salts of the alkaloids, $(RO)_2 Ca + 2NH_4 Cl = 2ROH + 2NH_3 + CaCl$] ether acts a solvent for narcotine and ethanol facilitates the separation of morphine as crystals. Cork the flask, shake for 15 min and allow to stand overnight. Decant the ethereal solution as completely as possible through a filter funnel retaining the morphine crystals. Wash the contents of the flask with another 10 ml of ether and filter. Now pour the aqueous liquor from the flask on to the filter and wash the flask and filter with morphinated water until the filterate is free from chloride. Displace the ammonia fumes from the flask by blowing with air.

Transfer the contents of the funnel back to the flask with water. Add 25 ml of N/10 HCl, boil gently to remove CO_2 and back titrate the excess of acid with N/10 NaOH to an orange shade end point using methyl red as an indicator. A correction of + 0.052 g must be added to the calculated amount of anhydrous morphine due to the solubility of morphine in the ether-water mixture.

EXERCISE 3. Determination of Ephedrine sulphate Injection

Method : Transfer the contents of six vials of ephedrine sulphate injection (50 mg/ml per vial) to a dry container. Then pipette exactly 5 ml of the combined injection into a clean separatory funnel. Add 5 ml of water and adjust the volume to 10 ml. Saturate the solution with 3 g of Nacl. Now , add 5 ml of NaOH solution and extract with four 25 ml portions of $CHCl_3$. Wash the combined chloroform extract with 10 ml of saturated solution of brine and filter through cotton. Extract the wash solution with 10 ml of $CHCl_3$ and add to the main chloroform extract. Add methyl red TS, and titrate with 0.1 N perchloric acid. Perform a blank determination. Each millilitre of 0.1 N $HClO_4$ is equivalent to 21.43 g of $(C_{10}H_{15}NO)_2\ H_2SO_4$.

The following reactions are involved in the above assay :

$$(C_{10}H_{15}NO)_2 . H_2SO_4 + 2NaOH \longrightarrow 2C_{10}H_{15}NO + Na_2SO_4 + 2H_2O$$

$$C_{10}H_{15}NO + HClO_4 \longrightarrow C_{10}H_{15}NO . HClO_4$$

8.4 Analysis of Volatile Oils

8.4.1 General

The volatile oils are complex substances composed of mixtures of compounds of widely differing chemical properties. They are also known as essential oils and are used for flavouring purposes. The essential oils contain a wide variety of organic compounds and can be classified as described below :

(i) Hydrocarbons : The important compounds belonging to this group are pinene, camphene limonene, bornylene, fenchene, dipentene, sylvestrene and phellandrene

(ii) Alcohols : They are present both in the free state and in combination with acids as esters. The well known compounds of this group are linalol, santalol etc.

(iii) Aldehydes : The examples of this class are citral, citronellal, salicyl aldehyde, benzaldehyde, cinnamic aldehyde.

(iv) Ketones : The important substance are camphor, fenchone, thujone and menthone.

(v) Phenols : The important examples are anethol, eugenol, carvacrol, chavicol, thymol, safrol etc.

(vi) Acids : The are present both in the free state e.g. acetic, propionic, butyric, valeric, benzoic, cinnamic, hydrocyanic acids and in combination with alcohols as esters like linalyl acetate, bornyl acetate, menthyl acetate.

(vii) Sulphur Compounds : The common example being allyl isothiocyanate (i.e. mustard oil).

The overall quality control of the essential oils is based on : (a) determination of certain physical characteristics, (b) quantitative estimation of the chief constituent i.e. alcohol, aldehyde or ester etc, and (c) the qualitative tests of substances that are used for their adulteration.

The quality and purity of the essential oils is also noted from their colour, odour, appearance, solubility, specific gravity, optical rotation, refractive index, solidifying power, boiling and melting points. These properties should be looked up in standard texts.

EXERCISE 1. Preparation and standardization of 0.5 N alcoholic potassium hydroxide.

Method : Dissolve 2.5 g of lead acetate in 5 ml of water and add the solution to 1 litre of ethanol contained in a glass stoppered bottle. separately dissolve 5 g of potassium hydroxide in 25 ml of warm ethanol, cool the solution and add it slowly with stirring to the alcohol solution of lead acetate. After 1 hr shake the mixture vigorously, allow it to stand overnight, decant the clear liquid and collect the ethanol by distillation.

Meanwhile dissolve about 35 g of KOH in 20 ml of water. Add sufficient aldehyde-free ethanol as prepared above and adjust the volume to 1 litre. Allow the solution to remain in the tightly stoppered bottle for 24 hr. Decant the clear supernatant and transfer it to another stoppered bottle. Pipette 25 ml of 0.5 N HCl, dilute with 50 ml of water, add 2 drops of phenolphthalein TS and titrate with alcoholic KOH solution to a pink end point. Calculated the normality

EXERCISE 2. Analysis of Peppermint oil for total esters.

Method : Weigh accurately 10 g of peppermint oil in a 250 ml conical flask. Add 10 ml of neutralized ethanol, 2 drops of phenolphthalein TS and 0.1 N NaOH until faint pink colour appears. Now, add 25 ml of 0.5 N KOH and reflux on a water-bath for 1 hr. Allow the mixture to cool, add 20 ml water, 3 drops of phenolphthalein TS and titrate excess of alkali with 0.5N HCl. Perform a blank determination under the same conditions but without the sample. Each millilitre of 0.5 N KOH consumed in the hydrolysis is equivalent to 99.15 mg of total esters calculated as menthyl acetate ($C_{12}H_{23}O_2$).

The reactions involved are :

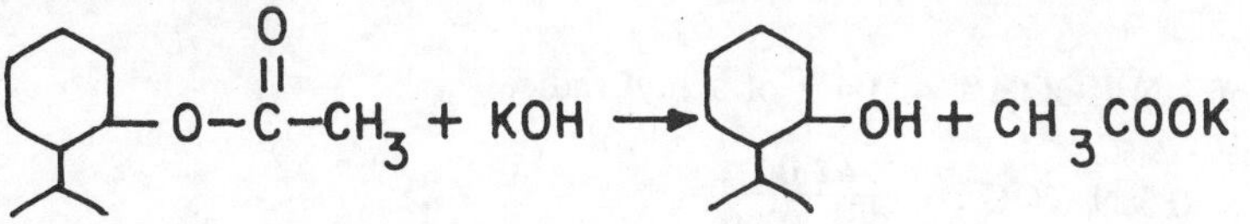

$$\text{(menthyl)}-O-\overset{O}{\overset{\|}{C}}-CH_3 + KOH \longrightarrow \text{(menthyl)}-OH + CH_3COOK$$

1 ml N/2 KOH ≡ 99.15 mg $C_{12}H_{23}O_2$

EXERCISE 3. Analysis of peppermint oil for total Menthol.

Method : Transfer 10 ml of peppermint oil in a 100 ml round bottom flask, add 10 ml of acetic anhydride and 1 g of anhydrous sodium acetate. Reflux the mixture for 1 hr, cool the solution and transfer it to a separatory funnel. Rinse the flask with three 5 fml portions of warm water and add them to the separatory funnel. Run off the water layer and wash the remaining oily layer with dilute sodium carbonate test solution until the last washings are alkaline to 2 drops of phenolphthalein TS. Dry the resulting oil with anhydrous Na_2SO_4 and filter, Transfer 5 ml of acetylated oil to a tared 100 ml flask and obtain the exact weight of the oil. Add 50 ml of 0.5 N ethanolic KOH to the oil. Attach a reflux condenser and reflux for 1 hr. Allow the mixture to cool, add 10 drops of phenolphthalein TS and titrate the excess alkali with 0.5 N HCl. Perform a blank titration under the same conditions but without the sample. Calculate the percentage of total menthol in the oil by the following formula :

$$\frac{A \times 7.813}{B - (A \times 0.021)} \times [1 - (E \times 0.0021)]$$

where A is result obtained by subtracting the number of millilitres of 0.5 N HCl required in the above titration from number of millilitres of 0.5 N HCl required in the blank titration.

B is the weight of the acetylated oil taken.

E is the percentage of esters calculated as menthyl acetate ($C_{10}H_{19}.\ C_2H_3O_2$).

The calculations and reactions involved in the above analysis are shown below :

(i) $$\text{(menthyl)}-OH + (CH_3-\overset{O}{\overset{\|}{C}})_2O \longrightarrow \text{(menthyl)}-O-\overset{O}{\overset{\|}{C}}-CH_3 + CH_3COOH$$

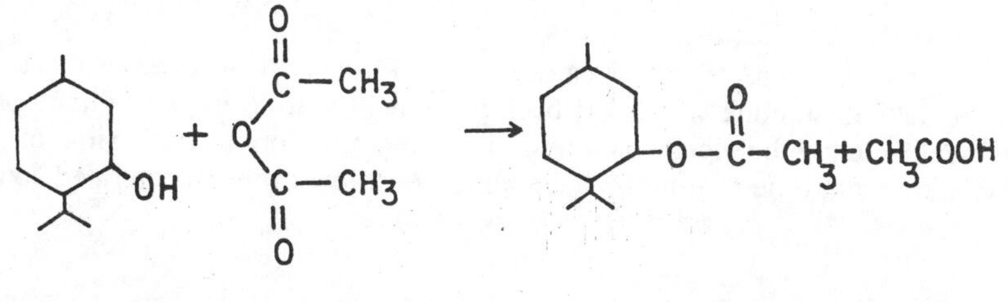

(ii) $-O-\overset{O}{\overset{\|}{C}}-CH_3 + KOH \longrightarrow -OH + CH_3COOK$

(i) The molecular weight of Menthol = 156.27 g

(ii) 1 millilitre of 0.5 N KOH $\equiv \frac{156.27}{2 \times 1000} = 0.07813$ g of menthol

(iii) To get the result in terms of percent we have $0.07813 \times 100 = 7.813$ g

(iv) The term B — (A × 0.021) corrects for the weight of acetyl radical in the sample of acetylised oil.

(v) The factor 0.021 is the amount of acetyl radical ≡ 1 ml of 0.5 N KOH.

(vi) The above is computed as follows :

Mol. wt of Menthyl acetate = 198.31 g

Mol. wt of Menthol = 156.27 g

∴ Mol Wt of Acetyl radical = 42.048

∴ 1000 ml of 1 N KOOH ≡ 42.04 g of acetyl radical

∴ 1 ml of 0.5 N KOH $\equiv \frac{42.04}{2 \times 1000}$

∴ A × 0.021 is the weight of acetyl radical deducted from B, the weight of the acetylised oil.

(vii) Because the original oil contained some menthol combined as ester, a correction for the weight of the acetyl radical in the original oil is applied by multiplying by [1– (E × 0.0021)]. This factor 0.0021 is the ratio of weight of acetyl radical to that of menthyl acetate i.e. 42.04/198.31 = 0.21

(viii) Suppose in the above analysis, E which is the % of total esters is found to be 5, then the correction will be 1– (0.05 × 0.21) or 1– (5 × 0.0021).

(ix) Thus the final formula arrived is

$$\frac{A \times 7.813}{B-(A \times 0.021)} \times [1-(5 \times 0.0021)] = \% \text{ Total Menthol}$$

Table 8.5
Ester content limits for Volatile oils

Oil	Amount	Official Requirement, %
Peppermint oil	10	$C_{19} H_{18} C_2 H_3 O_2 \geq .5$
Methyl Salicylate	2	$C_6 H_4$ (OH) COOH CH_3 .≥ 98
Lavender oil	5	$C_{10} H_{17} C_2H_3 O_2 \geq 35$ (as linalyl acetate)
Pine needle oil	10	$C_{10} H_{17} C_2 H_3 O_2$ = 3-10 (as bornyl acetate)

EXERCISE 4. Analysis of Caraway oil.

Method : Accurately measure 10 ml of caraway oil and place it in a cassia flask. Add 50 ml of saturated solution of sodium sulphite which has been made neutral to 2 drops of Phenolphthalein TS by means of a saturated solution bisulphite solution. Heat the solution by refluxing on a water bath, neutralizing the mixture from time to time by the addition of a few drops of saturated sodium bisulphite solution. When no colouration is obtained on further addition of Phenolphthalein TS heat for further 15 min. Cool the mixture and when the liquids have separated add more of sodium sulphite solution to raise the lower limit of the oily layer in the graduated portion of the neck of the flask. Note the volume of the residual oily liquid. The difference between the volume of the oil used as the sample and the volume of the oily layer that remains insoluble represents the carvone which dissolves in the aqueous layer.

Say in the above case if the volume of the residual liquid is 5 ml, the % of carvone in the oil will be :

$$\frac{10-5}{10} \times 100 = 50\%$$

The reactions involved in the analysis are given below :

$Na_2SO_3 + H_2O \longrightarrow NaHSO_3 + NaOH$

$HSO_3 + H_2O \rightleftharpoons H_3O^+ + SO_3^{2-}$

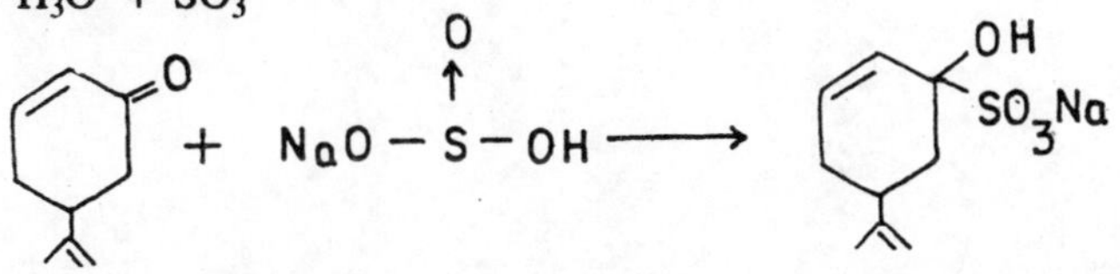

Carvone + $NaO-\overset{O \uparrow}{S}-OH \longrightarrow$ (OH, SO_3Na addition product)

Carvone, which is the chief constituent reacts with $NaHSO_3$ forming a water soluble addition product. The saturated solution of sodium sulphite acts to salt out from the aqueous phase those volatile oil constituents which do not react with bisulphite. Sodium sulphite is hydrolysed by water to produce sodium hydroxide which renders the solution basic and turns pink. On further addition of $NaHSO_3$ the reaction proceeds tó left rendering the solution acidic.

EXERCISE 5. Analysis of Benzaldehyde

Method : Place about 1 ml of benzaldehyde in a weighing bottle and weigh accurately. Transfer the weighed material into a 250 ml conical flask containing 25 ml of hydroxylamine HCl reagent. (This reagent is prepared by dissolving 34.7 g of NH_2OH. HCl in 160 ml of water and diluting to 1 litre with ethanol). Rinse the sides of the flask with additional 50 ml of the reagent. Allow the mixture to stand for 10 min, add 1 ml of bromophenol blue TS and titrate the liberated hydrochloric acid to a light green end point with 1 N NaOH. Perform a blank titration under the same conditions but without the sample. Each ml of 1 N NaOH is equivalent to 106.1 mg of $C_7 H_6 O$.

The reactions involved in the reaction is as follows :

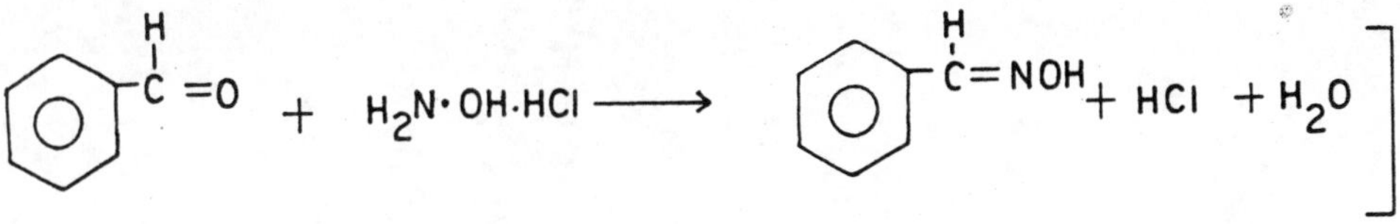

$$C_6H_5-\overset{H}{C}=O + H_2N\cdot OH\cdot HCl \longrightarrow C_6H_5-\overset{H}{C}=NOH + HCl + H_2O$$

Volatible oils containing very small quantities of oldehydes such as lemon oil or those which contain constituents that form water soluble addition products with Na HSO_3 cannót be assayed accurately by this method. They are therefore determined by hydroxyl-amine method as described above.

Table 8.6
Volatile oils Analysed for Aldehyde content

Oil	Amount used	Method	Official Requirement %
Benzaldehyde	1 g	Hydroxylamine	Benzaldehyde ≥ 98
Lemon oil	5 g	,,	Citral, 3-5.5
Cinnamon oil	10 ml	Bisulphite	Total aldehyde ≥ 80

SECTION-C
GENERAL PHYSICAL METHODS OF ANALYSIS

GENERAL PHYSICAL METHODS

Introduction

The general physical methods of analysis like the determination of specific gravity and density; solubility; molecular weights; viscosity and surface tension which are commonly available in other text books will not be dealt with in this book. On the other hand topics on refractometry, polarimetry and optical rotatory dispersion have been incorporated into this section.

9

Refractometry

9.1 General

Although the index of refraction is simply a physical constant but it can be used in the determination of purity and identity of drug substances. In some cases, it may be used to estimate quantitatively the strength and purity of solutions or proportions in which liquids are mixed ; e.g. percentage of alcohol in water.

9.2 Theory

When a ray of light passes from one transparent medium to another of different optical density, some of the light is reflected and the light which passes into the medium is refracted (bent). Light which enters perpendicularly to the surface of contact is not refracted and is called the normal. The extent and direction of refraction is dependent on the difference between the densities of the two substances. The angle between the ray in the first medium and the normal is called the angle of incidence i and the corresponding angle in the second medium is called angle of refraction r. The sine of i and sine of r are proportional to the velocity of light in the two mediums.

The index of refraction of a chemical or a drug substance can be defined as the ratio of velocity of light in air to the velocity of light in the medium or as the ratio of the sine of angle of incidence to the sine of angle of refraction. It may be written as :

$$n = \frac{V_{air}}{V_M} = \frac{\text{Sin } i}{\text{Sin } r} \quad \text{...} \quad (1)$$

It may be noted that when a ray of light passes from a less dense medium I to a more dense medium II, it will be bent so that the angle of refraction r will be less than the angle of incidence i and according to the law of refraction, the relationship between these two angles will be :

$$\frac{\text{Sin } i}{\text{Sin } r} = \frac{N}{n} \quad \text{...} (2)$$

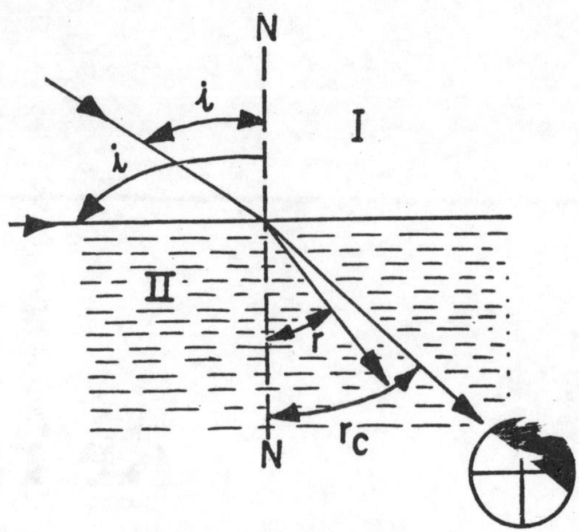

Fig. 9.1. Refraction of Light

Where n is index of refraction of less dense medium and N is the index of refraction for the more dense medium

Further, when the angle i increases, the angle r also increases and attains its maximum value r_c as the angle of incidence approaches 90°. This is called the *grazing incidence*. The maximum value of refraction is called the *critical angle* r_c and is defined as the angle of refraction when the angle of incidence equals 90°. This ray of refracted light forming the critical angle is called the *critical ray*. It forms the boundary defining the critical angle and it is this boundary which furnishes the refractive end point of a substance. In the practical work for the determination of refractive index for substances, the critical angle of the sample is related to the critical angle of a standard of known refractive index used in the calibration of the refractive index. The equation No 2 can be rearranged as :

$$n = \frac{\text{Sin r N}}{\text{Sin i}}$$ where n is refractive index of the substance and N is the refractive index of prism.

Because N is a constant and sin 90° = 1, measurement of r_c will be an estimation of the refractive index of the sample compound i.e. n = N sin r_c

The refractive index generally decreases with increase of the wavelength of light used therefore a monochromatic light source should be used. However, the refractometer should be able to compensate for the use of white light.

The variation of refractive index with wavelength when the medium does not absorb light is represented by Cauchy formula :

$$n = A + \frac{B}{\lambda^2} + \frac{C}{\lambda^4}$$ Where A, B and C are constants

The refractive index of a liquid decreases as the temperature increases, the percentage decrease ranging from 0.01 to 0.1% per degree depending upon the nature of the liquid. As the refractive index can be measured within ± 2×10^{-4}, temperature control is necessary. The refractive index is generally represented as n_D^{20} where temperature is represented as the superscript and the wavelength of light is used as subscript, here D refers to sodium D line.

The refractive index of a solvent changes if a solute is dissolved in it. This variation of refractive index is useful in following chromatographic separations. The specific refractive index increment dn/dc is the change of solute concentration, the latter being expressed in g/ml i.e.

$$\frac{dn}{dc} = \frac{n_{solution} - n_{solvent}}{\text{Concentration of Solute}}$$

The concentration of a solution can be determined by measuring its refractive index. According to Lorentz and Lorenz the specific refraction is given by :

$$[n] = \frac{n^2 - 1}{n^2 + 2} \cdot \frac{1}{p}$$

Where P is the density of liquid of refractive index n.

The molar refraction is given by :

$$R = \frac{n^2 - 1}{n^2 + 2} \cdot \frac{M}{p}$$

Where M is the molecular weight. It has the dimension of molar volume and is an additive property of groups or elements comprising the compound. This additivity is due to the property of polarisability of molecules when subjected to electromagnetic radiation. The incident radiation sets the electrons vibrating and induces dipoles in the molecule. The total polarisability of the molecule is related to the sum of all the induced dipoles and therefore to the number and type of constituent atoms. Thus, specific refraction is valuable in identification of a substance and as a criteria of its purity. If the empirical formula of a compound is known and its molar refraction is measured by adding the values for the atoms in the molecule the structure of the substance can be determined.

Table 9.1
Atomic Refractivities

Group	Mr_D	Group	Mr_D
		Br	8.865
H	1.100	I	13.900
C	2.418	N (NH_2)	2.322
		N (NHR)	2.499
		N (NRR)	2.840
C = C	2.398	N (NH_2, aromatic)	3.21
O (C = O)	2.211	N (NHR, ")	3.59
O (OH)	1.525	N (NRR, ")	4.36
O (ether, ester)	1.643	N (amide)	2.65
S (c = s)	7.97	NO_2 (aromatic)	7.30
S (S-H)	7.69	C ≡ N	5,459
F	1.0		
Cl	5.96		

9.3 Refractometers

There are three types of refractometers available, namely : (i) Abbe (ii) Immersion or dipping and (iii) Pulfrish. However, Abbe refractometer is commonly used because of its simplicity, ease of manipulation and the small amount of material required for analysis.

Abbe Refractometer

A schematic diagram of Abbe refractometer is shown in the Fig. 9.1b. Now models are available.

The sample is placed between the two prisms called diffusing prism (DP) and reflecting Prism (RP) respectively. Light rays which are reflected from the mirror enter the diffusing Prism DP where the rays are scattered in all directions. The scattered rays pass through the sample and then through the refracting prism RP at a grazing incidence of 89.99°. They are refracted at the critical angle r_c. The light rays which enter the refracting prism at angles less than 90° are refracted at smaller angles than the critical angles and are responsible for the light observed in the eye piece. The lens L in the telescope T collects the rays and eyepiece. The movable arm M, which is attached to the prisms is moved in the direction which gives a dark and light boundary in the field at exactly the position where the two hairs intersect i.e. view B. (The two other views A and C are given for comparison purpose and are not meant for the end point of measurement. Below the movable arm M is fixed the scale S. The value is read on this scale at the end point of measurement and gives the refractive index of the sample. Albee refractometer can be used with ordinary white light and has a wide range of indices from 1.3000 to 1.7000. For measurement with liquids only a few drops sufficient to form a thin film are placed between the poisons and even if the liquid is coloured or turbid, thinness of the film permits a determination of the refractive index without any problems.

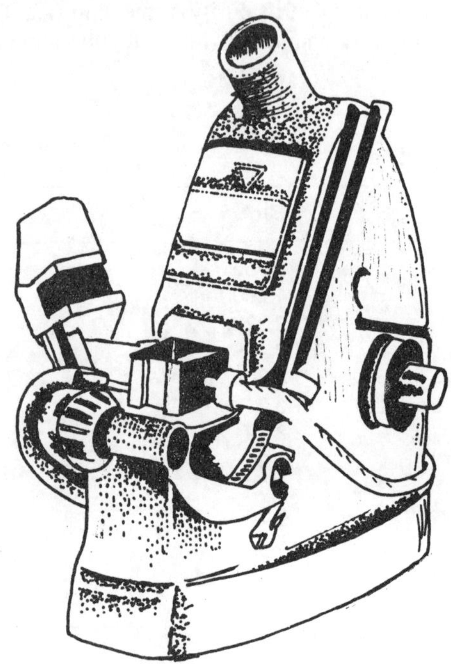

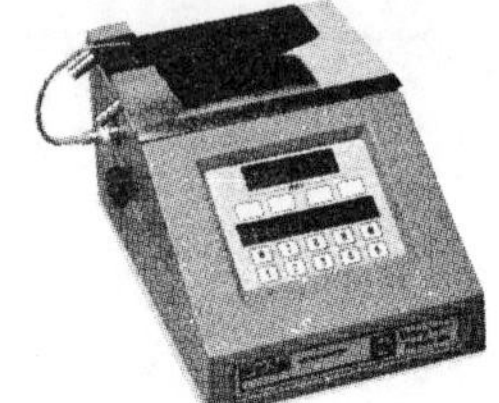

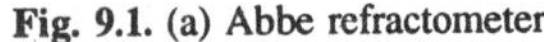

Fig. 9.1. (a) Abbe refractometer

Fig. 9.1. (b) A modern Refractomer, Model RFM-332 (Courtesy of Bellingham Stanley Ltd.)

EXERCISE 1. To determine the concentration of Dextrose in Dextrose Solution.

Method : Prepare accurately 1.0, 5.0, and 10% (W/V) dextrose solutions, each of 50 ml volume. Measure the refractive index of each of the solutions according to the following procedure. Attach the test plate to the refractive prism of the refractometer with the aid of monobromonaphthalene or other liquid provided with the test plate by moistening the test plate with the liquid and pressing it against the refracting prism. Focus the liquid on the test plate, adjust the instrument until the border line of the critical

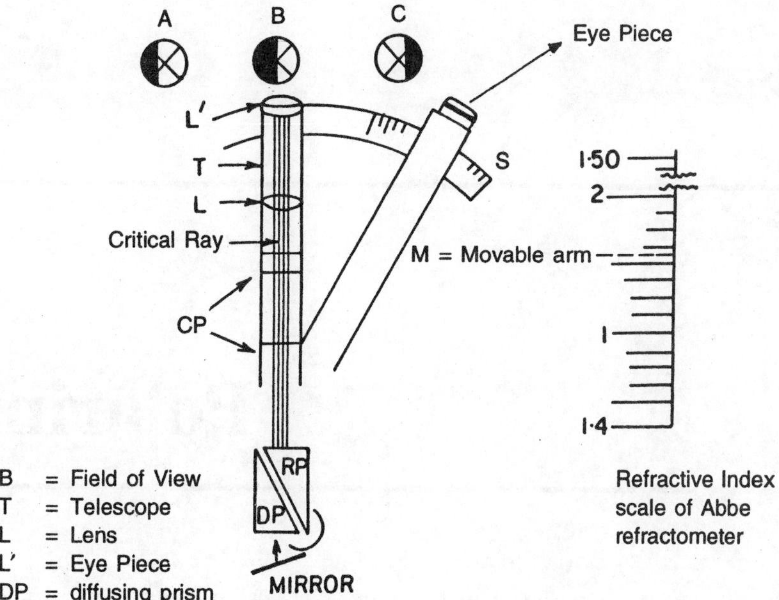

Fig. 9.1. (b) Abbe refractometer

angle coincides with the cross hairs in the telescope. Note the reading of the refractive index. The reading of the instrument should corespond to that given on this plate. If any adjustment of the instrument is required, correction should be applied to the readings (Water can also be used for the calibration of the instrument ; n_D^{25} = 1.3325). Remove the test plate, clean the prism with cotton soaked in ethanol. Place 2 to 3 drops of the dextrose solution on the prism and tighten the prisms firmly. Position the light source so that light is reflected through the prism and adjust the instrument until the border line between the dark and the light halves of the field of view coincide exactly with the cross hairs of the telescope by rotating the compensator prisms (CP) to obtain a sharp uncoloured border. Read the refractive index of the solution directly from the graduated scale to the 4th mean of the readings as the refractive index of the solution. Note the temperature at which readings are taken.

Prepare graph by plotting refractive index on the Y axis and molar concentration on the X-axis. Obtain an unknown sample from the instructor and measure the refractive index. From the graph determine molar concentration. Calculate the % W/V of anhydrous dextrose in the solution of unknown concentration.

EXERCISE 2. Determination of the Refractive index for Various organic liquids.

Method : 1. Obtain the following organic liquids : benzene, carbon tetrachloride, diethyl ether, ethyl alcohol and glycerine. 2. Set the abbe refractometer as per instructions by the instructor or as per operating manual 3. Turn the water circulation system so that temperature is 20°C. 4. Adjust the light source so that a clear field is obtained. 5. Clean the prisms with ethanol. 6. Measure the refractive index of water and then for the above stated organic liquids. 7. Determine their dispersions, ($n_f - n_c$). 8. From the refractive index and the density of each compound, calculate the specific refractivity of each compound. 9. With the aid of molecular weights, the molar refractivities of these compounds can also be determined. 10. Make a mixture of *unknown* quantities of benzene and carbon tetrachloride and measure its refractive index. 11. From the densities and values of the individual refractive indices, calculate the % weight of each component in the *unknown* mixture.

10

Polarimetry

10.1 General

There are many organic compounds which have ability to rotate the plane of polarized light. Such substances are called *optically active* or that they possess *optical rotary power*. The optical rotatory power arises due to the presence of structural asymmetry contained in any substance. This again may be because of symmetry of a plane or a centre of symmetry in the molecule, some examples of the origin of structural asymmetry inherent in the structure of molecules are (i) dextrose (ii) in the crystalline form like quartz but not in the liquid or gaseous state (iii) helical form of polypeptide. The other examples of asymmetrical molecules are; D + glyceraldehyde and 3–phenyl–2–butanol as shown below.

CHO
H—C*—OH
CH OH

D+GLYCERALDEHYDE

H, H_3C—C*—C*—CH_3, OH, H_5C_6, H

3-PHENYL-2-BUTANOL

Further, substances can be classified as "isotropic" when radiation coming into contact with them is affected in the same way regardless of direction of vibration or direction of propagation. For example, gases, liquids in absence of orienting field, isometric crystals (NaCl). When one direction is not optically equivalent to the other because of differences in the numbers of each kind of atoms encountered or in the spacing of units in the lattice patterns, such substances are called "anisotropic". For example, uniaxial crystalline solids, tetragonal, hexagonal etc. Let us consider the resolution of an incident radiation falling on a uniaxial crystal containing a single optic axis. The crystal will resolve the radiation into 2 rays having mutually ⊥ plane of vibration. One vibration will be in a principle plane i.e. plane formed by the optic axis and ⊥ to the main faces of the crystal. The other vibration will be in the plane ⊥ to the principal axis. The ray along the optic axis will establish the ordinary index of refraction (n_o) and is called "Ordinary ray". It travels with vibrations ⊥ to the principal plane at the same velocity. The other component i.e. ray with vibrations in the principal plane is called "extra ordinary ray". It has the index of refraction n_E and varies with the direction of propagation.

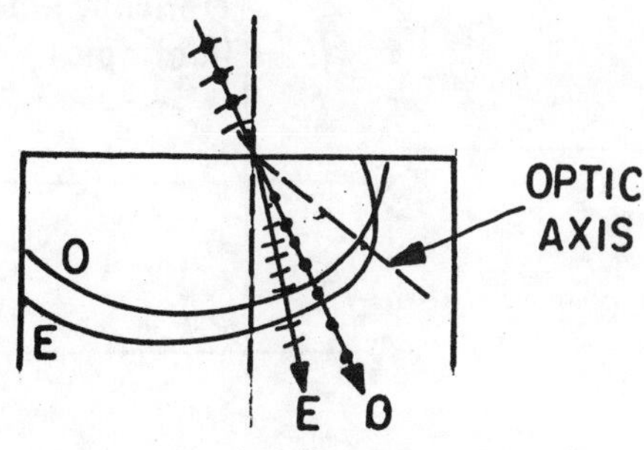

Fig. 10.1 Radiation falling on a uniaxial crystal

10.2 Theory

The subject of polarimetry involves the study of following two changes that may be produced in a polarized light when it interacts with an optically "anisotropic matters". (i) a change in the direction of vibration i.e. a rotation of a linear vibration perpendicular to the direction of propagation and (ii) a change in the state of vibration i.e. a transition of a linear vibration into an elliptic or circular vibration or vice-versa. Generally a change in the direction of vibration of linearly polarized light during passage through an anisotropic matter is called "optical rotation" i.e. when the effect is due to anisotropic refraction, but when effect is produced by anisotropic absorption or scattering it is called 'optical dichroism". Therefore, such substances which have an inherent ability to rotate the plane of polarized light are called "optically active."

Under normal conditions, the natural ordinary light is presumed to consist of a large number of electromagnetic waves vibrating in all possible directions around the direction of propagation. If from this natural wave front, only those rays vibrating in one particular plane are separated out by some means, it is called "plane polarized light". Similarly, a circularly polarized light would comprise a wave in which electrical component (also the magnetic component) would travel either clockwise (left handed) around the direction of propagation e.g. α, β — helix and screw nail etc.

Let us consider a linearly polarized beam of monochromatic light travelling along the plane of this paper along the direction of arrow as shown in Fig. 10.2 and 10.3.

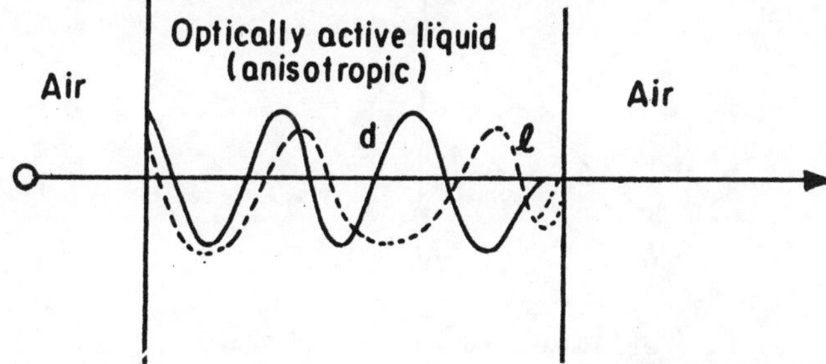

Fig. 10.2. Resolution of a beam of linearly polarized light into two components by an optically active liquid.

The beam is supposed to be resolved into two circular components around after it enters the liquid. The velocity of the two components in the liquid will be different from that of air. This is represented as follows :

$$V_d = V_l = V_2 \text{ because } V_1 : V_2 = n_2 : n_1$$

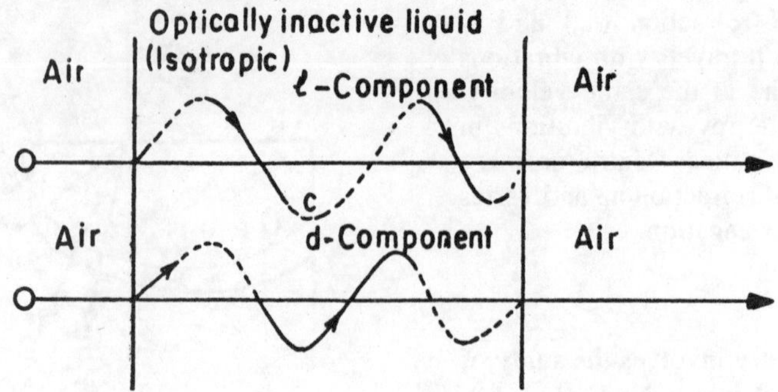

Fig. 10.3. Resolution of a beam of polurized light into two circular components by an isotropic liquid.

Where n_1 is the refractive index of air and n_2 is refractive index of liquid. V_2 is velocity in liquid and V_1 is velocity in air.

But refractive index $n = \frac{c}{v}$

Where c is velocity in vacuum, v is the frequency i.e. no of vibration per second (It is constant)

$$\therefore \quad n_1 = \frac{c}{v_1} \text{ and } n_2 = \frac{c}{v_2}$$

$$\text{But } \nu = \frac{V}{\lambda}$$

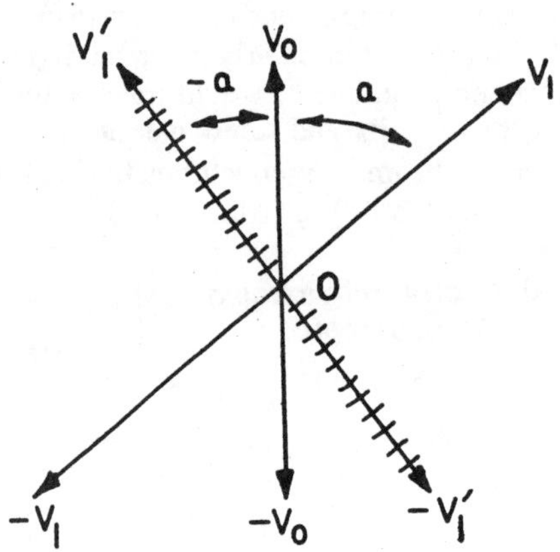

Fig. 10.4 Beam of linearly polarized light.

Further, $\lambda_1 : \lambda_2 = V_1 : V_2 = n_2 : n_1$ where λ_1 is wavelength in air and λ_2 is wavelength in the liquid, consequently light wave become contracted on entering in a liquid.

In figure 10.4. the beam of linearly polarized light is represented to intersect the plane at 0. Normally, the beam will vibrate along – V_o O V_o but it will vibrate along – V_1OV_1 or – $V_1'OV_1'$ after traversing an optically active substance. Rotation α will be positive if the direction is clockwise (i.e. – V_o OV_o → – V_1OV_1) and negative if the direction of vibration changes to — V_1' O V_1'. Substances that cause a positive rotation are termed *dextrorotatory* while that cause a negative rotation are termed *levorotartory.*

Let b be the length of the column of material travelled by the beam, λ the wavelength of light, υ is the velocity in vacuum, then the phase difference ϕ between the two rays will be given by :

$$\varphi = \frac{2\pi b v}{V_r} - \frac{2\pi b v}{V_l}$$

Where r and l are right and the left component of the plane polarized beam.

or $$\varphi = \frac{2\pi b v c}{V_r c} - \frac{2\pi b v c}{V_l c}$$

We know $$v = \frac{c}{\lambda} \quad \therefore \quad \frac{1}{\lambda} = \frac{v}{c}$$

Also $$n = \frac{c}{v} \quad \therefore \quad \bar{v} = \frac{1}{\lambda} = \frac{v}{c}$$

or $$= \varphi = \frac{2\pi b n_r}{\lambda} - \frac{2\pi b n_l}{\lambda}$$

$$\varphi = \frac{2\pi b}{\lambda}(n_r - n_l) \text{ or } \lambda = \frac{\pi b}{\lambda}(n_r - n_l)$$

Where α is the angle of rotation because α = 1/2 of phase difference.

10.3 Instrumentation Aspects

The main components of a polarimeter are : (i) The light source, (ii) a polarize, (iii) an analyzer, (iv) a graduated scale to measure the amount of rotation. (v) sample tubes. A block diagram of a manually polarimeter is given below. However, automatic digital type models are available in the market but are expensive.

A = Light source, B = Collimating lens, C = half-shadow prism D = Lever to adjust half-shadow

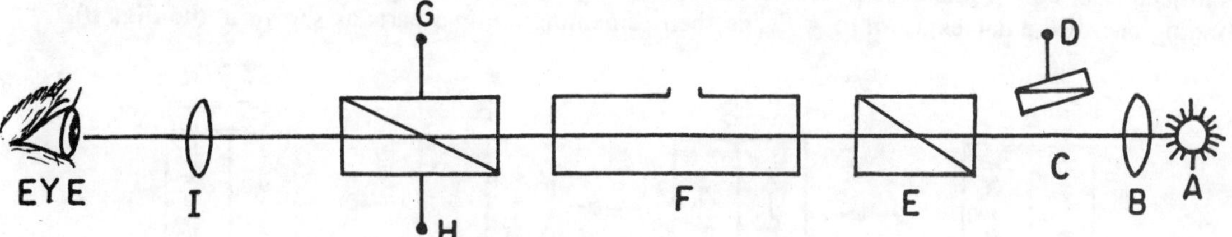

Fig. 10.5. A visual polarimeter (half shadow type)

angle,

E = Polarizing Prism, F = Sample tube, G = graduated scale, H = analyzing prism, I = eye piece.

The details concerning the main components are discussed below.

Light Source : The Common source of light used in polarimetry work are (i) sodium vapour lamp and (ii) mercury vapour lamps. The sodium vapour lamp emits light at wavelengths of 5890 A° and 5896 A°. The mercury vapour lamp emits light of wavelengths at 4358, 4916, 5461, 5770 and 5791 A°. Suitable type of filters can be used to isolate required lines.

Polarizer: Several different types of polarizing prisms are known. They differ in the angles of the faces of the prism and of the cut diagonally through the prism. The Nicol prism and the Glau-Thompson prism are most commonly used polarizers. The Nicol prism is cheaper but not as good as the Glau-Thompson prism. The make up and mechanism of the Nicol prism is explained below :

Nicol prism is prepared from calcite crystals with a minimum of alteration of natural crystal faces.

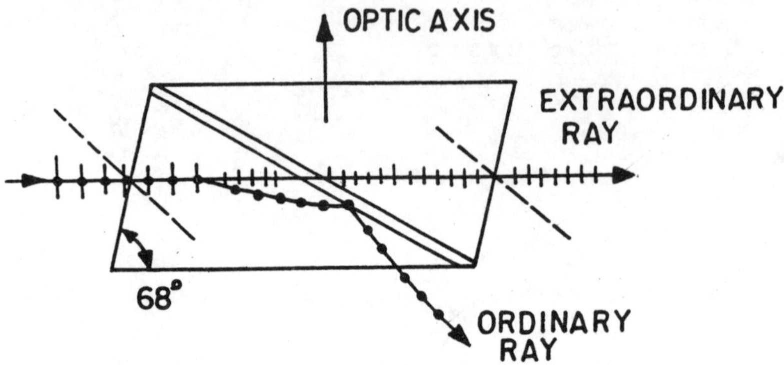

Fig. 10.6. Nicol Prism

The crystal is cut diagonally into two halves at such an angle so that one component of the light is totally reflected. The second component of the light passes through the second half of the crystal in the same direction as the original beam. The two halves of the crystal are cemented together by means of Canada balsom which has an index of refraction of 1.4865. The calcite is uniaxial crystal having n_e of 1.4865 and n_o of 1.6584. Thus the light emerging from the Nicol prism is displaced from the original and will revolve in a circle as the prism is rotated. Nicol prism can be used only in Visible range since Canada balsam is opaque to U.V. light. It also has certain other disadvantages like as dispersion and complete extinction cannot be obtained. The Glau-Thompson prism has many advantages over the Nicol prism and can also be used in UV region. The other polarising prisms available are Wollastan and Rochon prisms.

Analyzer : One of the simplest types of analyzers used in visual polarimeters is the Cornu modification of Jellett prism. It is constructed by sawing a Glau-Thompson prism into half along A B grinding one of the halves down to A C and then cementing the two parts as shown in the Fig. 10.7.

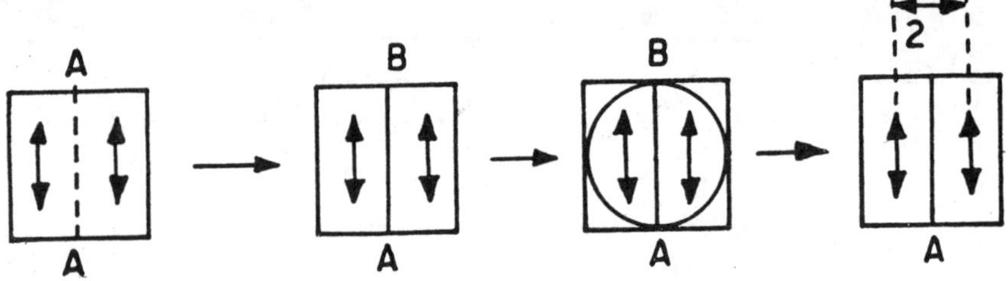

Fig 10.7. Jellett–Cornu Prism (arrows Indicate the direction of extinction).

When light passes through polarizing prism the two halves will produce polarized light beams tilted slightly with respect to each other. The rotation of the analyzer prism in front of such a polarizing prism would produce a complete extinction, first of one-half of the field and then the other-half. At some intermediate position, the two halves of the field would appear of equal brightness. This point is taken as the balance point (Fig. 10.8)

Lippich Prism : It is an another type of half-shadow device used for matching of two half-fields for a balance point. In this type of set up a small polarizing prism (A) precedes the large prism (B). With this kind of arrangement (Fig.10.9) one-half of the field can be rotated slightly with respect to other half. The analyzers must be at some intermediate position in order to achieve equal illumination of both halves of the field. The small prism is arranged in a slightly slanting position, (1 – 2°) in order to obtain a well illuminated and sharp dividing line of two fields. For this purpose, the faces of the small prism are corrected by 6-7°.

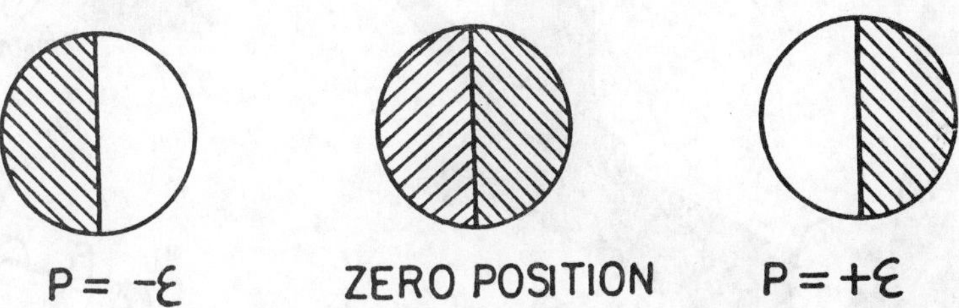

Fig 10.8. Fields of view (search for field intensity)

Polarimeter tubes : Two types and two sizes of polarimeter tubes including a jacked type for the purpose of cooling the sample are available. They are made of plane glass with a length of 1 dm or 2 dm and internal diameter 10 mm. Polarimeter tube is covered at both ends by plane parallel glass discs which are held in place by holders. For a tight, an elastic ring of rubber is inserted between the disc and the holder. The tube is placed in the light path normal to the beam.

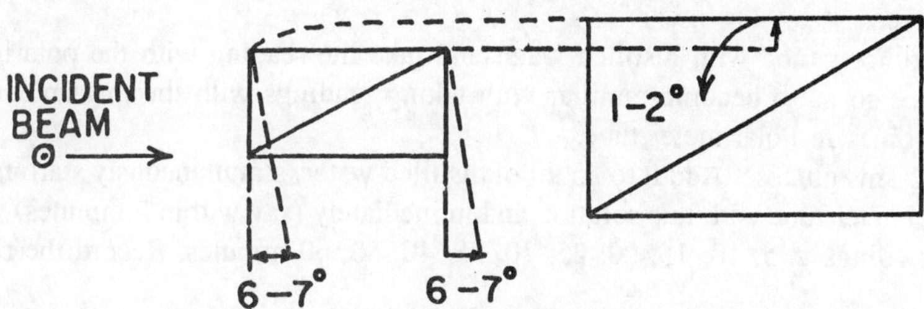

Fig. 10.9. Lippich Prism

10.4 Calculations : The results of polarimetric measurements are calculated under a set of standard conditions. If b is the layer thickness in decimeters, c is the concentration of solution in grams per 100 ml of solution α is the observed rotation in degrees and $[\alpha]_x^t$ is the specific rotation under standard conditions:

Thus $$[\alpha]_x^t = \frac{100\,\alpha}{bc}$$

Temperature is important, will cause contraction and expansion of the liquid.

Measurements of optical rotation are made with sodium D light (5890 A + 5896 A) at 25°. Temperature, solvent and concentration can have effect on the results.

EXERCISE 1. To investigate by half time method, the order of reaction of mutarotation of glucose using 5% and 10% solutions.

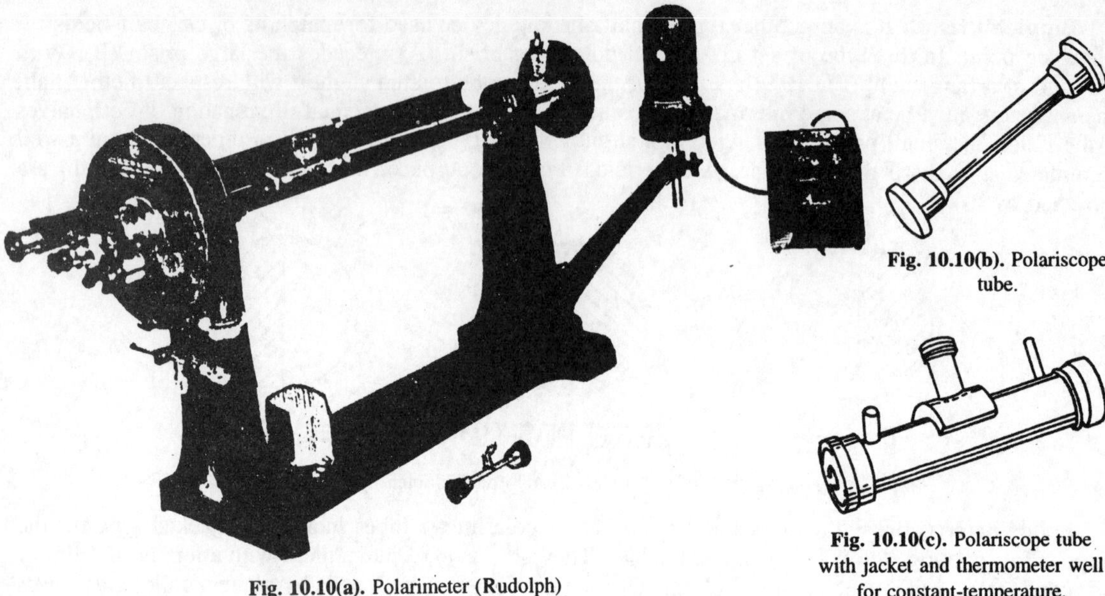

Fig. 10.10(a). Polarimeter (Rudolph)

Fig. 10.10(b). Polariscope tube.

Fig. 10.10(c). Polariscope tube with jacket and thermometer well for constant-temperature.

PROCEDURE

1. Check the zero setting of the instrument by taking the reading of the polarimeter without the polarimeter tube.
2. Fill the polarimeter tube with distilled water and take the reading with the polarimeter. Repeat it twice or thrice so as to become familiar with taking readings with the instrument. See that there are no air bubbles in Polarimeter tube.
3. Weigh 2.50 grams glucose. Add it to 25 ml of distilled water, simultaneously starting the stop-clock. Fill the polarimeter tube with this solution and immediately (say within 2 minutes) take the reading. Repeat the readings at 5, 10, 15, 20, 25, 30, 35, 40, 50, 60 minutes. Record the readings on your notebook.
4. Weight 1.25 grams of glucose, Add it to 25 ml of distilled water, simultaneously starting the stopclock. Fill the polarimeter tube with this solution first rinsing it carefully with the solution. Take the reading immediately (say within 2 minutes). Repeat the readings at 5, 10, 15, 20, 25, 30, 35, 40, 50, and 60 minutes. Record the readings in your notebook.

S.No.	Time	Rotation

5. Draw a graph between time and angular rotation for both the solution using the same scale on the

same graph sheet. Extrapolate to zero time. Half of the difference of zero and infinity reading in each case gives the value of glucose half reacted and corresponding time for both solutions is noted. Record them in your notebook.

6. Verify your result using the equation:

$$\frac{t_1}{t_2} = \left(\frac{r_2}{r_1}\right)^{n-1}$$

where

r_1 = rotation at halftime t_1 for 5% solution.

r_2 = rotation at halftime t_2 for 10% solution.

n = order of reaction.

Interpretation of Results

The times of or half inversion of glucose for both 5% and 10% solutions should be same, as the reaction is of first order.

Precautions

1. Do not move the source when it is hot.
2. When filling the polarimeter tube, see that there are no air bubbles in it .
3. While using the instrument, see that the lenses are clean. Do not unnecessarily touch them with your hands. Clean them with tissue paper only. See that the glass covers of the polarimeter tubes are not dirty. The slightest strains on optical glass will hamper accurate readings.

EXERCISE 2. Determination of specific Rotation of Rochelle salt (Potassium sodium tartrate)

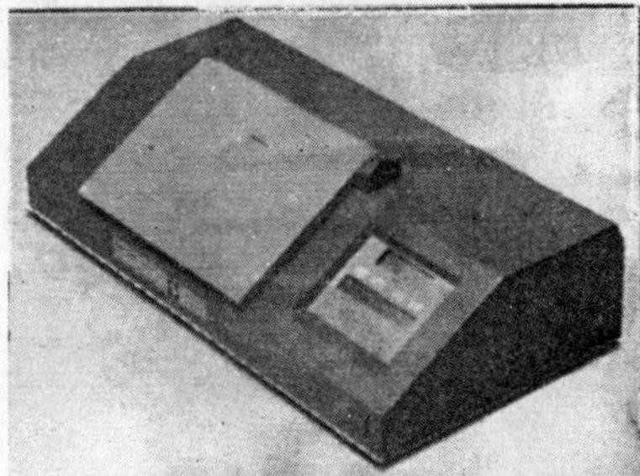

Fig. 10.11. The ADP-220 Polarimeter (Courtesy of Bellingham Stanley Ltd.)

Method: 1. Set up the polarimeter as per instructions of the instructor or as per instruction manual. 2. Prepare a standard solution of the given sample by dissolving 30.0 gm in 70 ml of water. 3. Place distilled water in the polarimeter tube and obtain a zero reading. 4. Replace the water in the polarimeter tube and measure the angle of rotation for the standard salt solution. 5. Calculate the specific rotation for this compound. 6. Now, obtain a solution of the *unknown* concentration from the instructor and measure its optical rotation obtained previously, calculate the concentration of the *unknown*.

11

Optical Rotatory Dispersion and Circular Dichroism

11.1 GENERAL

In the previous chapter, it has been pointed out that a beam of light has associated with it electrical and magnetic field vibrating at right angles and perpendicular to the direction of the propagation of the beam. If one selects one particular wavelength from the beam will oscillate sinusoidally along the direction of propagation and the wave will become a monochromatic plane polarized beam.

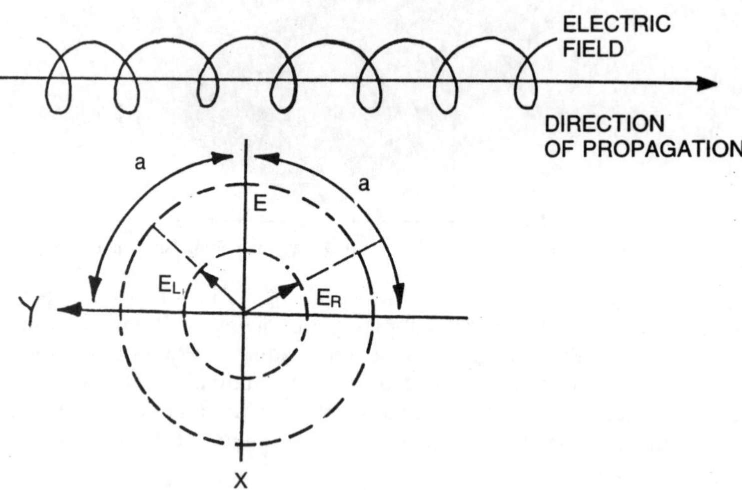

Fig. 11.1 Plane polarized light and its resolution into components

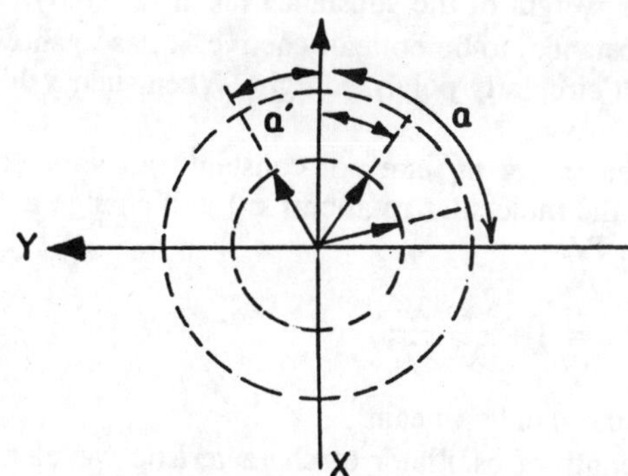

Fig.11.2 Plane polarized light after passing through an optically active material. A phase difference has occurred corresponding to angle α.

In this beam of polarized light (Fig. 11.1) the vector E is the resultant of 2 vectors of equal length E_R and E_L which correspond to the right and left circularly polarized components and a and a′ are the two equal angles. The direction of vibration is along the axis x.

Theory

Suppose the waves associated with E_R and E_L in the Fig. 11.1 rotate at different speeds, the angles a and a′ will be different and in the process the electric vector E or the plane of polarization will be rotated through on angle α. Further, if the right circularly polarized ray E_R travels faster i.e. a > a′ and α is positive, the medium is dextrorotatory. When a < a′ and the plane makes α as negative the medium is levorotatory. It is to be understood here that the speed of the light travelling through a medium is a function of its refractive index (n) and the medium will be optically active if it has different indices of refraction for the right and the left circularly polarized light. Consequently n_L will be different from n_R. This can be stated by means of a Fresnel equation as :

$$\{\alpha = \frac{\pi}{\lambda}(n_L - n_R) \qquad \text{(I)}$$

where α = rotation in radians per unit of length

λ = wavelength of incident light n_L and n_R are indices of refraction

When a is changed to degrees per decimeter one can obtain specific rotation [α] as

$$[\alpha] = \frac{\alpha}{c} \cdot \frac{1800}{\pi} \qquad \text{(II)}$$

where c = concentration in g/ml of solution.

1800/π is conversion factor.

The molecular rotation [ϕ] can be obtained by the equation III shown below :

$$[\phi] = \frac{[\alpha] . M}{100}$$

Where M, is the molecular weight of the substance taken for study.

In order for a material (substance) to be optically active, it has to show different indices of refraction (n_L and n_R) for the left and right circularly polarized light. When such a thing exists, the medium is called "circularly birefringent".

As the indices of refraction (n_L & n_R) are not constant, but vary differently with wavelength, the specific rotation [α] and also the molecular rotation [ϕ] will change as a function of wavelength. This can be represented by equation IV.

$$n = 1 + \frac{\kappa . \lambda^2}{\lambda^2 - \lambda_0^2} \qquad \text{(IV)}$$

where λ = wavelength of the incident beam .

κ = constant of strength of oscillator of characteristic wavelength λ_0.

The variation of optical activity with the wavelength give an "optical rotatory dispersion curve" (ORD curve, unequal velocity of transmission between left and right circularly polarized light). For a compound containing no chromophore, the optical activity will decrease in magnitude as the wavelength increases. Therefore, a *plain positive* or *plain negative* dispersion curve will be obtained depending on whether it rises or falls with decreasing wavelength (Fig. 11.3). Drude equation (V) is used the express the dependence of optical rotation of a substance on wavelength

$$[\alpha] = \frac{A}{\lambda^2 - \lambda_0^2} \qquad \text{(V)}$$

where A = constant (from experimental rotations)

λ_0 = wavelength of the closest absorption maximum.

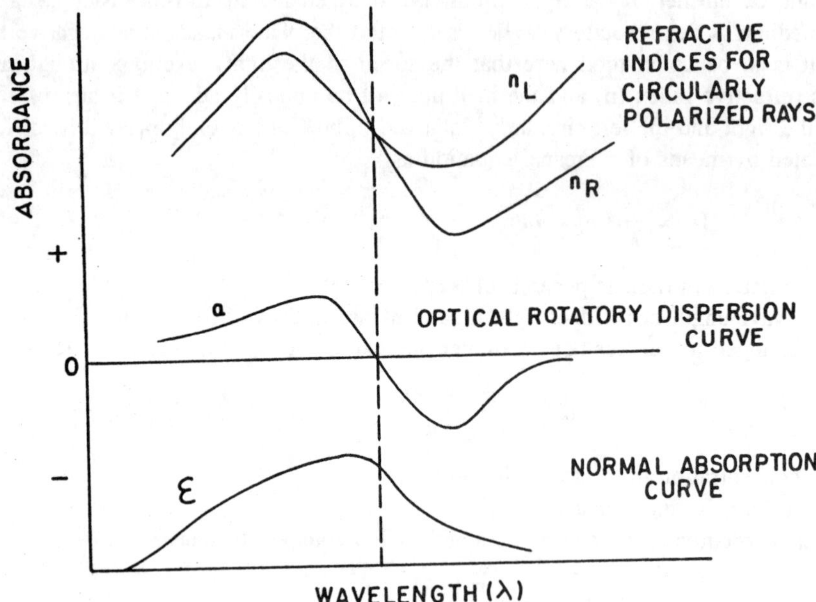

Fig. 11.3. Set of curves for refractive index, ORD and absorption for a compound

In terms of molecular rotation the above can be changed to :

$$[\phi] = \frac{K}{\lambda^2 - \lambda_0^2} \qquad \text{(VI)}$$

where k is equal to A multiplied by molecular weight of the optically active compound divided by 100 i.e.

$$K = \frac{A \, . \, M}{100}$$

When λ_0 cannot be found experimentally then λ will be much greater than λ_0 and VI will change to

$$[\phi] = \frac{K}{\lambda^2} \qquad \text{.................(VII)}$$

The above equation shows decrease in molecular rotation with increasing wavelength.

In case a compound shows two absorption maxima, then a following two term equation can be used :

$$[\phi] = \frac{k_1}{\lambda^2 - \lambda_0^2} + \frac{k_2}{\lambda^2 - \lambda_1^2}$$

Where the first term gives ORD contribution at λ_0 due to one chromophore and the second term at λ_1 due to a second chromophore.

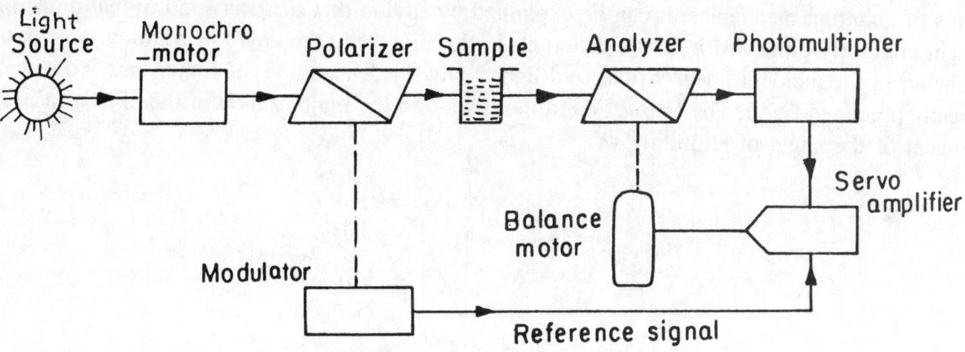

Fig.11.4. Spectropolarimeter, Block diagram

11.2 Instrumentation Aspects

The block diagram of a spectropolarimeter used for the measurement of ORD curve (spectra) is shown in Fig.11.4.

The light source consists of a xenon arc lamp which emits light continuously from 190 to 700 nm. The light passes through a monochromator and then through a polarizer, sample cell and analyzer like in the visual polarimeter. Two methods have been employed for determining the position of the analyzer which gives the extinction. Both methods use the photomultiplier to detect the transmitted light. In the first method, the polarizer is made to oscillate mechanically through a small angle of about 2^0 and in this way the plane of polarization of the beam passing through the sample is thus modulated by the same angle. The analyzer is then rotated until the intensity of the light reaching the photomultiplier is the same for extreme positions of the polarizer. In the second method, the modulation of the plane of polarization is obtained not mechanically but by interposing in the light path between the polarizer and the analyzer a ''Faraday cell''. It consists of a silica cylinder surrounded by a coil through which is passed an a.c current (60 Hz). The magnetic field of the coil induces in the silica optical rotation whose sign depends on the direction of the current through the coil. The plane of polarization of the beam which passes through the Faraday cell gets modulated. When the analyzer is not in its extinction position, this causes an asymmetric a.c. current in the photomultiplier which is detected and used to drive the analyzer to its extinction position.

11.3 Circular Dichroism

Theory

The two components E_L and E_R of a circularly polarized beam on passing through an optically active medium shows ''circular birefringence'' i.e. different speeds due to inequality between the refractive indices n_L and n_R. At the same-time the two components (E_L & E_R) are also differently absorbed. Therefore, in the spectral region in which optically active absorption bands are present, the length of the vector E_R is no longer equal to E_L and their resultant E will no longer oscillate along the circumference of a circle. Instead, the head of the resultant vector now describes an ellipse. Thus we can say that when an optically active medium is traversed by a plane polarized light in the spectral region in which optically active chromophore absorbs, the plane of polarization not only rotates at an angle α but also the resulting light is elliptically polarized the medium exhibits ''Circular Dichroism'' i.e. unequal absorption (Fig.11.5). In terms of quantum mechanics, it can be explained by saying that the transition probabilities of the left and right circularly polarized light are different. In the Fig. 11.5, the angle of rotation α is given by the angle between the incident linearly polarized light along the X-axis and the major axis b of the emergent elliptically polarised light.. The ratio of the minor axis a to the major axis b of the ellipse (a/b) measures the tangent of the angle of ellipticity ψ.

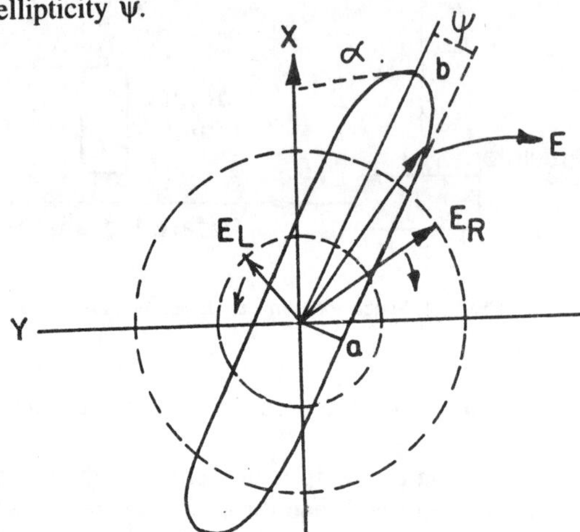

Fig. 11.5 Circular dichroism. Vector E now describes an ellipse. The ellipticity is the angle ψ. α is rotation angle.

As the major axis b and minor axis a of the ellipse are the sum and difference of the amplitude P of both circular components, upon emerging form the optically active medium the tangent of the angle of ellipticity ψ will be given by :

$$\tan \psi = \frac{(P_R - P_L)}{(P_R + P_L)} \qquad \text{(I)}$$

while absorption law can be defined :

$$P = P_0 \, e^{-\frac{2\pi k}{\lambda}} \qquad \text{.... (II)}$$

where k = absorption indices

λ = wavelength of the incident light

The angle of ellipticity when measured in radians per unit of length is given by:

$$\psi = \frac{\pi}{\lambda}(K_L - K_R) \qquad \text{.... (III)}$$

where K_L and K_R are absorption coefficients for left and right circularly polarized light. ε_L and ε_R can be substituted for K_L and K_R as molecular coefficients.

Thus $K \cong 2.303 . \varepsilon . c$

where c is concentration in moles/litre. By analogy with specific rotation [α], the specific ellipticity [Ψ] can be given by:

$$[\psi] = \frac{\psi}{l . c}$$

where ψ is in degrees, l = length in decimeters, c = concentration in gms/ml of solution

Similarly, molecular ellipticity [θ] can be written as :

$$[\theta] = \frac{[\psi] . M}{100} = 2.303\left(\frac{4500}{\pi}\right)\left(\varepsilon_L - \varepsilon_R\right) = 3300\left(\varepsilon_L - \varepsilon_R\right)$$

But $\varepsilon_L - \varepsilon_R$ differential dichroic absorption = $\Delta\,\varepsilon$

$$\therefore [\theta] = 3300. \Delta\,\varepsilon$$

The combination of unequal absorption (i.e. CD) and unequal velocity of transmission (i.e. optical rotation) of left and right circularly polarized light in the region in which optically active absorption bands are observed is a phenomenon known as "cotton effect". It was observed by cotton that an optically active compound showed an abnormal behaviour in this spectral region.

An ideal chromophore which is optically active and responsible for anomalous dispersion is the low intensity carbonyl band. It has a characteristic U.V. maximum at 270—300 nm with an extinction coefficient of 100.

The amount of the resulting angle of rotation is dependent upon the degree of asymmetry of the molecule and on the relationship of the wavelength of the absorption maximum of a chromophore in the vicinity of the asymmetry. As the wavelength of the polarized light is decreased, an increase in the numerical magnitude of the angle of rotation usually occurs. If the compound under study shows no selective absorption in either the near UV or visible regions the curve obtained on plotting the wavelength against angle of rotation is called "*plain curve*". If a curve increases to a peak (P) and then to a trough (T) or the reverse it is known as "*Cotton effect curve*". Entrance into wave of the curve is in an increasing positive direction the curve shows "*positive cotton effect*". If the enterance into wave of the curve is in the negative direction from the longer wavelength is called "*negative cotton effect*" (Fig. 11.6 and 11.7).

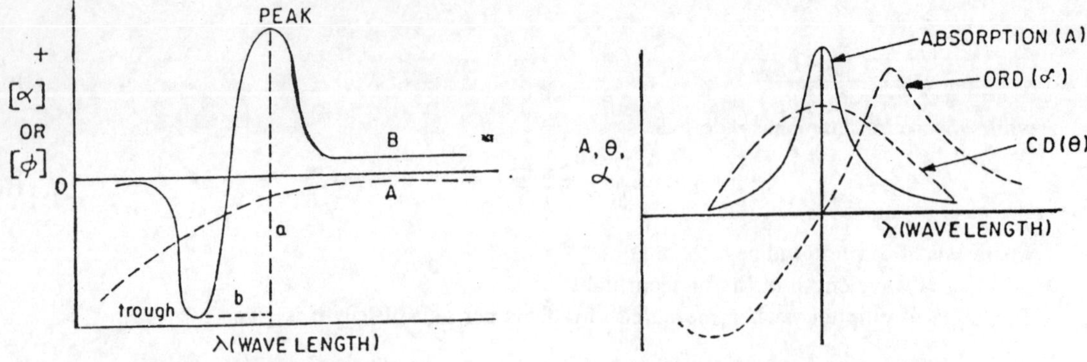

Fig.11.6. ORD curve, A = negative plain curve; B = positive cotton effect with peak & trough; a = amplitude: b = breadth.

Fig. 11.7. U.V absorption, CD and ORD spectra of a compound.

11.4 Instrumentation Aspects

The block diagram of a circular dichrometer are shown in the figure 11.8.

First the beam of radiation must be plane-polarized, second, the polarized beam must be passed through a device that will resolve into its right and left-circularly polarized components. Then one component is retarded by one-quarter of wavelength from the other. One of common circular resolvers is the Pockels electrooptic modulator, where it undergoes two internal reflections, introducing a phase retardation of 1/4 of wavelength. These are passed through a circularly dichroic.sample. The electrical system process the alternating component so as to record the circular dichroism of the sample. The Pockels modulator consists of a plate of crystalline KH_2PO_4 where electric field induces birefringence, so that the initially plane polarized radiation becomes circularly polarized. The retardation can then be produced by choice of a potential.

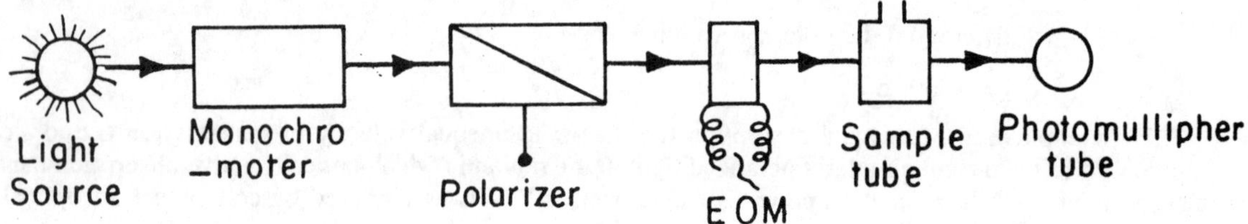

Fig. 11.8. Optical Components of a Circular dichrometer

11.5 Uses of CD

The CD measurements are meant for the purpose of structure determination for establishing stereochemistry and conformation.

EXERCISE 11.1 Determination of optical Rotatory Dispersion for nicotine.

Method : 1. Set up the polarimeter as per instructions of the instructor or as per operating manual. 2. Dissolve 10.0 gm of nicotine in 90 ml of ethanol. 3. Fill the polarimeter tube with water and determine the zero reading. 4. Replace the water in the polarimeter tube with ethanol and obtain optical rotation. 5. Place nicotine solution in the polarimeter tube and measure the optical rotation for the solution. 6. Replace the sodium lamp with mercury vapour lamp and obtain optical rotation for water ethanol, and nicotine solution. 7. Obtain various filters and measure optical rotations for water, ethanol and nicotine solution. 8. Calculate the constants for the Drude equation.

SECTION-D
ELECTROCHEMICAL METHODS OF ANALYSIS

12

Electroanalytical Methods

12.1 General

Electroanalytical methods are based on various phenomena which occur in an electrochemical cell. They incorporate a number of different techniques that involve the detection of the amount of concentration of a component in terms of (i) effect of the component upon and electrode (ii) The effect of that component upon an impressed voltage (iii) The effect of passage of current through the sample in changing the chemical state of the component.

The various electroanalytical methods available today can be classified as follows :

(a) When the quantity measured involves resistance the method is called *conductometric titration.* (b) when the quantity measured is in terms of current-voltage, the method is called *Polarography* (c) when the quantity measured is EMF versus concentration, the produce is called *potentiometric titration* (d) when the quantity measured is EMF versus time, the method is called *chronopotentiometry.* (e) when the quantity measured involves current versus concentration the method is called *amperometric titration.*

12.2 Principles Of Electrochemistry

An electric current is the flow of electric change. In metals this charge is carried by electrons and electrical conduction of this type is called *electronic conduction*. The current moves as a result of the application of electric force supplied by a battery or some other force of electric energy.

In an electrochemical cell, the current results from a chemical reaction in which electrons are taken up at one electrode and released at the other. The reaction is made up of 2 parts, an oxidation reaction taking place at the anode where electrons are given up by a reduced form to produce an oxidized form;

$$\text{Red} = \text{Ox} + ne$$

e.g. $$Zn = Zn^{2+} + 2\,e$$

and reduction reaction at the cathode consisting of an another set of oxidized and reduced forms

$$ne + \text{Ox}' = \text{Red}'$$

e.g. $$2e + Cu^{2+} = Cu$$

The overall or net reaction is

$$\text{Red} + \text{Ox}' = \text{Red}' + \text{Ox}$$

or

$$Zn + Cu^{2+} = Zn^{2+} + Cu$$

The emf of the cell or difference in electrical potential between the two electrodes depends on the equilibrium constant for the chemical reaction that takes place in the cell and the *activities* of the reactants and products. Thus we should know that in both dry cell and lead storage battery chemical energy is converted into electrical energy, but in the charging of the lead storage battery, electrical energy is used to bring about chemical reaction.

In this text book we will be discussing only potentiometric and polarographic methods of analysis because these are commonly used.

12.3 Potentiometric Titrations

Potentiometry is one of the volumetric techniques of electroanalytical chemistry. It consists of determination of the potential difference between an indicator electrode and a reference electrode. The two electrodes i.e. half—cells and a salt bridge form the electrochemical cell that is immersed in the solution to be analysed. The important characteristic of the reference electrode is that it maintains constant potential which is not affected by a change in the composition of the solution that is being estimated. On the contrary the potential of the indicator electrode is a function of the concentration of one of the ions in the solution. If during a titration, the reference electrode output is constant, the changes in the EMF of the cell will reflect the changes in the concentration in the solution.

12.4 Electrode Potentials

As explained under principles of electrochemistry, in potentiometry the potential of an indicator electrode is related to the *activity* i.e. effective concentration of the species that is being determined. for a general equilibrium reaction like a A + b B = c C + d D this can be obtained by means of a *Nernst equation* explained below :

$$E = E^o - \frac{RT}{nF} \ln Q$$

E = Potential observed

E^o = potential when all species are in the standard state, defined as the activities of all ionic species are 1 M, metallic and non-metallic species are 1 mole fraction; the pressure of any gas is 1 atmosphere and temperature 25°.

R = gas constant = 8.3144 joules/mole/deg.

T = Temperature, degree, Absolute

n = no of electrons transferred in the redox reaction.

F = faraday = 96500 coulombs

Q = activity quotient.

The constant RT/F and factor 2.303 is evaluated at standard temperature.

$$\frac{RT}{F} \times 2.303 = 0.0591$$

$$\therefore \quad E = E^o - \frac{0.0591}{n} \log Q$$

The above equation is valid at only 25°C.

With aid of Nernst equation it is possible to calculate potential of any half cell or electrode or any cell from the electrode potential at standard conditions.

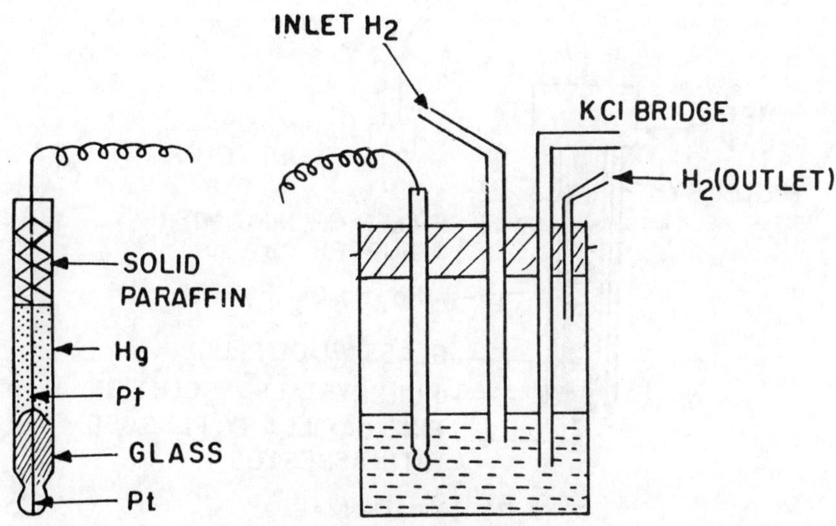

Fig. 12.1 Standard Hydrogen Electrode

12.4.1 Hydrogen Electrode

A hydrogen electrode is universally used as the standard of reference for the determination of relative half-cell potentials but it is difficult to construct and maintain. It consists of a Pt electrode coated with Pt black. The electrode is made of a small plate of Pt (2 × 3 mm) welded to a Pt wire. The wire is melted into a glass tube in such a way that it is entirely surrounded to a length of at least 5 mm by glass. This glass tube should have a thermal expansion coefficient equal to that of Pt to avoid any leak between the wire and the glass. The interior of the glass is filled with Hg, a copper wire is inserted and the top is sealed with paraffin. The Pt electrode is placed in a cylindrical glass vessel that is fitted with a rubber stopper having several holes, one for each electrode, one as an inlet for H_2, another as an outlet, one for KCl bridge and one for a thermometer. Hydrogen gas maintained at 1 atmosphere is continuously bubbled across the surface of the Pt to keep the electrode in constant contact with both the solution and the gas The Pt which takes no part in the electrochemical reaction aids in the transfer of electrons.

The half-cell reaction involved in the hydrogen electrode electrode is :

$$H_2 \text{ (gas)} \rightleftharpoons 2H^+ + 2e \quad E° = 0.000 \text{ Volt}$$

When coupled to another half-cell, the hydrogen electrode can reverse its behaviour. When it behaves as an anode, hydrogen gas is oxidized to H ions and when it acts as a cathode reverse is the case.

12.4.2 Calomel Electrode

The most common reference electrode used in potentiometric work is the calomel electrode shown in the

Fig 12.2. The outer tube contains a KCl solution whereas the inner tube, a mercury - mercurous chloride paste. The two tubes are connected through a small pinhole in the inner tube. A porous fibre is fixed to the end of the outer tube and is used for connecting the second half-cell to which it is coupled.

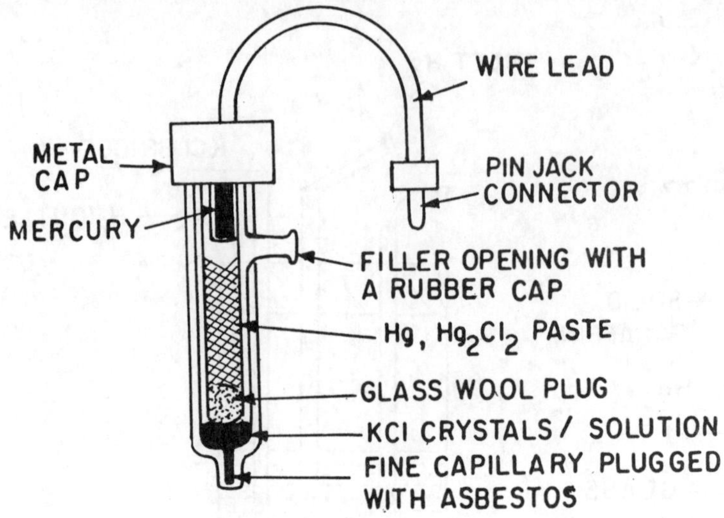

Fig. 12.2. Calomel Electrode

Calomel half-cell is represented as follows :

$$Hg_{(l)},\ Hg_2Cl_2\,(s)\,/\,Cl^{-}_{(xM)}$$

Where the vertical line denotes the boundary across which a potential develops, xM indicates the concentration of Cl^- in the solution and must be specified.

The electrode reaction is given by the equation :

$$2Hg + 2Cl^- \rightleftharpoons Hg_2Cl_2 + 2e^- -$$

The concentrations of KCl solution that can be used are 0.1 M, 1.0 M and saturated solution. In each of these three types, the solution is saturated with mercurous chloride. Their standard oxidation potentials with respect to standard hydrogen electrode at 25°C are 0.334 volt, – 0.280 volt and – 0.242 volt respectively. They will behave as cathodes when used with respect to hydrogen electrode.. The most commonly and widely used one is saturated calomel electrode as a reference electrode.

12.4.3 Silver - Silverchloride Electrode

The silver - silverchloride electrode (Fig. 12.3) is used as an inner reference electrode in the glass indicator electrode. It is similar to the calomel electrode. It consists of a silver wire immersed in a solution of KCl that is saturated with AgCl. The half-cell is represented as,

$$Ag_{(s)}\,/\,AgCl_{(sat)},\ Cl^{-}_{(xM)}$$

and the half reaction is as ;

$$Ag + Cl^- \rightleftharpoons AgCl + e$$

The potential of the electrode is dependent on the activity of the Cl^- ion in equilibrium with AgCl. The electrode is usually prepared with saturated Kcl solution and its oxidation potential is 0.197 Vol (at 25°C) with respect to hydrogen electrode. The emf of the eletrode is not affected by diffuse light or artificial light of ordinary intensity.

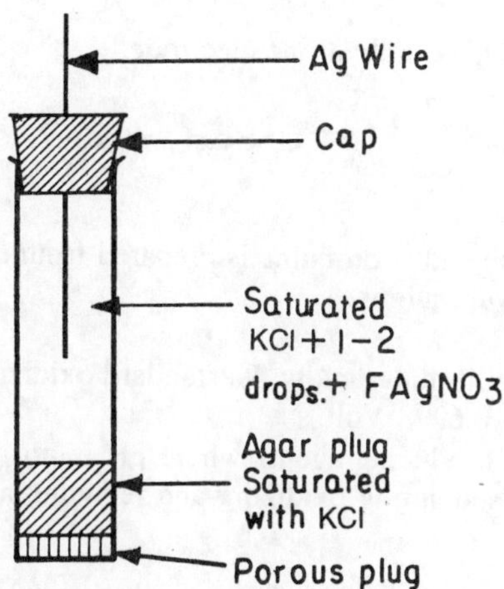

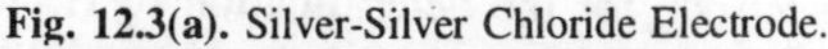

Fig. 12.3(a). Silver-Silver Chloride Electrode.

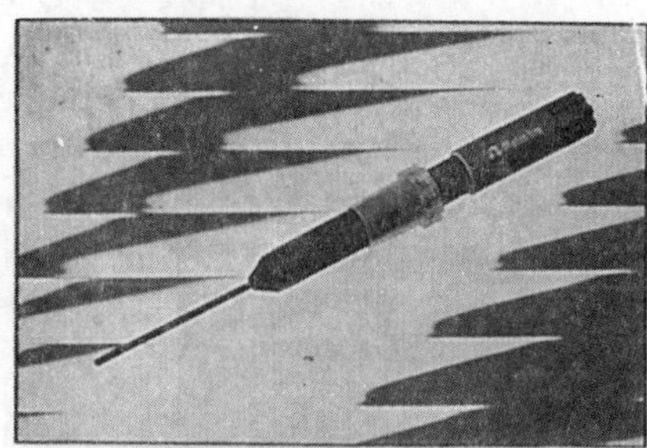

Fig. 12.3(b). A modern Ag/AgCl electrode

12.4.4 Liquid Junction (Salt Bridge)

In potentiometric titration work a separate reference electrode and an indicator electrode are usually connected by a junction that allows ions to pass but does not permit solutions to mix. The common type of electrolyte junction is a wick of asbestos fiber sealed into glass as in a fiber - type calomel electrode.

The electric potential generated by separation of charges at the boundary between two dissimilar solutions is known as the "*Junction Potential*". Whenever two solutions of two different compositions are in contact, there is a tendency for diffusion of ions from one solution to the other to equalize the concentrations. Further, because the positive and negative ions have unequal mobilities, on diffusing across the boundary, one side accumulates an excess of positive ions. Depending upon which side of the boundary becomes positive the junction potential adds to or subtracts from the potential of the reference electrode. This junction potential will be less when the ions of the electrolyte have nearly the same mobilities.

Reduction of the liquid junction potential can be obtained by interposing a salt bridge containing a concentrated electrolyte solutions. A saturated (4.2 M) KCl or NH_4 NO_3 solution is generally used because the mobilities of K^+ and Cl^- are nearly the same and are not affected by the temperature. The salt bridge provides the electrical contact between the electrodes of the electrochemical cell. The current passes by ionic migration without any effect upon the potential of the cell itself.

Indicator Electrodes

12.4.5 Hydrogen Electrode

The hydrogen electrode can be used as an indicator electrode in acid - Base titrations. But its use is limited, this is because many solutions which contain substances like permanganate, iodine, ferric iron easily reduce organic substances. They react directly with H_2 gas and consequently alter the pH of the solution. Substances like proteins, H_2S and CN^- poison the platinum electrode and cause it to transfer electrons erratically and slowly. The other factors restricting its use is the inconvenience and hazard involved with H_2 gas.

12.5.6 Quinhydrone Electrode

The hydroquine - quinone system indicated below forms the quinhydrone electrode.

$$HO-C_6H_4-OH \rightleftharpoons O=C_6H_4=O + 2H^+ + 2e$$

$$H_2Q \rightleftharpoons Q + 2H^+ + 2e^-$$

A solution containing equal concentrations of quinone and hydroquine is prepared from quinhydrone which is a molecular addition product of quinone and hydroquinone.

$$2\,QH \rightleftharpoons Q + H_2Q$$

The electrode is simple to construct and comes to equilibrium rapidly. Its standard oxidizing potential with respect to standard hydrogen electrode at 25°C is – 0.6998 Volt.

It is employed in the presence of mild oxidizing and reducing agents where pH is not greater than 8. It is sensitive to high concentrations of salt solutions and strong oxidizing and reducing agents.

12.5.7 Glass Electrode

The glass electrode is the most commonly used indicator electrode for the determination of H^+ ions. It does not function on any electron transfer reaction, but involves an ion-exchange reaction. A diagrammatic sketch of the glass electrode is shown in the Fig. 12.4.

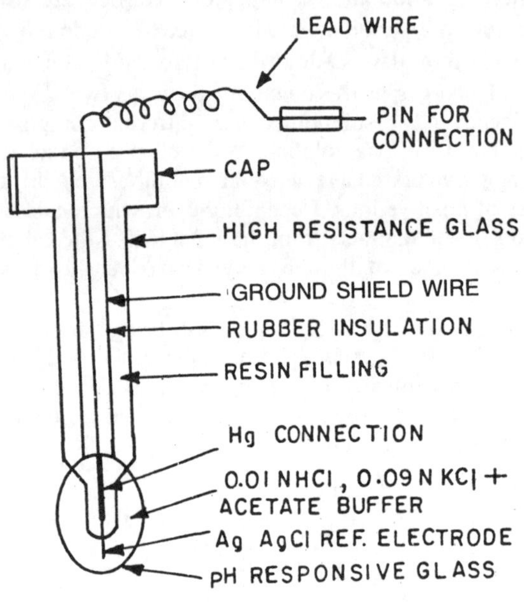

Fig. 12.4(a). A Glass Electrode

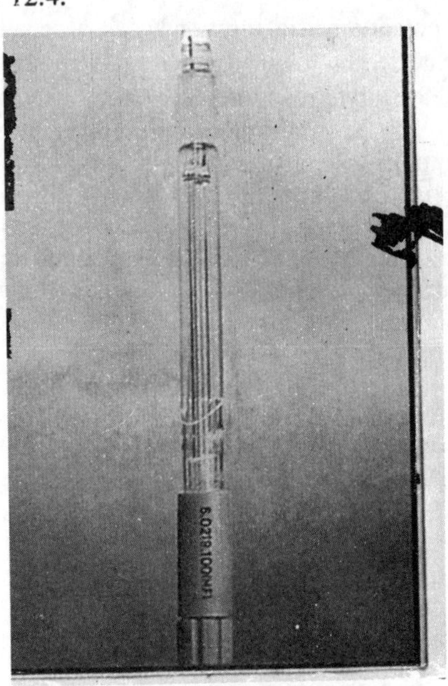

Fig. 12.4(b). A modern Glass Electrode (Courtesy of Metrohm Ltd.)

The tip of the electrode is made in the form of a bulb or thin-walled membrane is made of a special glass (SiO_2, Na_2O and Al_2O_3, and is selectively permeable to the H^+ ions).The glass bulb is filled with a reference solution of 0.01 N HCl, 0.09 N KCl and acetate buffer. Silver coated with AgCl dips into the reference solution and functions as the internal reference electrode.

In the potentiometric determination of pH, a glass electrode is generally coupled with a saturated calomel electrode. When silver - silverchloride is the internal reference electrode in the glass electrode, the glass - saturated calomel electrode system is represented by :

Ag/AgCl, 0.01 N HCl Internal reference electrode	Glass membrane	Test Solution	Saturated Calomel as External Electrode

Each vertical line in the electrochemical cell above denotes a boundary across which a potential develops. The inner surface of the glass membrane remains in contact with 0.01N HCl solution and the outer surface with the test solution for which pH is to be measured.

At both inner and outer surfaces the glass membrane absorbs water and forms hydrated layers in the glass structure. The H^+ ions diffuse through the hydrated layers in the direction of the lesser concentration and in the process replace (ion - exchange) Na^+ ions or other metal ions contained in the structure of the glass membrane.

$$\underset{\text{glass}}{SiO^-Na} + \underset{\text{solution}}{H^+} \longrightarrow \underset{\text{glass}}{SiO^-H^+} + \underset{\text{solution}}{Na}$$

As a result of this diffusion and exchange process, a phase boundary potential is set up on each side of the glass membrane. The magnitude of the potential is determined by the pH of the test solution. It should be noted that the glass membrane must contain water in its structure for the glass electrode to maintain its pH sensitivity.

At 25°C, the potential of the cell comprising glass - saturated calomel electrode system is represented by the equation :

$$E = K + 0.0591 \text{ pH}$$

Where K is a constant and takes into account the following aspects; (a) the sum of the internal and external reference electrode potentials, (b) the junction potential between the two reference electrodes and the solutions in which they are immersed, and (c) the asymmetry potential which is produced in the glass surfaces of the electrodes because of the strains set up during their manufacturing process. The asymmetry potential is affected by dehydration in the glass surfaces of the electrodes and also possibly by chemical attack on one glass surface and not the other. As the asymmetry potential changes slowly, K must be reestablished at regular intervals by measuring the potentials for electrode system in a solution of known pH or in a buffer.

A glass electrode will not perform properly as a pH indicator if its membrane is dehydrated. Therefore a glass electrode should be stored in distilled water to avoid dehydration. The glass saturated calomel electrode system measures pH under of wide variety of conditions because it is not affected by oxidants, reductants, proteins and gases like the other electrode systems and therefore do not interfere with its performance.

12.6 pH Measurements

A common example of potentiometric determination is the measurement of pH. The pH of a solution can be obtained either (i) by measuring the potential difference between the combination of an electrode pair with a potentiometer or (ii) directly with the aid of a pH meter. Both these methods are explained below.

By Combination of Electrodes : If a hydrogen (indicator) electrode and a saturated calomel (reference) electrode are combined, the potential of the resultant electrochemical cell is related to the pH of the reaction taking place at 25°C. The electrode reactions taking place are :

$$\text{Hydrogen : } H_2 \rightleftharpoons 2H^+ + 2e \quad E^\circ = 0.000 \text{ Volt}$$

$$\text{Calomel : } 2Hg + 2Cl \rightleftharpoons Hg_2Cl_2 + 2e \quad E^\circ = -0.242 \text{ Volt}$$

In the above cell, actually reduction occurs at the calomel electrode while oxidation occurs at the hydrogen electrode. The net cell reaction can be written as :

$$H_2 + Hg_2Cl_2 \rightleftharpoons 2H^+ + 2Hg + 2Cl^- \quad E^\circ = 0 + 0.242 \text{ Volt}$$

Using the Nernst equation the potential of the cell i.e. E_{cell} can be calculated by the following relation:

$$E_{Cell} = +0.242 - \frac{0.0591}{2} \log \frac{(a_H^+)^2 (a_{Hg})^2 (a_{Cl}^-)^2}{(a_{H_2})(a_{Hg_2Cl_2})}$$

In the above relation, the activities of all the reactants and products are unity and H^+ concentration is the only variable quantity, hence we can write :

$$E_{Cell} = 0.242 - \frac{0.0591}{2} \log (a_H^+)^2$$

But by definition we know,

$$pH = -\log (a_H^+)$$

So we can write :

$$E_{Cell} = +0.242 \text{ Volt} - 0.0591 \text{ pH}$$

$$\therefore \text{ pH} = \frac{E_{cell} - 0.242 \text{ Volt}}{0.0591}$$

Similarly, we can relate pH to the potential for any other combination of a cell or electrode pair.

Measurement of pH by Direct Method : pH measurements can be performed directly by the combination of the glass-saturated calomel electrode system. The pH meter may be null detector type or a direct reading type. However, now-a-days direct reading digital type pH meters are available and can

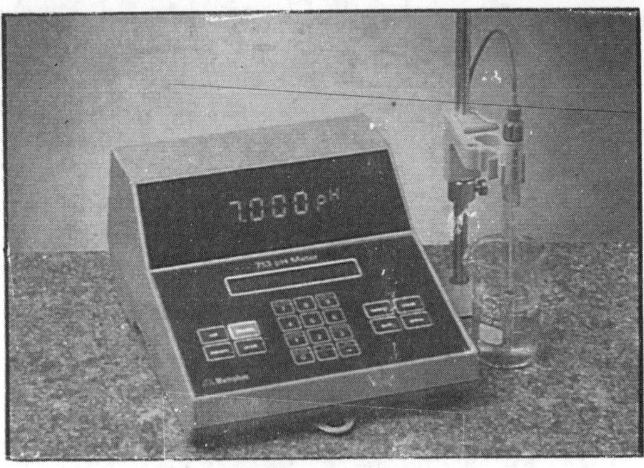

Fig. 12.5 Digital pH Meter Model-713
(Courtesy of Metroham Ltd.)

be used for potentiometric titrations.

Basically, a pH meter consists of an amplifier and associated circuits to connect the glass and the reference electrodes to either an indicating meter calibrated in pH units or to a recorder. The glass electrode is connected to the amplifier input and the reference electrode to the amplifier output. In addition a "*standardized control*" is also fixed in series with the electrodes to *buck out* any voltage produced by the electrodes so that the meter will read changes in potential from an initial meter reading that is adjusted to a solution of known pH.

12.7. Potentiometric Titrations

The object in the potentiometric titrations is to obtain the precise location of the equivalence point. Potentiometric titrations can be applied for acid-base, precipitation, complexometric and oxidation-reduction reactions in aqueous or non-acqueous media. The cell potential pH is recorded after each addition of the reagent.

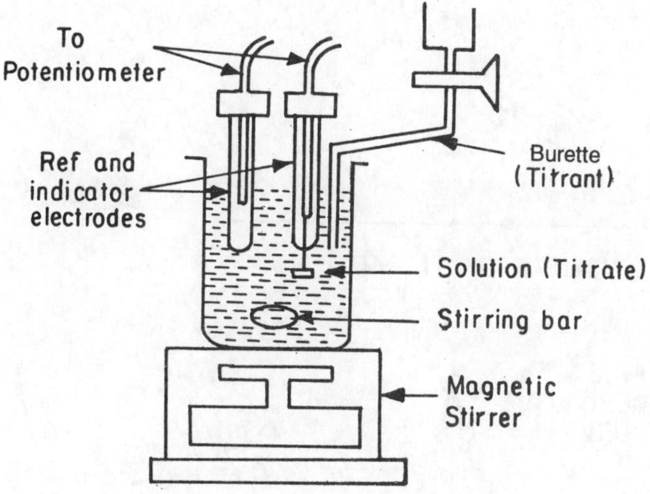

Fig. 12.6 Apparatus for Potentiometric Titration

In the beginning of the titration, large amounts of titrant can be added but as the end point is approached, each addition of the titrant is decreased until the equivalence point is obtained. The equivalence point can be obtained by various ways, a few are described below.

12.7.1 Graphic Determination of the End Point

In a potentiometric titration, a plot of the emf or pH of the solution as ordinate versus the volume of the titrant added as abscissa is constructed. From this titration curve, the mid point around the steeper portion of the curve is estimated visually as the equivalence point of the titration. At this point the imf and or pH and the volume of titrant added at the end point are estimated.

In a second graphic procedure a plot of the change in potential or pH per volume increment of titrant $\Delta E/\Delta V$ or $\Delta pH/\Delta V$ as ordinate versus volume of titrant as abscissa, is constructed. The titration curve obtained in this manner shows a maximum slope i.e. a maximal value of $\Delta E/\Delta V$ or $\Delta pH/\Delta V$. This maximal value corresponds to an inflection point on the normal titration curve. At this maximum the volume of the titration at the equivalence point is determined.

A third graphic approach for locating accurately the equivalence point is from the second derivative $\Delta^2E/\Delta V^2$ or $\Delta^2E/\Delta V^2$ titration curve. The curve is traced by plotting the second derivative as ordinate versus volume of titrant as abscissa. In this plot the 2nd derivative of titration curve is zero at the point where the first derivative $\Delta E/\Delta V$ or $\Delta pH/\Delta V$ is a maximum. The curve also shows that the 2nd derivative changes sign (+) to (–) and passes through zero between volume readings around the equivalence point. The equivalence point volume lies within this interval. The shape of these graphs are shown below.

The other methods for locating the volume of titrant at the equivalence point in a potentiometric titration are (i) analytical method and (ii) titration to a fixed potential.

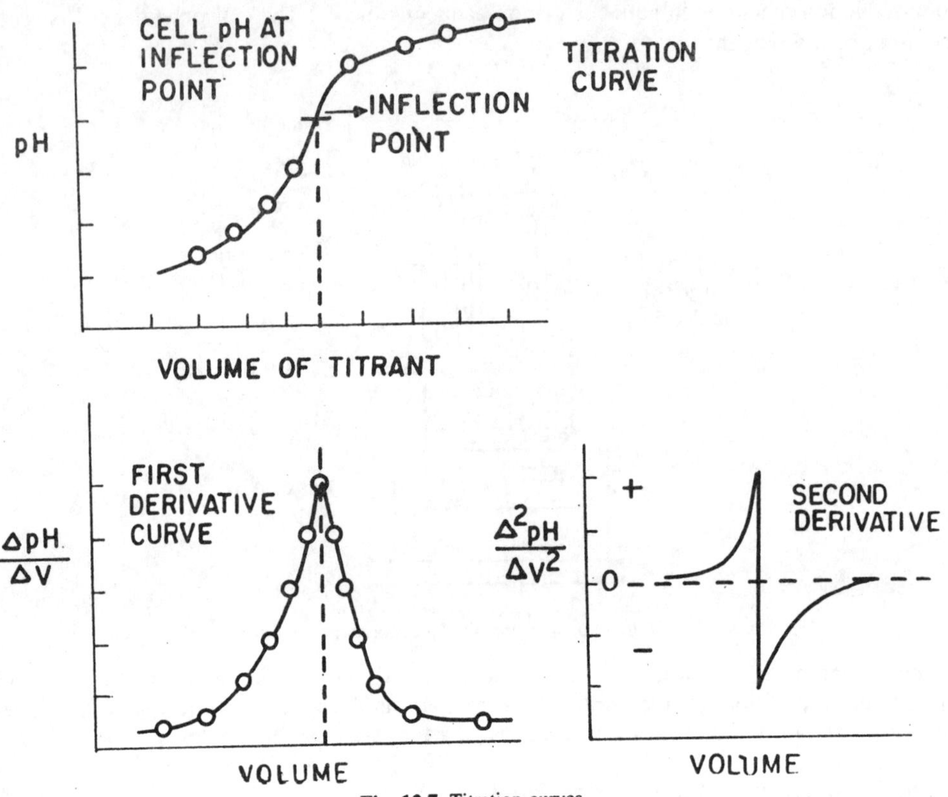

Fig. 12.7. Titration curves.

The applications of potentiometric titrations are for example in the assay of caffeine, phenobarbitone, thonzylamine hydrochloride and tetrahydrozoline hydrochloride etc.

EXERCISE 1. Potentiometric titration of an acid.

Method 1. Receive the pH meter with glass electrode and reference electrode from the instructor, read the operational manual or the sheet and ready the instrument. 2. Collect your sample in a 250 ml volumetric flask, dilute to mark with distilled water and mix well. 3. Transfer a 25 ml aliquot of the sample solution to the titration vessel and insert the electrodes, adding distilled water to ensure their adequate immersion. 4. Perform the titration against 0.1 N sodium hydroxide solution as described in section 12.7 of this chapter. 5. Locate the end point as per the techniques of the section 12.7.6. Report the results as directed by the instructor.

EXERCISE 2. Potentiometric titrations with Hydrochloric acid.

Method : Take 20 ml quantities of sodium carbonate or sodium borate or triethyl-amine (all 0.5 N) and titrate with 0.5N HCl as described in the above procedure.

EXERCISE 3. Determination of Calcium chloride.

Method : 1. Prepare 0.1M calcium chloride standard solution with dilutions of 1 : 5, 1 : 10 1 : 50 and 1 : 100. 2. Prepare an electrode potential vs concentration calibration curve using the standard solution thus prepared. 3. Prepare an unknown calcium chloride solution (about 10^{-3} M solution adjust to pH 10 with ammonium hydroxide). 4. Determine the concentration of the *unknown* calcium chloride solution by measuring the potential obtained when electrodes are immersed in above solutions and using the calibration curve.

EXERCISE 4. Determination of hardness of water.

Method : 1. prepare the assembly and apparatus as already described in previous exercises. 2. Examine the tap water and estimate its hardness. 3. Now boil and cool the tap water and determine hardness again. 4. Now take the laboratory distilled water and determine its hardness.

For the last two exercises specific ion electrodes are used along with a reference electrode and connected to a conventional pH meter having expanded pH scale. A calibration curve is prepared first in such estimations.

13

Polarography

13.1 General

Polarography is an electroanalytical method in which small amounts of substances are reduced or oxidized (less commonly) at microelectrode in an electrolysis cell. The procedure can be used for qualitative and quantitative analysis of electroreducible and electro-oxidizable substances or ions. The commonly used electrolysis cell in the polarographic work consists of a dropping mercury electrode as the analytical microelectrode and a saturated calomel electrode as the reference electrode. The method is based on the polarization of the microelectrode. This condition is produced when the cell current is no longer dependent upon the equilibrium potential of the microelectrode but is dependent upon the diffusion rate of the reducible species in the test solution. A gradually increasing voltage is applied to the electrodes of the cell, corresponding current measured and a plot of the current versus voltages is constructed either manually or recorded automatically. In the curve obtained there is a plateau region where the cell current is proportional to the concentration of the reducible species in the solution being analyzed. The polarographic method can be applied to metals and also to organic compounds. Oxygen can be determined in water samples to detect pollution. Drugs and metabolites can be determined polarographically.

13.2 Apparatus and Method

An apparatus used for the polarographic measurement is shown in the figure 13.1.

It consists of a potentiometer connected to two electrodes through a microammeter. One electrode is polarizable and the other is not. The non-polarizable electrode (anode) is the reference electrode. It is usually a saturated calomel electrode (SCE). The reference electrode has to be larger than analytical electrode so that its electrical resistance is low and potential remains unchanged during electrolysis.

The polarizable electrode (cathode) is kept small and is called microelectrode. As it is small it is easily polarized and also the electrolysis is kept slight. The commonly used analytical electrode is the dropping mercury electrode (DME). The DME consists of small droplets of mercury emerging by gravity from a piece of small bore capillary tubing attached to bottom of a stand tube and a mercury reservoir. The mercury droplets issuing out from the capillary are of constant diameter (0.05 mm) and of constant drop rate which is controlled by adjusting the height of the mercury reservoir. Thus DME provides a constant fresh surface to the reducible species contained in the test solution.

A suitable voltage is applied to the polarographic cell by adjusting the standard resistor & the slide wire. The electrolysis currents (10^{-8} to 10^{-4} amp) which flow in the cell are measured by a potentiometer. However they can also be measured or recorded automatically in the more modern instruments.

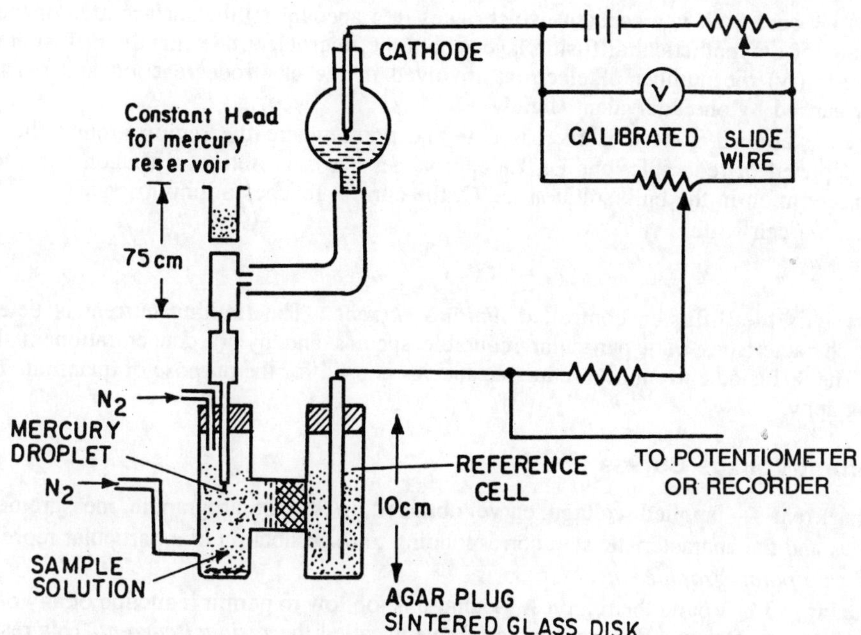

Fig. 13.1. Polarographic H-Cell

13.3 Electrolysis Process in Polarography

To start the electrolysis process, the applied voltage is gradually increased so that the potential of the DME becomes progressively negative. When sufficient voltage has been applied to the cell to start the electrolysis, reduction will occur at DME (i.e. when the applied emf exceeds the back emf of the cell). As long as there is a supply of reducible ions at the electrode surface, an increase in the applied voltage will increase the rate of electrolysis and consequently the cell current. when the supply of the reducible ions adjacent to DME has been depleted a saturation or limiting current is reached. As a result of this localized decreased concentration, any further increase in the applied voltage will cause polarization of the microelectrode. This polorization of DME is produced due to difference in concentration gradients between the reducible ions at the electrode surface and in the bulk of solution. The only way the reducible ions can be replinished is by diffusion. Since the rate is proportional to the concentration gradient through which the diffusion occurs, it can be written as :

$$\text{rate of diffusion} \propto (C - C_0)$$

where C = concentration of the reducible ions in the bulk of the solution. and C_0 is the concentration in the immediate vicinity of the electrode.

But, the rate of reduction at the electrode is a function of the rate at which the ions reach the electrode surface by diffusion and as the rate of reaction is proportional to the current of the cell, the following equation can be written :

$$i = k\,(C - C_0)$$

where i = current, k is a constant which takes into account (i) the surface area of the electrode, (ii) the thickness of a hypothetical diffusion layer about the microelectrode (iii) the diffusion constant of the reducible ion (iv) the number of electrons involved in the electrode reaction and (v) the quantity of electricity carried by one equivalent (farady).

When the applied voltage is increased to the point where the region around the microelectrode becomes depleted of reducible ions i.e. C_0 approaches zero, the rate of diffusion becomes proportional to the concentration in the bulk solution i.e. C, the current reaches a limiting value.

Hence, we can write:

$$i_d = k\,(C)$$

where i_d is the diffusion controlled *limiting current* . The limiting current is determined by the diffusion characteristics of a particular reducible species and by its concentration in the bulk of the solution. The diffusion current of a reducible species is used for the purpose of quantitative determination in polarography.

13.4 Current Voltage Curves

The cell current — applied voltage curve obtained in the polarographic measurement is called a *polarogram* and the characteristic step corresponding to the reduction of a particular reproducible species is known as a *polarographic wave.*

In the Fig. 13.2, around the region A, potential is too low to permit reduction of any of the substances known to be present. A small current which flows is called the *residual current.* This residual current is due to the charging of the mercury drop surface by the supporting electrolyte and to the trace impurities in the test solution. In the region A to B electrolysis occurs and is accompanied by an increase in the current. In this region of the curve, DME is in equilibrium with the residual species and is independent of the applied voltage. When B is reached concentration polarization occurs and the diffusion — controlled limiting current is reached. An increase in the applied voltage B along the plateau will cause a resumption in the residual current gradient. The "polarographic wave height" is obtained from the polarogram by deducing the evaporated residual current in the plateau region of the polarographic wave. It is also the diffusion current i_d. The half wave potential, E 1/2 is a constant characteristic of a reducible species and is used for its qualitative identification. This potential is half way to the reduction step i.e. the potential at a point on the polarogram where the cell current i, is equal to 1/2 of the diffusion, i_d . It is measured by extrapolation of the polarogram.

13.5 Concentration Determination In Polarography

The polarographic diffusion current at DME is obtained by Ilkovic equation $i_d = 607\ nCD^{1/2}\ m^{2/3}\ t^{1/10}$ where i_d is the average diffusion current (in micro ampreres) during the life of the droplet of mercury, 607 is a numerical constant, (706 is used when i_d expresses the maximum diffusion current) n is the number of electrons involved in the reduction at DME, C is the concentration of reducible species in millimole/litre, D is the diffusion current of the reducible species in cm^2/sec, m is the flow rate of the mercury from the DME in mg/sec, and t is the mercury drop time in seconds.

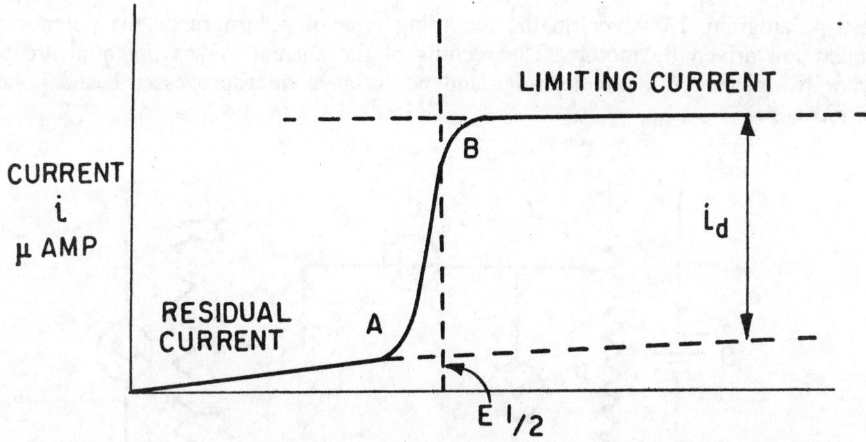

Fig. 13.2. A simple Polarogram; A = decomposition potential, B = concentration polarization, i_d = diffusion current, E 1/2 = half wave potential.

In order to obtain quantitative results, it is important to control variables from one polarographic determination to another. For example, changing capillaries in the DME will change m, a change in temperature will affect D while adjusting the height of mercury reservoir will alter the drop time t.

If the same supporting electrolyte and solvent system is used and all the above stated factors are kept constant (evaluated as k), the Ilkovic equation for a particular species can be written as $i_d = k(C)$

13.6 Applications

1. The majority of heavy metals ions, some non-metals like O_2, O_3, Cl, Br, can be determined by polarography in trace amounts.
2. In biological fluids, O_2 can be determined (both invivo and invitro).
3. For the analysis of organic compounds, the following functional groups; azo, diazo, nitroso, dioxy can be determined by polarography. Simple functional groups on conjugated systems like α, β — unsaturated, aromatic aldehydes, ketones carboxylic acids, lactones, nitriles can also be reduced in this method.
4. We may determine any substance quantitatively by polarography if it can be reduced at the dropping mercury electrode. However, it must be soluble in a solvent appropriate for reduction.

13.7 Instrumentation Aspects

Several different types of polarographs from manual to recording type have been available in market. Now microprocessor controlled polarographs have become available. To understand all the essentials of a commercial polarograph the circuit diagram of simple polarograph is explained in Fig. 13.3

The circuit consists of a battery or an accumulator B (3—4 V) which is connected to a potentiometer and a switch. The apparatus is started by first connecting the electrodes of the polarographic cell C. The meter is set to a minimum sensitivity range by means of the shunt R and then apparatus switched on by means of the switch S. Initially a low potential, say about 0.1 V is applied to the electrodes by adjusting the potentiometer P. The meter sensitivity is increased and the corresponding current is measured and recorded. The polarizing potential is then adjusted to a higher value (e.g. 0.2 V) and the corresponding current is measured. This processes is repeated until sufficient number of readings are taken to be able to produce a polarogram. However, in the recording type of polarographs the potentiometer and the recording chart are driven by motors. The records of the current verses potential are plotted photographically or by means of a pen recorder and now-a-days microprocesser based polarographs. are available world wide.

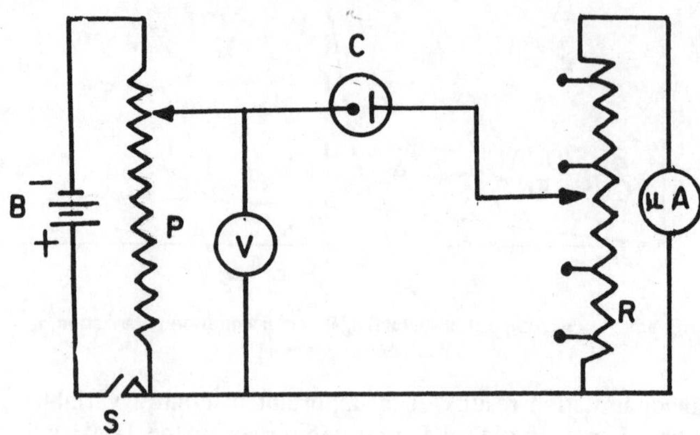

Fig 13.3 Circuit diagram of a simple Polarograph, B = battery, C = Polarographic cell, R = shunt, S = switch, V = voltmeter, P = Potentiometer

13.8 General Experimental Method

The following procedure should be followed in performing experiments on polarography: 1. Adjust the height of the reservoir to give a drop time of about 3-4 seconds with the mercury tip immersed in water. 2. Deoxygenate the test solution by passing N_2 through it for 10-15 minutes. 3. Rinse the electrode with a little of the solution and immerse the electrode tip in the solution. 4. Standardise the potentiometer and set the galvanometer or recording pen to zero. 5. Connect the electrodes to the polarograph and adjust the galvanometer to the minimum sensitivity. 6. The correct sensitivity is found by increasing the polarising voltage to about –1.8V and then adjusting the sensitivity control to get a less than full-scale deflection 7. For a manual type of polarograph, now, set the potentiometer to zero and observe the meter reading. 8. If the meter reading is negative, increase the applied potential in 0.1V increments until a positive value is obtained. 9. Record the average current values by increasing 0.1 increments of the applied voltage until current changes begin to increase. 10. Now, reduce the voltage increments to about 0.02V until the current changes are lowered. 11. Finally, continue to change the potential until it is about -2.0V. 12. Draw the polarogram graphically and read the diffusion current from the curve.

For the case of an automatic recording polarograph the following modifications should be noted. 1. After standardising the potiometer, the potiometer is set to a desired initial value and the recorder pen to a zero line. 2. The controls for driving the potentiometer slide wire and recorder pen are switched on and if the sensitivity setting is correct a polarogram will be plotted automatically. 3. When the experiments are completed the DME is washed thoroughly with water and then placed in water. 4. The mercury reservoir is lowered down to a point where the mercury stops to emerge from the capillary.

EXERCISE : 1. Determination of cadmium by polaragraphy.

Method : 1. Set up the polaragraphic apparatus. 2. Prepare the following three solutions : a standard cadmium chloride solution (0.01 N) in a 100 ml volumetric flask, 1N KCl and Triton X-100 (0.2% in water). 3. Place the given cadium chloride sample in a 100 ml volumetric flask and label the flask as ''sample''. 4. Prepare three 100 ml volumetric flasks and mark them as ''standard'', ''sample and residual''. 5. To the above three flasks add 10 ml of 1N KCl and 1.0 ml of Triton X-100 ml solution. 6. In the ''standard'' flask place 10.0 ml of standard cadmium chloride solution. 7. Dilute the contents of the three flasks up to the mark & mix well. 8. Allow the flasks to attain the temperature of the polarograph. 9. transfer some of the solution from the ''residual'' flask to the polaragraphic vessel and deacrate the vessel by a stream of nitrogen as per instructions in the manual. 10. Then remove the nitrogen tube without disturbing the solution. 11. Adjust the applied voltage so that the dropping mercury electrode is at – 0.8 V versus S.C.E and note the current. 12. Remove the solution from the polaragraphic vessel and rinse with distilled water. 13. Repeat the steps 9, 10 with the solution from ''sample'' and ''standard'' flasks. 14. Calculate the mg of cadmium in the total sample.

SECTION-E
SPECTROSCOPIC METHODS OF ANALYSIS

14

Visible Spectrophotometry

14.1 General

Absorption spectrophotometry can be defined as the measurement of absorption of radiant energy by various substances. It involves the measurement of absorptive capacity for radiant energy in the visible, UV and infra-red (IR) regions of the spectrum. As the techniques of visible and UV are different from those of I.R. therefore each one of them will be dealt with in separate chapters. The present chapter will discuss visible absorption methods. By selecting proper techniques and instruments one can estimate the drugs manufactured in the industry and study their amounts or concentrations. Thus one can say that quality control or drug analysis is not complete without spectrophotometry.

14.2 Electromagnetic Radiation

Soon after the structure of atom was established it became clear that light is produced by oscillations of electrons within atom and that light is electromagnetic (EM) in nature. It was also realized that the electric

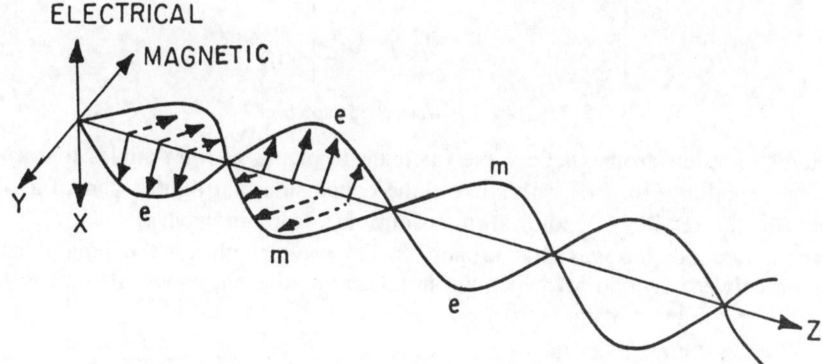

Fig. 14.1. EM Wave showing electric and magnetic components.

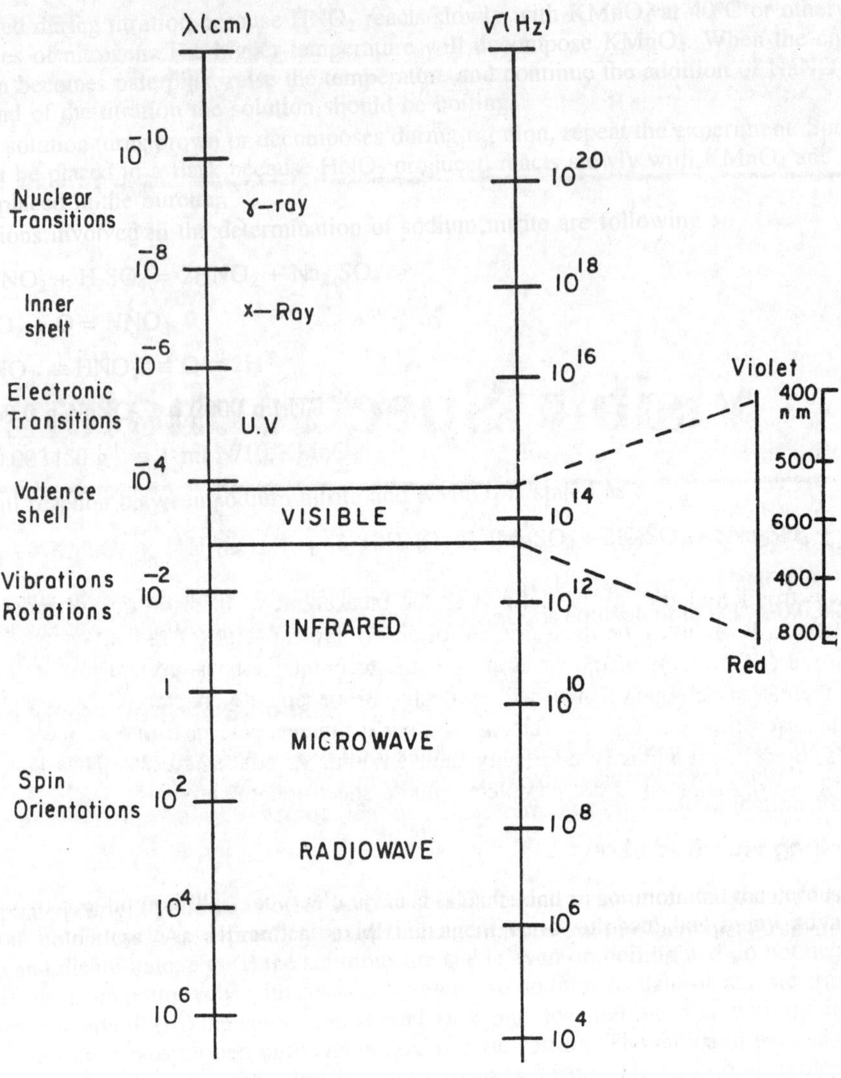

Fig. 14.2. Electromagnetic spectrum

and magnetic fields in an electromagnetic wave fluctuate in planes at right angles to each other and to the direction of propagation (Fig. 14.1). This led to the conclusion that light is part of a whole range of electromagnetic radiation (EMR) extending from cosmic rays to radio waves.

Electromagnetic radiation has wave like properties. The wavelength λ is the linear distance along the line of propagation between two points which are in phase on adjacent waves, its unit is A° where

$$1A^\circ = 10^{-1} \text{ nm} = 10^{-4}\mu = 10^{-8} \text{ cm}$$

$$1\mu = 1000 \text{ nm}$$

$$1 \text{ cm} = 10^{-4}\mu = 10^{-7} \text{ nm} = 10^{8} A^\circ$$

The frequency ν is the number of cycles (CPS) occuring per second (Hertz, Hz).

or $\nu = \frac{c}{\lambda}$ where c is the velocity of light (3.0×10^{10} cm/sec.)

Frequency units are large and cumbersome to use, therefore wave number $\bar{\nu}$ i.e. no of waves/unit of length or reciprocal of wavelength in cms is used or $\nu = \frac{1}{\lambda}$

Radiant energy also behaves as if it is made up of packets of energy or photons. The energy of a photon depends on the frequency of radiation.

$$E = h\nu \quad \text{or} \quad E = \frac{h \cdot c}{\lambda}, \; h = \text{planck's constant} = 6.62 \times 10^{-27} \text{ erg/sec.}$$

14.3 Absorption of Radiant Energy

We have learnt that molecules are energetic, that they can rock, twist and bend and if right frequency of energy is used, the electrons within the molecules move from the ground to the excited state. Further, the overall contribution to the kinetic energy of a molecule is made up of (i) translational (ii) rotational (iii) vibrational and (iv) electronic motions of the molecules or the electrons and the nuclei in the molecule. The translational energy is associated with the motion of the molecule as a whole or due to free motion in space. It can specify the position of the centre of mass of the molecule. The rotational energy is due to the rotation of the molecule i.e. rotating about the axis through its centre of gravity. It can give the orientation or number of angles of a molecule in space. The vibrational energy is due to the movement of atoms within the molecule. It is because molecules are made up of atoms bonded together and they can vibrate and rotate simultaneously. The electrons move around the nuclei and are involved in electronic excitations. When a molecule absorbs visible or ultraviolet energy, an electron or electrons will be raised to a higher energy level if the energy of requirement for that transition is equal to the energy of the incoming photon. The electrons in the inner shells of atoms and those that are shared by two adjacent atoms are not affected to the same extent by in coming radiation as those that cannot be localised within the molecules. It is these electrons that are not localised, give rise to spectra in the visible and ultraviolet regions of the electromagnetic spectrum.

14.4 Laws of Photometry

When a beam of radiant energy strikes a solution of an absorbing substance contained in cuvette or a cell, several things may happen to it : (i) it may pass through the matter with little absorption taking place and therefore little energy loss; (ii) the direction of propagation of the beam may be altered by reflection, refraction, diffraction and some scattering due to the particulate suspended matter may also occur; (iii) the radiant energy may be absorbed entirely or in part. This absorption will involve a transfer of energy to the medium and will be related to the characteristic molecular structure of the substance.

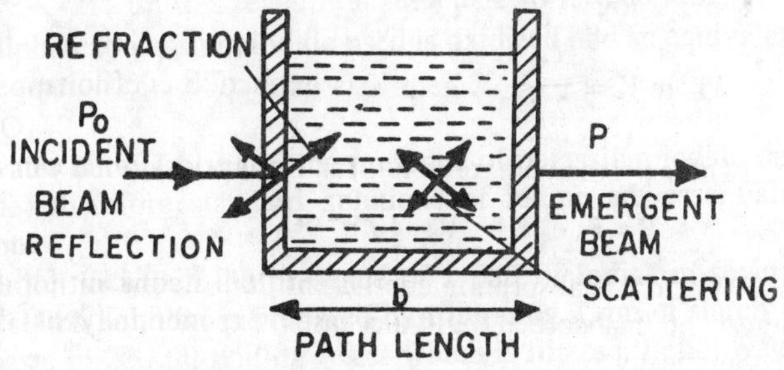

Fig. 14.3 Derivation of Beer's Law.

The rate at which energy is transported in a beam of radiant energy is denoted by P_o for incident beam and by P for the quantity remaining unabsorbed after passage through a sample. The ratio of the radiant energy transmitted by sample to the radiant power incident on the sample is called transmittance T i.e.

$$T = \frac{P}{P_0}$$

The logarithm to the base 10 of the reciprocal of transmittance is known as absorbance i.e.

$$A = \log_{10} \frac{1}{T} = \log_{10} \frac{P_0}{P}$$

The above phenomenon is further explained in terms of two laws which are called *laws of photometry.* These are described as follows : (i) Bouguer or Lambert law which states that when a beam of monochromatic light previously rendered plan parallel enters an absorbing medium at right angles to the plane, parallel surfaces of the medium, the rate of decrease in radiant power with the length of light path through absorbing medium b is proportional to the radiant power of the beam. In other words the light will be diminished in geometric or exponential progression or if a certain thickness absorbs half the light, then the thickness which follows the first and is equal to it will not absorb the entire 2nd half but only the half of this half and consequently reduces it to 1/4.

Let dP represent each increament of beam of monochromatic radiation and db represent each increament of the medium.

$\therefore -\frac{dp}{db} \propto P$ where P is the incident power and b is the thickness of the medium or container for a solution

or $-\frac{dp}{db} = Kp$, rearranging we have

$\int_0^{P_b} \frac{dp}{P} = K \int_0^b db$, on integration and changing logarithm to base 10 we have

$-\log P = Kb + C$ (For convenience common logarithm is used here).

Initially P_o is incident power reaching a given area per second, b the thickness is equal to zero and C is equal to $-\log P_o$

$$\therefore \quad -\log P = Kb - \log P_o$$

$$\text{or} \quad \log . \frac{P}{P_0} = -Kb \qquad \text{.............(1)}$$

Where $K = \frac{k}{2.303}$ where K is extinction coefficient

The eq. 1. is an expression for Bouguers low. It can also be written in its exponential form as :

$$P = P_o e^{-kb} = P_o . 10^{-0.434kb}$$

Where k is absorption coefficient. It is a constant for a given wavelength and temperature i.e. radiant power of unabsorbed light deceases exponentially as the thickness of absorbing medium increases arithmatically.

(ii) Bernard and Beers law states that the radiating power of a beam of parallel monochromatic radiation decreases as the concentration of the absorbing constituent increases or the fraction of light transmitted by a given thickness of solution decreases exponentially with increasing concentration of solute or density increases linearly with concentration.

Similarly, each increment of beam of monochromatic radiation can be represented by dp and each concentration increasement by dc

$\therefore -\frac{dp}{dc} \propto P$ where P is incident power

$$\text{or } -\frac{dP}{dC} = k'P \text{ or } -\int_{o}^{pc} \frac{dp}{P} = k' \int_{o}^{c} dc$$

integrating and changing logarithm to base 10, we have $-\log P = k'C - \log P_o$

$$\text{or} \quad \log \frac{P}{P_o} = -k' c$$

The eq. (2) can also be written in exponential form $P = P_o e^{-k'c}$

The eq. (1) and (2) can be combined since both are proportional to P the radiant power.

$$\text{Thus } \log \frac{P_o}{P} = k'' \, b \, c \qquad \text{.....(2)}$$

Where $k' . k = k''$, k'' is molar absorption coefficient and dependent on solvent and temperature

By substitution of A for $\log \frac{P_o}{P}$ and $\underline{a}$ for k''

$$\text{we have } A = a \, b \, c \qquad \text{.....(3)}$$

The eq. (3) is called Bouguer - Beers law or Beers Lambert law. This is an equation of a straight line with an intercept of zero and slope value of *ab* as shown in Fig. 14.4.

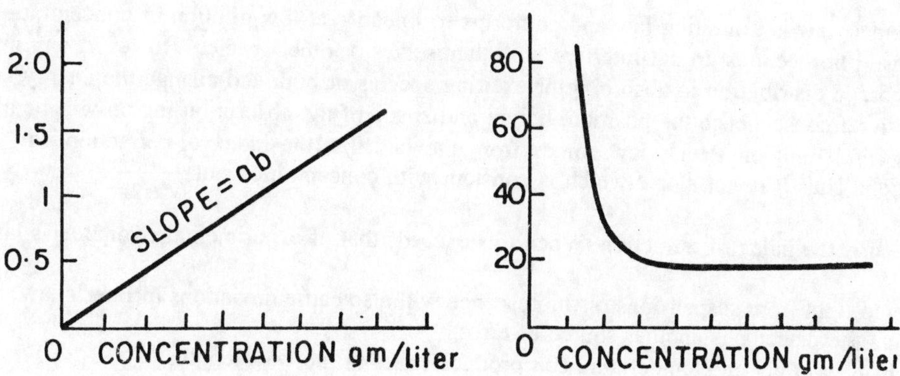

Fig. 14.4. Comparison in scale between absorbance and transmittance

In the equation A = abc the concentration c = gm/litre and thickness b is in cm. The eq. 3 can also be written as $A = \varepsilon \, bc$ ------(4)

Where ε is molar extinction coefficient and then c = moles/litre.

The eq. (3) can also be written as :

$$a = \frac{A}{bc} \text{ i.e. absorbtivity.}$$

Further, one can write $\varepsilon = q \times$ molecular weight and

$$\varepsilon = E_1^1 \times \frac{\text{MolecularWeight}}{10} \quad \text{where } E_1^1 = E\,(1\,\%,\ 1\text{ cm.})$$

Where ε is called molar absorptivity.

$$\text{Also the percent } T = 100\,T = 100 \times \frac{P}{P_o}$$

The presentation of visible and UV spectra is done in terms of A, log A, a, ε, log ε or T against wavelength (mμ) and the spectra will look like as shown below (Fig. 14.5).

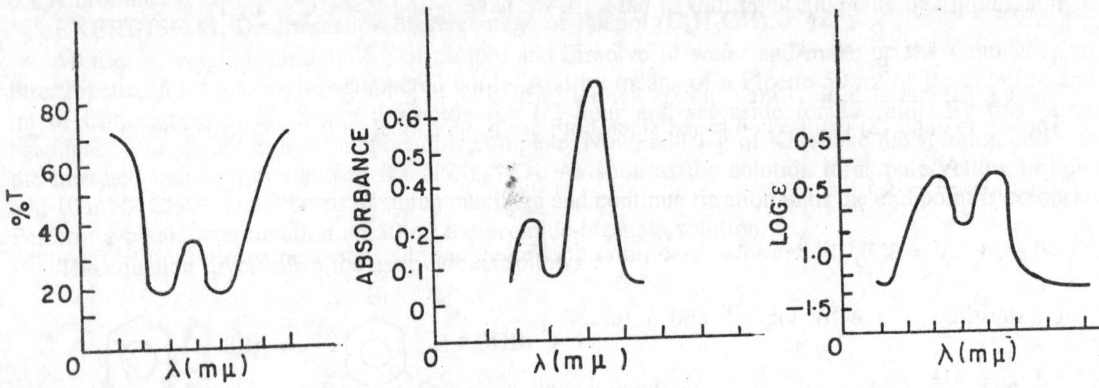

Fig. 14.5 Presentation of spectral data.

14.5 Deviations and Sources of Error

Beer's Lambert law is a limiting law and conforms to linearity at low dilution or concentration (10^{-2}M) because absorption centres do not interfere with themselves or other species. However, any interference will alter charge distribution in absorbing or exciting species or both and change the energy content for excitation. As a consequence the position, height and shape of the absorption region will be altered.

The second limit on Beer's law comes from the fact that the index of refraction will alter with concentration. Thus it is not a or ε which is constant with concentration but $\frac{an}{(v^2+2)^2}$.

Where n is the index of refraction. When this exceeds that of experimental error, Beer's law will not hold.

Scattered light from suspensions or fluorescence will also cause deviations in Beer's law. Stray light which enters the detector is another source of error.

The changes in pH and temperature can produce shifts in the wavelengths.

14.6 Determinations of Mixtures

In the analysis of substances one encounters mixtures of two or more substances. Rather than trying to separate the individual constituents, it is possible to analyse the mixture using simultaneous spectrophotometric determinations. What is needed, is that there be available absorption peaks for each component and that these should be free from absorptions by the other constituents. Further, it is assumed that the absorbances for each component are additive, but at the sametime the experimental errors also mount up rapidly. Thus, one can write for a mixture :

$$\text{Log}\ \frac{P_o}{P} = A = \varepsilon_1 b_1 c_1 + \varepsilon_2 b_2 c_2 \ldots\ldots = b\,\Sigma_i\ \varepsilon_i\ c_i .$$

If the mixture has two constituents (Fig.. 14.6) one can write :

$$A\lambda_1 = (c_1\,\varepsilon_1)_{\lambda_1} + (c_2\varepsilon_2)_{\lambda_1}$$
$$A\lambda_2 = (c_1\,\varepsilon_1)_{\lambda_2} + (c_2\,\varepsilon_2)_{\lambda_2}$$

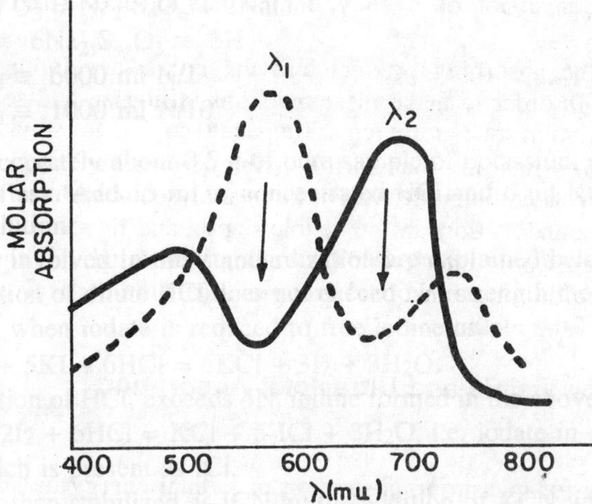

Fig. 14.6. Simultaneous Determination (Two components).

Where c_1 and c_2 are concentrations and ε_1 and ε_2 are molar absorptivities at λ_1 and λ_2 respectively, the path length b being constant.

The equations are solved by substituting the known values and required data is obtained.

If the two substances contribute to absorption at each wavelength, the calculations can be performed by the alternative method given below :

Let component a have E_1' values of a_1 at λ_1 and a_2 at λ_2. Let component b have E_1' values of b_1 at λ_1 and b_2 at λ_2. The extinction of a solution of mixture is determined at λ_1 and λ_2 and the E_1'' values are calculated — S_1 and S_2 at λ_1 and λ_2 respectively.

Then

$$100S_1 = a_1 X + b_1 Y$$

and

$$100S_2 = a_2 X + b_2 Y$$

Where X = concentration (% W/W) of component a and Y = concentration (% W/W) of component b. Solving the simultaneous equations for X and Y :

$$X = 100\left(\frac{b_1S_2 - b_2S_1}{b_1a_2 - b_2a_1}\right) \text{ and } Y = 100\left(\frac{a_1S_2 - a_2S_1}{a_1b_2 - a_2b_1}\right)$$

For mixtures of three constituents the calculations become more difficult and care must be taken for analysis if precise results are to be obtained.

In case of analysis of a single constituent in a mixture, the determination can be performed provided the absorption due to other components is ignored.

14.7 Colorimetry

When a specimen or a substance does not possess suitable chromogenic properties, it may be made to react with an absorbing reagent and converted to an absorbing species.

There are many instances of the above stated approach being adopted and measurements being made in the visible region. For example, though alcohols do not absorb between 200 to 1000 nm but treatment with phenyl isocyanate produces the corresponding phenyl alkyl carbamate which absorbs at 280 nm. Ferric ion (Fe^{2+}) is very weakly coloured material but a reaction with 1, 10-phenanthroline produces a stable deep red complex. Conversion of carbonyl compounds to semicarbazones shifts the spectra by 30 to 40 nm.

It is necessary that the absorbing product and the colour-developing reagent are stable for a reasonable period of time. In order to make these reactions utilitarian and selective it may be necessary to control pH, or adjust oxidation state or use a masking agent so that any kind of interferents are removed.

In colorimetry, measurements are done in the visible region but colorimetric methods are applied even though a compound or its coloured derivative to be analysed absorbs in the UV region. The reasons being that : (i) fewer compounds absorb in the visible region and therefore this technique is used in the presence of substance which would interfere if UV region were used, (ii) chemical reactions utilized to prepare derivatives are specific for a functional group and (iii) the derivative formed is conjugated thus increasing the sensitivity of the method.

14.8 Instrumentation for Visible and Ultraviolet Absorption

14.8.1 General

The instruments developed for measuring absorption of radiant energy by substances in the visible and ultraviolet portions of spectrum have been given various names as photometers, spectrometers spectrophotometers etc. Various types of models and designes have been evolved down these years and are commercially available in various price ranges.

Photometer : It is a simple instrument for measuring radiant power or some function of this quantity by means of a photocell.

Spectrometer : It is an instrument which comprises an entrance slit, a dispersing device, one or more exit slits and measurements are made at selected wavelength within a spectral range. The quantity detected is a function of radiant energy.

Spectrophotometer : It is a spectrometer with further sophistication and furnishes the ratio or a function of ratio of the radiant power of two beams as a function of spectral width.

14.8.2 Principle Components

The most important components of a photometer consist of : (i) a source of radiant energy, (ii) some type of filter for isolation of a band of radiant energy, (iv) an optical system for producing a parallel beam of filtered light for passage through an absorption cell, (v) a detector for unabsorbed energy, and (vi) a read out system. In sophisticated spectrophotometers a prism or a grating is used in place of a filter as a dispersing device for isolation of required spectral band of radiant energy. The arrangement for the above components is shown in the Fig. 14.7.

A generalised idea of the main components required for the design spectrophotometer are summarised in the table below :

Table 14.1

Radiant Energy Source	Associated Optics	Dispersing Elements	Detectors
W – Lamp,	Lenses	Absorption Filter	Barrier layer Cell
Xe, Hg arc,	Mirrors		
H_2, D_2	Slits	Interference Filter	Phototube
Discharge tube	Cuvetts	Prisms, grating	Photomultipher tube

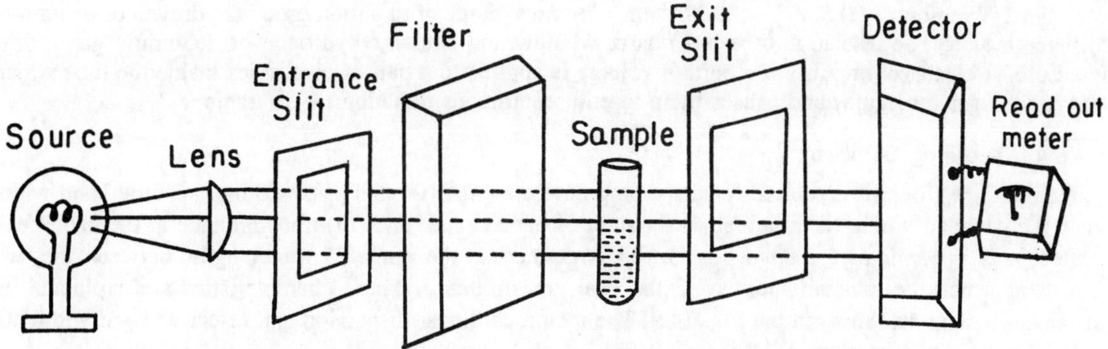

Fig. 14.7 Schematic diagram showing various components of a Filter photometer.

The specific properties required for the various components are discussed below.

14.8.3 Radiant Energy Sources

The function of a light source is to provide the incident light of sufficient intensity for measurement. The sources selected must have the required range of spectral distribution and stability within the operating period and operating temperature. As far as work in the visible and near UV region is concerned common radiation sources used are : (i) tungsten lamp or (ii) ω-filament and (iii) tungston-iodine lamp. The size and shape varies from a 100 watt projection lamp to a 6 volt automobile lamp. However, it should be noted that the tungsten lamp emits the major portion of its energy in the near infrared region. Only about 15% of its energy falls within the visible region curve at an operating temperature of 2600 — 3000°K as shown in the Fig 14.8. Generally, a heat absorbing filter is inserted between the lamp and the sample holder to absorb most of the IR radiation without lowering the energy of the other required wavelength.

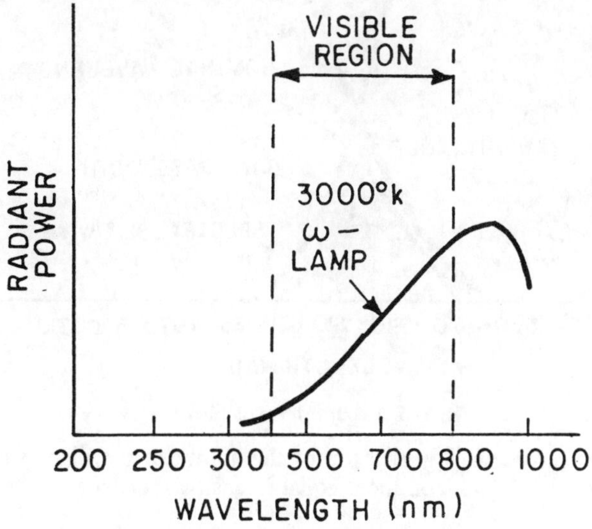

Fig. 14.8. Spectral distribution of w-lamp..

For UV region i.e. 1850A° — 3900A° the common source of radiation used is hydrogen or deuterium discharge tube. The discharge tube has quartz window and contains hydrogen or deuterium gas at low pressure. A electrical impulse of a certain voltage is applied to a pair of electrodes inside the tube which excites the gas molecules and causes them to emit continuous radiation in UV region.

14.8.4 Dispersing Devices :

The important properties required for dispersing device are its: (i) band pass width or spectral band width or effective band width, (ii) nominal wavelength of band centre, and (iii) transmittance at the band peak called *peak transmittance* . *Band pass width* is defined as the range of wavelengths between the two points at which the transmittance is 1/2 the peak transmittance. These characteristics are explained by means of a diagram shown in the Fig. 14.9. The reciprocal linear dispersion and effective band width are related by:

$$D^{-1} = \frac{\Delta \lambda}{\Delta y}$$

where D^{-1} is reciprocal linear dispersion. $\Delta \lambda$ and Δy are finite intervals of wavelength and linear distance repectively.

When $\Delta y =$ slit width w, $\Delta \lambda$ is effective band width i.e. $\Delta \lambda = W D^{-1}$

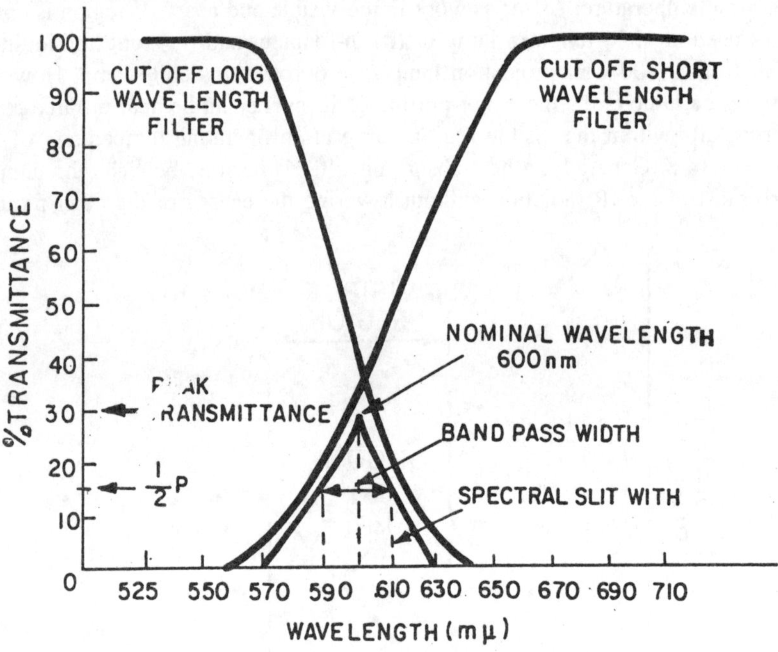

Fig. 14.9 A composite glass filter.

The *resolving power* or resolution is a measure of the ability of the dispersing device to separate distinctly two closely spaced wavelengths of about equal intensity, therefore we can say:

$R = \frac{\lambda}{d\lambda}$ where λ is the average wavelength of two images, and $d\lambda$ is their difference.

Filters: The function of a filter is to absorb, reflect or deviate all frequencies from an optical path except for one band i.e. the band pass width. The selection of a filter is based on a compromise between peak transmittance and band pass width; the former should be as high as possible while the latter should be as narrow as possible. The following four types of filters can be classified : (i) gelatin filters, (ii) liquid filters, (ii) tinted glass and (iv) interference filters. The first three types function by selective absorption of unwanted wavelengths while the fourth type depend upon constructive interference of light rays. The essential characteristics of these filters are described below :

Gelatin filter : It consists of a layer of gelatin impregnated with suitable organic dyes sandwiched between two sheets of glass. Gelatin filter is now seldom used because it tends to deteriorate with time due to alteration in gelatin and bleaching of dyes.

Liquid filter : These are solutions of appropriately absorbing components.

Tinted glass filter : It consists of a solid sheet of glass that is coloured by a pigment which is either dissolved or dispersed in the glass.

Interference filter : It consists of an evaporated coating of transparent dielectric spacer of low refractive index sandwiched between the semi-transparent silver films (Fig. 14.10) Magnesium fluoride (MgF_2) is a common dielectric because of its hardness. The light incident upon the face of the filter is reflected back and forth between the metal films. Each silver film reflects half and transmits the other half of any radiation that strike it. These filters have band widths of 10-27 mμ and peak transmittance of 40-60 %. They can be used with high intensity light sources since they remove unwanted radiation by transmission and reflection and not by absorption (Fig 14.11).

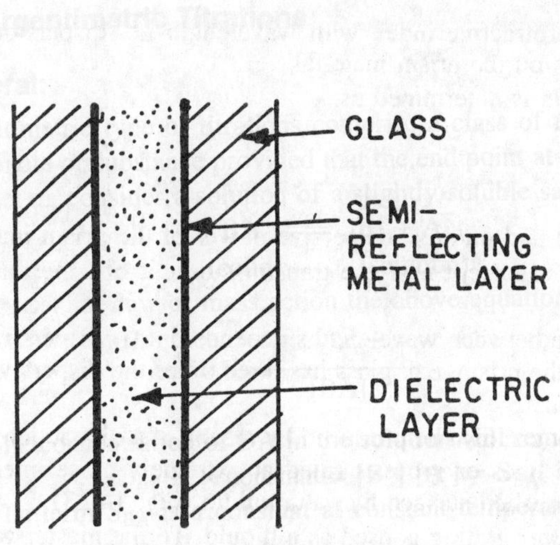

Fig. 14.10. Interference filter.

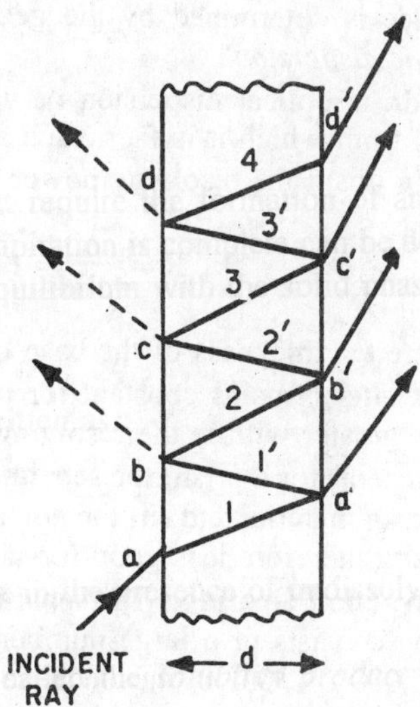

Fig. 14.11. Action of an interference filter.

Prisms : In a spectrophotometer, light from the source is directed through a convergent lens into a entrance slit at the focal point of the lens, then through a prism and a second convergent lens. The dispersion of radiation involves angularly separating the different frequencies in a wavefront. The mechanism involved is the process of refraction by the prism, e.g. the two wavelengths present in the incident beam (Fig. 14.12) are refracted through different angles and are separated by $\theta_2 - \theta_1$ on leaving the prism. The angular dispersion of prism is given by $d\theta/d\lambda$ where $d\theta$ is the angular separation of wavelengths differing by $d\lambda$ in magnitude. This angular dispersion of a prism can be resolved into two

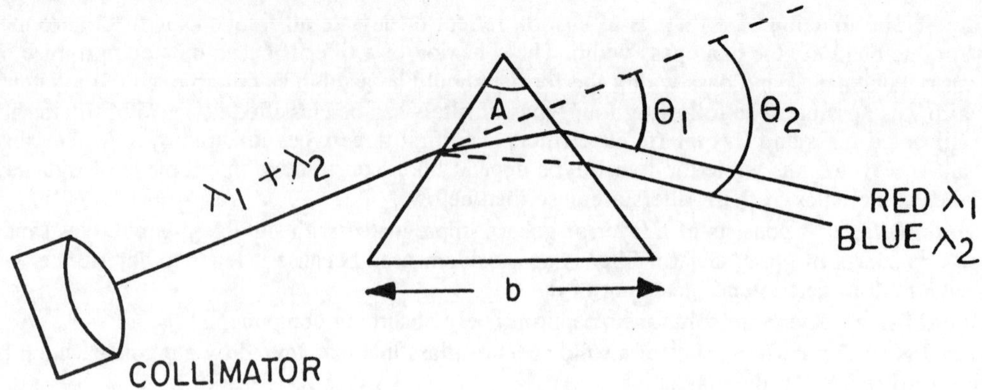

Fig. 14.12. Action of a prism.

components as :

$$\frac{d\theta}{d\lambda} = \frac{d\theta}{dn} \cdot \frac{dn}{d\lambda}$$

Where $d\theta/dn$ is change in refractive angle θ as a function of refractive index n of the prism. Its magnitude is determined by the geometry of the prism and the angle of incidence i. It is called the *geometric dispersion.*

$dn/d\lambda$ is optical dispersion or variation of refractive index with wavelength i.e. dispersion of the material from which it is fabricated and depends on the prism material.

For a prism the resolving power of resolution is determined as:

$$R = \frac{\lambda}{d\lambda} = t\left(\frac{dn}{d\lambda}\right)$$

where t = thickness of the base of the prism and $dn/d\lambda$ = dispersive power of the prism material.

The latter remains constant for prism material except near the transmission cut off, the thicker the base, the greater will be the resolving power.

In general for a prism the separation in space between wavelengths depends on: (i) dispersive power of the prism material and (ii) the apical angle of the prism, e.g. glass has three times the dispersive power than quartz therefore it is good for visible region.

Diffraction Grating : The separation of light can also be produced by means of a diffraction grating. A grating consists of a large number of parallel lines or grooves ruled at extremely close intervals — about 15,000 — 30,000 lines/inch on a highly polished surface like aluminium (Fig. 14.13)

In the preparation of a *replica* grating, a *master* grating is used as a mould. To the master grating is applied a film of a parting compound. The film is aluminized, the crevices are filled with an epoxy resin. Thereafter an optical flat is bonded to the aluminium replica by the epoxy resin or cement. When the epoxy resin has hardened and the replica grating completely aluminized, it is separated. Each groove in the grating functions as a scattering centre for the light rays impinging on it by the mechanism explained below (Fig. 14.14).

Let us say the grating is illuminated by incident rays R_1 and R_2 making an angle i with the normal. But R_2 must travel farther than R_1 by distance dsin i (d = distance between adjacent grooves and i = incident angle).

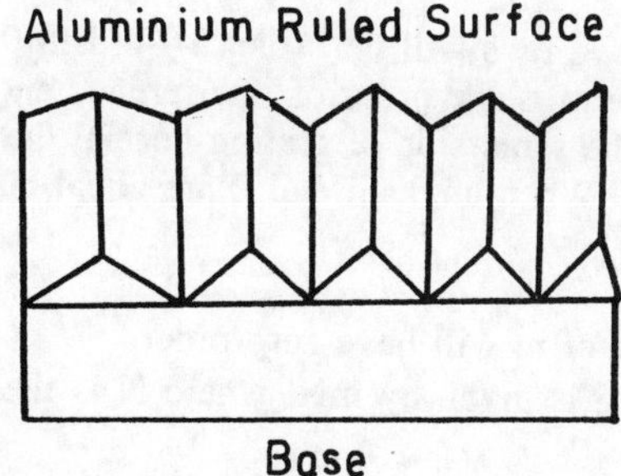

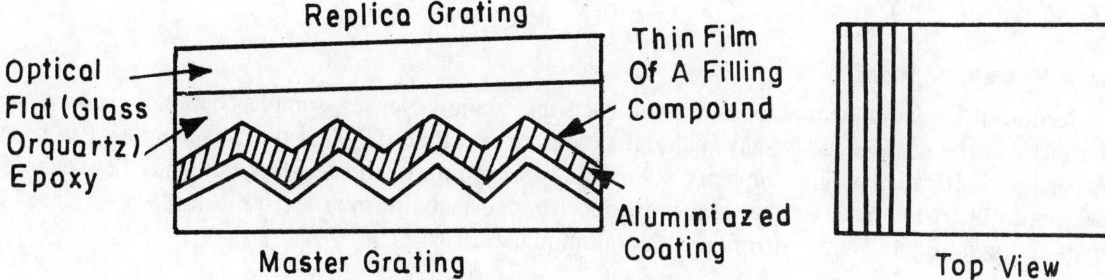

Fig. 14.13. Preparation of diffraction grating..

Similarly R_1 must go farther by d sin θ (θ = angle of reflection).

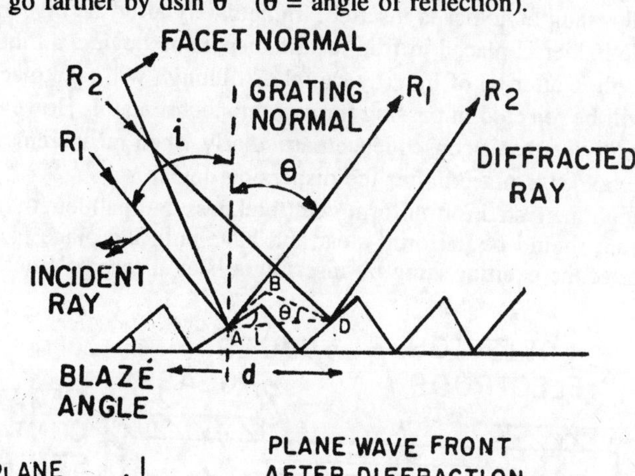

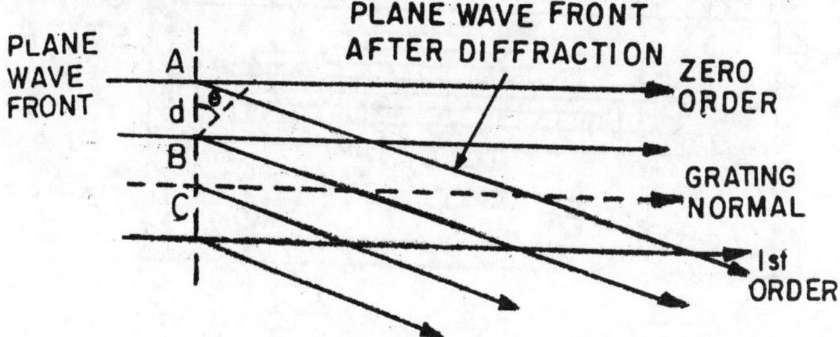

Fig. 14.14. Action of a Diffraction grating.

The net path difference for the two rays will be : (dsin i) – (dsin θ) = integral multiple wavelength mλ. or mλ = d(sin i ± sin θ) where m is the order of interference and will have values 1, 2, 3 .... : If incident and emergent beam are on the same side of grating normal the sign will be (+) i.e. rays will be in phase and combine constructively. When angles i and θ are equal but of opposite sign the equation

$$m\lambda = d(\sin i - \sin \theta) = 0$$

i.e. the grating acts as a plane mirror or m will have zero order.

The resolving power of a grating is given by mN, where N is the number of rulings and m is the order Number.

$$\therefore \quad R = \frac{\lambda}{d\lambda} = mN$$

14.8.5 Associated optics

The selection of transmittance material that are used for windows lenses, sample containers is governed by the fact that the absorbance by any material should be less than 0.2 % at the wavelength of use, e.g. quartz or fused silica is suitable for work below 300 nm, ordinary silicate glass transmits between 350 to 300 nm. In order to cut down the losses of light, front surfaced mirrors are used in place of lenses to focus or *collimate* light. These mirrors are also aluminized.

14.8.6 Sample Holder

In a spectrophotometer a provision is made for placing the sample solution between the light source and the detector. In general, the sample holder is inserted. immediately after the dispersing device in front of the detector. If the sample holder is placed in front of the dispersing device, all the light from the source will pass through the sample scattering of light by sample. Although will take place but will not produce any error because light will be rejected in passing through monochromator. However, in situations where fluorescence and photsensitivity are of consequence particularly when measurements are made in UV or visible range, the sample holder is placed after the dispersing device.

The sample tubes should be tested for uniform wall thickness and pathlength. Glass or quartz is used for the sample material, but should be uniform, clear and have polished plane faces. The sample holder is protected from the heat of the exciting lamp by inserting a heat absorbing filter between the lamp and the sample.

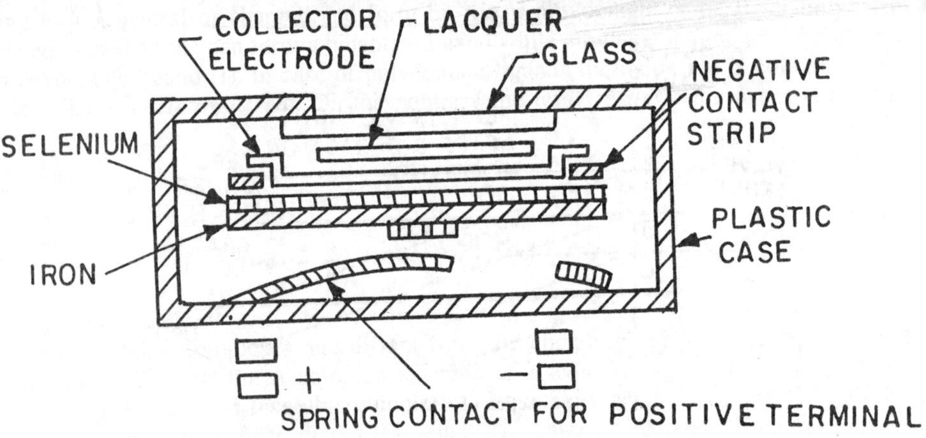

Fig. 14.15. Photovoltaic cell.

14.8.7 Detectors

After the radiation has been absorbed by the sample it must be detected. A detector system should possess the following characteristics : (i) should be sensitive (ii) should have linear response (iii) its noise level should be low (iv) should have short response time and (v) should be stable.

The detection of radiation may be done (i) atomically (ii) thermally or (iii) photoelectrically, but for studies in visible or UV any photosensitive device may be used.

The most commonly used detectors in the UV and visible spectrophotometers are (i) Photovoltaic cell or Barrier-layer cell (ii) Phototube and (iii) Photomultiplier tube these are described in detail below.

Photovoltaic cell : It consists of a plate of metal made of iron on which has been deposited a thin layer of semiconductor like selenium to form a rectifying junction. A very thin transparent layer of Ag is sputtered over semi-conductor to act as the collector electrode. The metal base acts as the second electrode. When radiant energy falls upon the semi-conductor surface, the electrons are excited at the Ag-Se interface.

They are released and pass on to the collector electrode. A hypothetical barrier region appears to be generated near the interface across which electrons pass easily from the semi-conductor to the collector electrode whereas a moderate resistance opposes the electron flow in the reverse direction. In this manner, photovoltaic cell generates its own emf and no external power supply is needed to be applied to observe the current. The current produced is an high as 0.08 μ amperes per μ watt.

The disadvantage with this cell is its low impedence, consequently the output cannot be amplified. It is generally used in filter photometers where high levels of illumination exist and there is no need to amplify a signal. Further, the photovoltaic cell shows fatigue because photocurrent rises to a value above equilibrium value and then falls-off with time. A gravity controlled shutter is used which permits light to strike the cell only while readings are taken.

Phototube : It consists of a negative electrode which is hemihedral in shape and coated with a light sensitive layer of silver or alkali metal or alkali metal oxide. An anode consists of a axially centered wire or a rectangular wire that frames the cathode. The two electrodes are sealed within an evacuated glass envelope. The anode is maintained at a positive potential by means of a battery. When the radiant energy falls on photosensitive cathode surface, electrons are emitted. These electrons pass over to the anode where they are collected and returned via external circuit.

Photomultiplier tube : The most commonly use detector in the UV visible spectrophotometers is the photomultiplier tube. It consists of an alkaline — earth oxide coated semi-cylindrical cathode, an anode made up of metal wire to collect electrons. The quartz window allows the radiation to fall on the cathode surface. A small number of electrons proportional to the intensity of the incident radiation are emitted from the oxide that is coated on the cathode. If these few electrons are allowed to flow directly to the anode they would produce only a small current (10^{-10} amperes). But the dynodes cause the current to be amplified by a factor of about 10^6. As the electrons are emitted, they are accelerated as they pass from dynode to dynode. Each dynode consists of a plate of material coated with a substance having a force of attraction for the escaping electrons. The high energy electrons strike with sufficient energy to dislodge and eject the secondary electrons. There are about 9 to 16 such dynodes in a photomultiplier tube.

14.9 Commercial Instruments

Various models and designs of single beam and double beams spectrophotometers are commercially available. They differ in price based on their design and sophistication. The schematic diagrams for the arrangement of main components in (i) a single beam and (ii) a double beam instrument are described

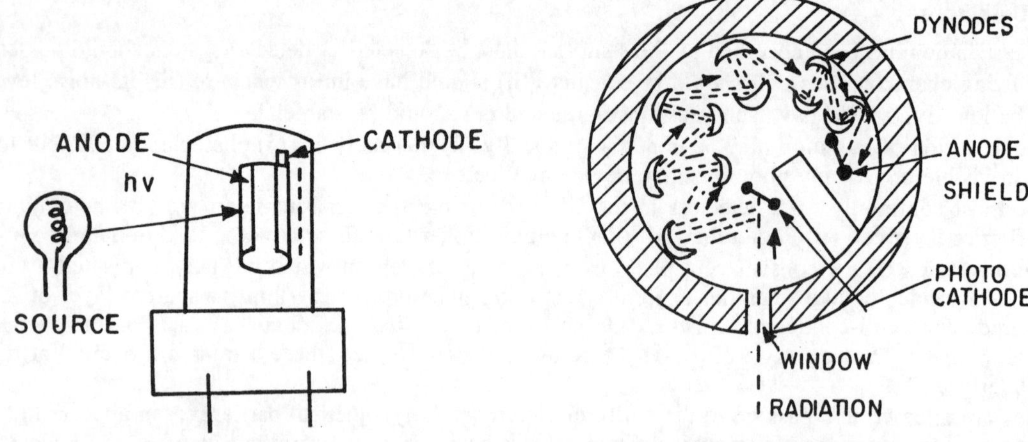

Fig. 14.16. A Phototube.

Fig. 14.17. Photomultiplier tube (a cross-section)

(i) Single Beam Instrument : The measurement with a single beam instrument involves three steps which are separated in time namely : (a) determination of zero % T with shutter in place, (b) measurement of 100% T (or P_0) and lastly (c) measurement of P. Thus it comprises only one beam of radiation.

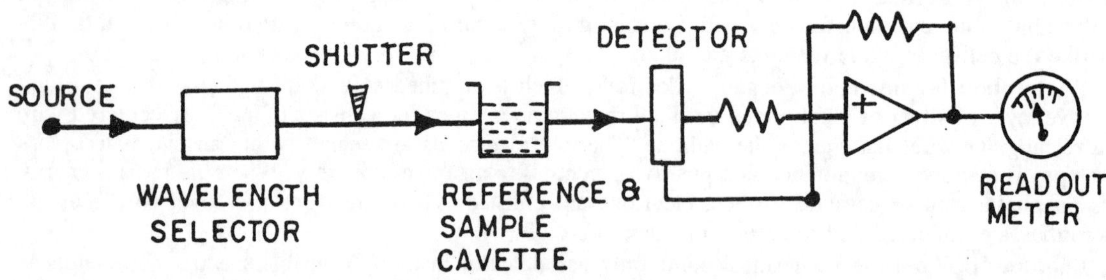

Fig. 14.18. Single beam Photometer.

A popular single channel grating type of spectrophotometer is Bausch and Lomb Spectronic — 20 colorimeter the schematic optical diagram of which is shown in the Fig. 14.19. The range of the spectrophotometer is 375 nm to 750 nm with a red sensitive phototube. A second phototube is located at the rear of light source to monitor fluctuations in the source.

(ii) Double Beam Instrument : As far as double beam or two channels instruments are concerned one can obtain two beams of radiation where (a) two paths are separated in space, simultaneous in time or (b) alternate in time and coincide in space. In case of arrangement (a) a V - shaped mirror is used as a beam splitter so that the two beams pass through the reference and the sample cuvettes simultaneously and reach the two detectors at the same time. It furnishes the ratio of the radiant power of two beams.

On the contrary, in case of arrangement (b) a rotating sector mirror is used which directs all of the radiation from the selector to the reference and sample alternatively in time. A grid mirror is used to recombine the pulses so that they fall on a single detector. The output of the detector is an alternating sgnal whose amplitude is proportional to the difference in intensities in the two channels. No shutter is

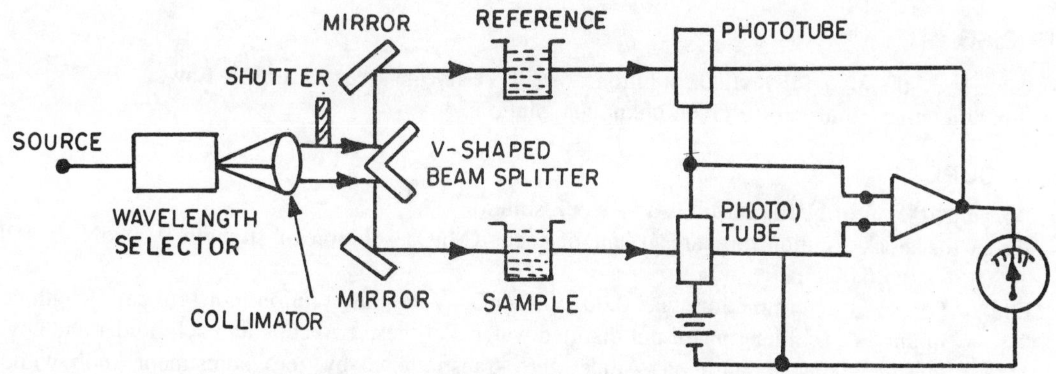

Fig. 14.19a. Double beam spectrophotometer (Simultaneous in time)

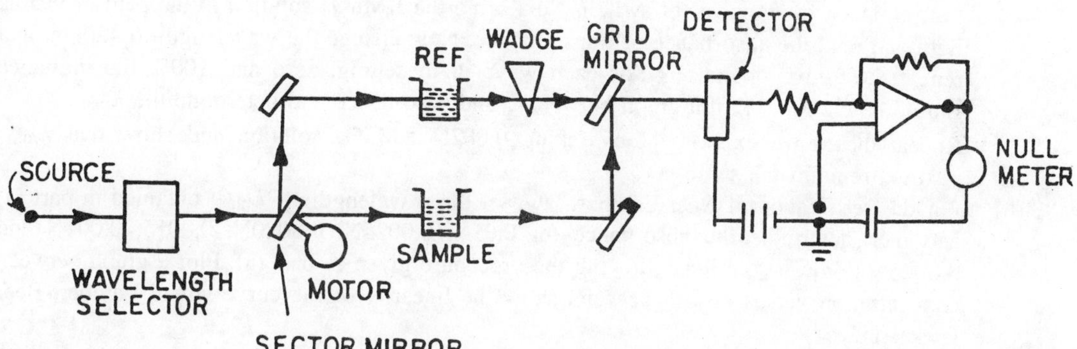

Fig. 14.19b. Double beam spectrophotometer (Alternate in time)

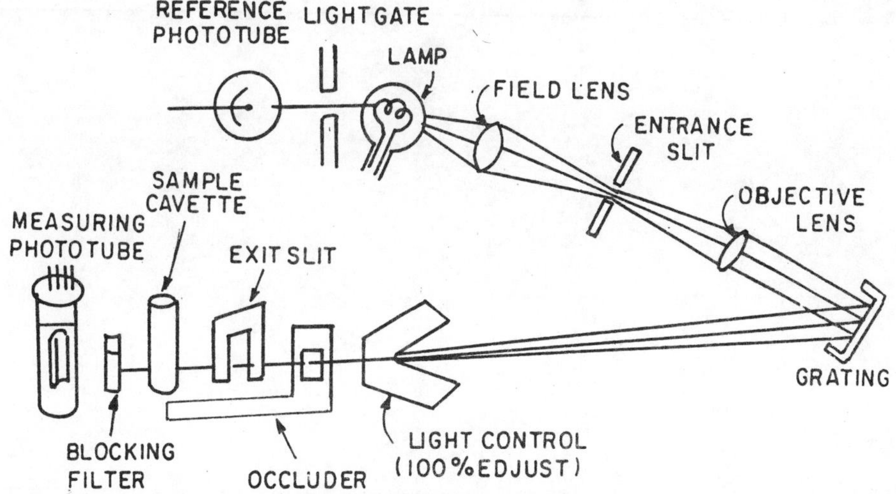

Fig.. 14.20. Optical diagram for Bausch and Lomb spectronic--20 colorimeter.

used in this arrangement. The reference signal is maintained constant by an automatic slit servo system which widens or closes the slit to achieve a 100% transmittance baseline.

EXERCISE 1

(a) Determine the λ_{max} for $KMnO_4$ solution. (b) Verify the Beer - Lambert Law.
(c) Find the concentration of a given unknown solution.

PROCEDURE :

(i) Prepare 100 ml of N/100 $KMnO_4$ as a stock solution
(ii) From the stock solution, prepare 100ml of each $KMnO_4$ solution of strength 0.0025N. 0.002N, 0.0015N, and 0.0005N.

PART (a) : For λ_{max} determination, take 0.001N $KMnO_4$. Take this solution in a 1cm path length cell. In another 1cm length cell put distilled water. Put these two cells in a cell holder and cover. Put the tungsten lamp on. Adjust zero transmittance by zero adjustment knob without opening the shutter of the phototube. Adjust the wavelength at 400 nm and bring the distilled water cell in the path of visible light and open the phototube shutter. Adjust 100% transmittance by the selector switch. Next bring the $KMnO_4$ solution in the path of visible light and read the absorbance or transmittance. Now change the wavelength to 420mm and repeat the above operations For each wavelength setting, zero and 100% transmittance should be checked. Plot a graph between c and absorbance and determine the λ_{max}.

Repeat the above experiment by taking 0.002N $KMnO_4$ solution and show that λ_{max}' position remains the same.

PART (b) : For the verification of Beer-Lambert law, set the wavelength at λ_{max}' obtained in part (a) and then determine the absorbance for 0.01N, 0.0025N, 0.0020N, 0.0015, 0.001N and 0.0005N $KMnO_4$ solution following the procedure given in part (a). Plot a graph between concentration versus absorbance and show the linearity of the curve where Lambert-Beer law is obeyed.

Observation table for part (a)

λ (nm)	0.001 N $KMnO_4$ Absorbance	0.002N $KMnO_4$ Absorbance
400		
420		
440		
460		
480		
500		
520		
540		
560		
580		
600		
620		
640		
660		
680		
700		
720		

Observation table for Part (b)

S.No.	Concentration (x-axis)	Absorbance (y-axis)
1.	0.0100N	
2.	0.0025N	
3.	0.0020N	
4.	0.0015N	
5.	0.0010N	
6.	0.0005N	

PART (c) : Fill the *unknown* given solution and determine the absorbance. From the graph, obtained in part - (b), determine, the concentration of the *unknown* given solution.

EXERCISE 2. Determination of a mixture of cobalt and nickel.

Method : 1. Prepare a standard solution (0.15M) of nickel by dissolving 4.36g of nickel nitrate hexahydrate in 100 ml of water.

2. Prepare a standard solution of cobalt (0.15M) by dissolving 4.36g of cobalt nitrate hexahydrate in water.

3. Prepare five different concentrations by diluting the standard solution of each of the compound.

4. Nickel absorbs at 395, 660 and 710 nm, therefore measure the absorbance of nickel at any of the wavelengths and also at 510 nm where cobalt absorbs.

5. Now, measure the absorbance of cobalt at 510 and 395 nm in the same manner.

6. Calculate the λ_{max} at each wavelength.

7. Now, prepare an *unknown* mixture from the two dilute solutions and measure the absorbance of the mixture at 395 nm and 510 nm.

8. Calculate the concentration of each component present in the mixture.

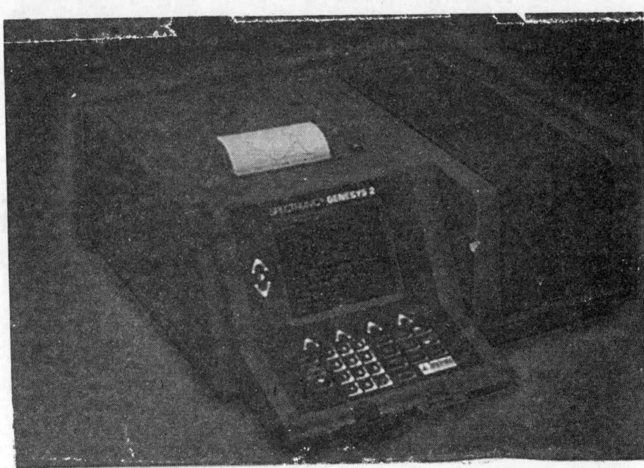

Fig. 14.21. Spectronic Genesys-2 UV/VIS Spectrometer (Courtesy of Spectronic Instruments).

15

Ultraviolet Spectrophotometry

15.1 General

UV radiation is that portion of the electromagnetic spectrum (EMS) which bridges the gap between the longest wavelength X-rays and the shortest wavelength visible light as shown in the chart below (Fig. 15.1)

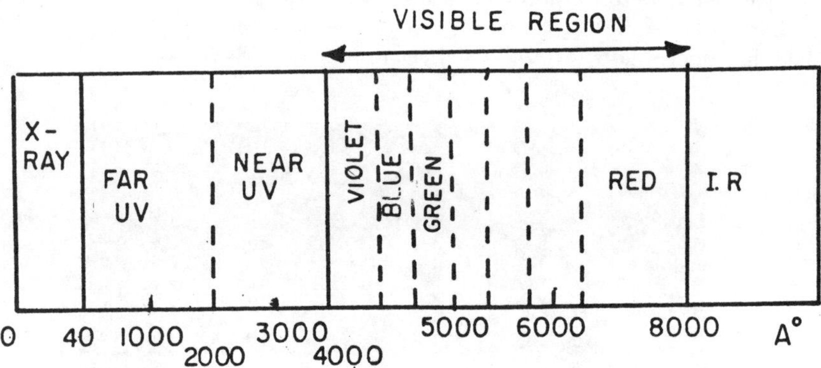

Fig. 15.1 UV region of EMS.

The UV region extends from 40 — 4000 A° and can be divided into *near* (2000 – 4000 A°) and *far* (40 – 2000 A°) regions. The far UV radiation is absorbed by air and also produces electronic transitions in atmospheric O_2, N_2 and CO_2. Therefore one must use vacuum apparatus to study far UV radiation. It is called the Vacuum UV. Further, glass absorbs radiation of wavelength less than 3000 A°. The instruments to study far UV must use quartz optics and quartz sample holders. Therefore, the region between 2000 – 3000 A° is called *quartz* region.

It takes radiation of higher energy to effect electronic transitions than to effect rotational and vibrational transitions. Electronic states in a molecule are thus always associated with a large number of vibrational and rotational states leading to a broad UV peak (Fig. 15.2). The electronic levels E_1 and E_2 of two electronic states (Fig. 15.2) are shown to be composed of a series of vibrational states V_o, V_1 V_2 etc and corresponding series of rotational states r_0 , r_1 , r_2 etc.

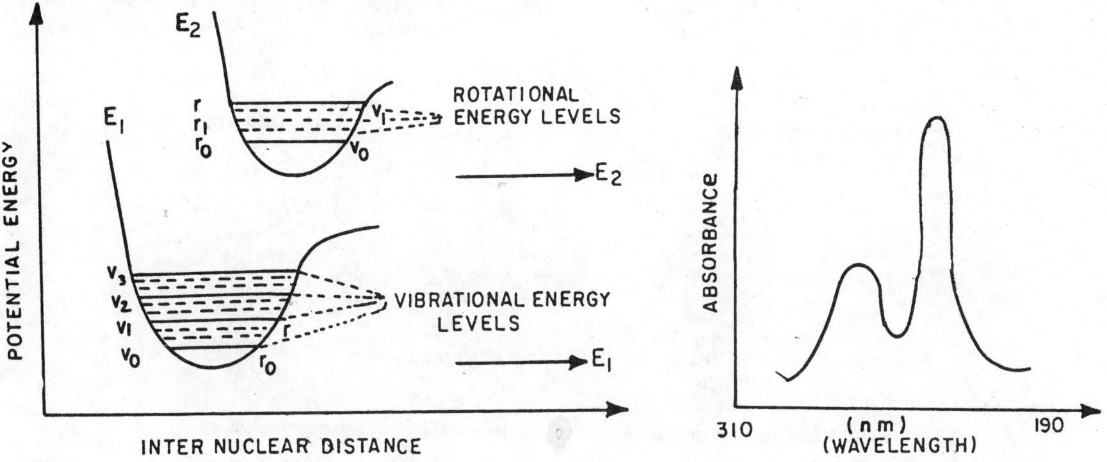

Fig. 15.2 Potential energy diagram.

Fig. 15.3 UV absorption Spectrum.

The energy associated with each photon in UV radiation is powerful in the range of 6.62×10^{-12} ergs whereas in case of microwaves energy per photon is 6.62×10^{-18} erg and can bring about only rotational transitions.

UV spectrum is a plot of *absorption intensity* (ordinate) VS wavelength in A° or nm (abscissa). Absorption intensity is plotted as ε or log ε and reported as ε_{max} meaning *maximum* molar extinction coefficient. The wavelength of absorption is reported as λ_{max} meaning maximum absorption.

The quantitative aspects of absorption spectrophotometry has already been dealth with in Chapter 14 and the same are applicable to the quantitive UV.

In case of an unknown substance where molecular weight (M) and hence molar concentration can be determined, the absorption intensity of 1 % solution of the substance is determined in a 1 cm cell. This is reported as $E|_{1\%}^{1cm}$ where E is the numerical value of the absorbance in a 1 unit cell of solution containing unit volume solution. E is called specific extinction coefficient, its relation to ε is

$$E|_{1\%}^{1cm} = \frac{10 \times \varepsilon}{\text{molecular weight}}$$

or $\quad \varepsilon = E|_{1\%}^{1cm} \times 0.1M$

15.2 Instrumentation

As already stated in the previous chapter sophisticated types of spectrophotometers for studies in UV and visible are commercially available alongwith operational details. There main components are : (i) a source of radiation (ii) a monochromator (iii) a dectector and (iv) a read out system. The properties and other requirement as well as design aspects have already been described . A schematic optical diagram of a double beam UV - Visible spectrophotometer is shown below (Fig. 15.4)

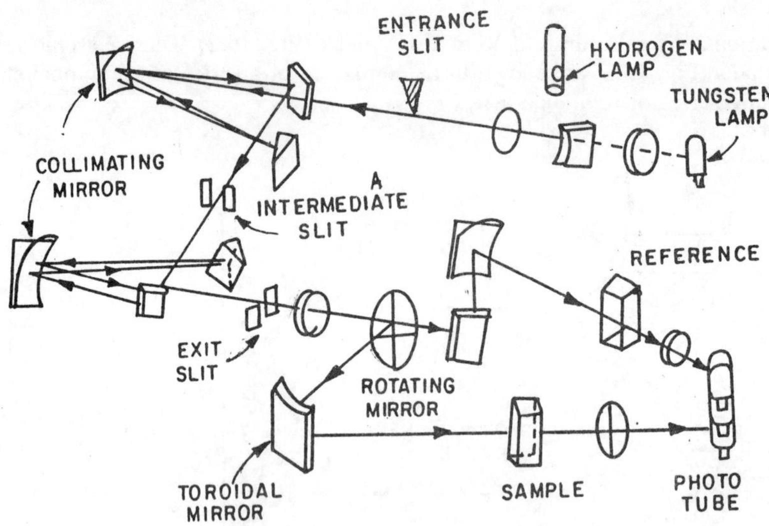

Fig. 15.4 Schematic optical diagram of double beam-in-time spectrophotometer.

In the operation of a spectrophotometer called double beam in time, a single beam of energy leaves the prism or grating monochromator and is alternately switched between the reference and sample paths to provide a double beam system within the sample compartment. The two beams are then recombined to fall on a single detector. The output of the detector is an alternating signal whose amplitude is proportional to the difference in intensities in the two channels. A slit servo continuously adjusts the slit opening of the monochromator to keep the energy through the reference cell constant at a 100% setting when the reference solution is in the light beam. A rotating half-sector mirror system is used to switch the reference and the sample paths. It is placed either before the entrance slit or after the exit slit of the monochromator.

In case of automatic recording spectrophotometers the measuring sequence is carried out automatically to provide the recorded data of the analysis. The sample - beam energy is compared automatically with reference beam energy and the ratio is the transmittance of the sample. Thus time consuming adjustments are eliminated and fast and accurate spectrograms are obtained.

15.3 Selection of Solvent

Pure water and ethanol shift the position and tend to broaden the bands. Highly pure non-polar solvents e.g. saturated hydrocarbons do not affect absorption bands. The solvents should have the ability to transmit radiation in the region of wavelength under study. They should not absorb in the same region as the solute.

The concentration of solutions should be in the range of $10^{-2} - 10^{-5}$ moles. The quantity of substance available for analysis should be in the range of 0.1 to 100 mg. The % transmittance should be between 20-65%, at high concentration the transmittance is low.

15.4 Absorption by Organic Molecules

It has been recognized that many substances appear coloured because they contain functional groups which are capable of absorbing radiation of certain wavelengths when ordinary light shines on them. Such functional groups which confer colour on substances are known as *chromophores*. They generally contain unsaturated bonds like C = C, C = O, N = N etc. The functional groups like — OH – NH_2, – Cl, – Br etc do not confer colour but have the ability to increase the colouring power of a chromophore and are called *auxochromes.* In other words the auxochromes do not absorb radiation longer than 200 nm, but when attached to a chromophore cause a shift in the absorption to a longer wavelength and also increase the degree of absorption; e.g. benzene has λ_{mas} at 254 nm whereas in case of phenol it shifts to 270 nm with ε_{max} at 1450 nm. A shift in the absorption peak of a chromophore from a standard position to longer wavelength is called *bathochromic shift* (blue shift) whereas to a short wavelength is called *hypsochromic shift* (red shift). When the degree of intensity is increased, it is called *hyperchromic shift* and when the intensity is decreased or lowered, it is called *hypochromic shift.*

(i) **Saturated Hydrocarbons**: In order to understand as to how substances absorb UV radiation one has to recall the fundamentals such as that the valence electrons are of three types namely : σ, π and non-bonding (n), and that the bond formation involves overlap of two orbitals each containing an electron. When two atomic orbitals overlap, the nature of the molecular orbital depends on whether the overlap occurs between two regions having the same sign or opposite sign. When the former occurs, the result is bonding orbital, whereas when the latter occurs the result is an anti-bonding orbital. In bonding orbitals, the electron charge is concentrated in the region between the two nuclei thereby holding the two nuclei together. On the other hand in anti-bonding orbitals electron charge is withdrawn from the region between the two nuclei thereby resulting in increased repulsion between the two nuclei. This is represented by the energy diagram (Fig. 15.5) below :

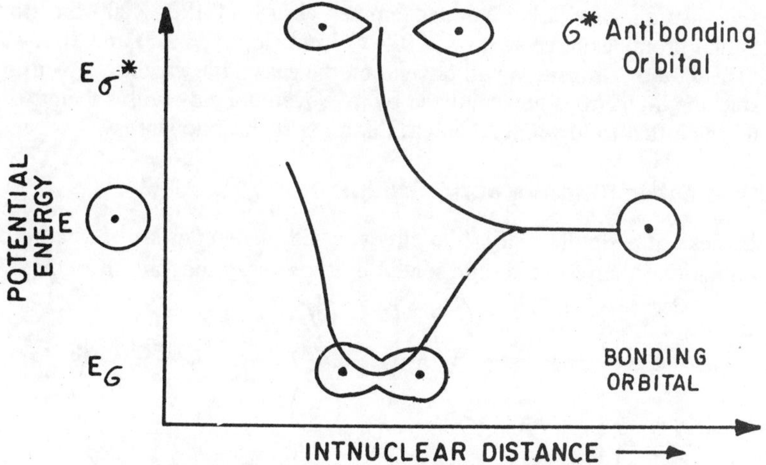

Fig. 15.5. Sigma (σ) bond in saturated hydrocarbons.

In the electronic state called ground state, both the electrons in the bonding orbital have opposite spin (↑↓) and no electrons are contained in the antibonding orbital. When energy absorbed equal to $\Delta E(\sigma \longrightarrow \sigma^*)$, takes place, the electronic transition from bonding to antibonding state occurs with retention of spins — this excited state is called *singlet state.* Since $\sigma \longrightarrow \sigma^*$ energy change is very high, it is found in vacuum UV region. Saturated hydrocarbons have C – C or C – H single bonds only (i.e. σ bonds) therefore they do not absorb in UV–Vis regions. However, the exception being cyclopropane, alicyclic compounds with small ring strain absorb at slightly longer wavelength at 190 nm.

15.4.1 Effect of Auxochromes on the Position of U.V. Bands

The functional groups like –ÖH, NH_2 and halogens possess a pair of non-bonded (n) electrons in addition to some sigma electrons. The n - electrons can be excited to σ^* energy level and since they are already at a higher energy level than the σ electrons in the molecule, the energy required for the n →σ * transition is less than that needed for σ → σ * i.e· $\Delta E_{(n\rightarrow\sigma)} < \Delta E_{(n\rightarrow\sigma)}$. This means that n→σ* transition occurs at longer wavelength than σ→σ* (Fig. 15.6).

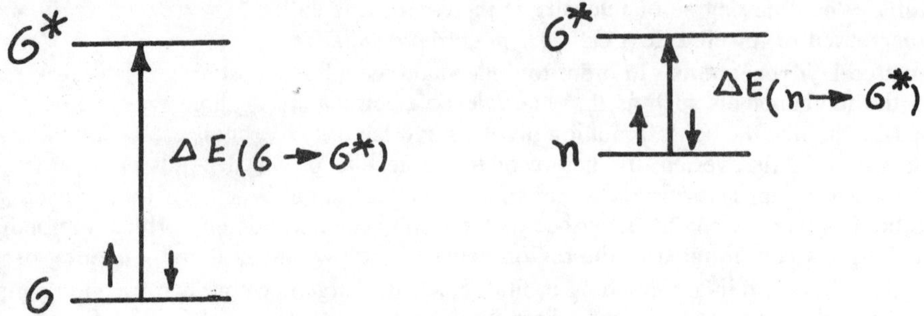

Fig. 15.6. σ → σ* and n → σ* *transitions.*

For example, saturated alcohols or epoxides absorb UV radiation at 180 — 185 nm (log ε = 2.5) involving n → σ^* transition. Similarly saturated amines absorb at 190 – 200 nm (log ε = 3.4). The saturated chlorides and bromides have λ_{max} of 170 – 175 nm (log ε = 2.5) and 200 – 210 nm (log ε = 2.6) respectively. The n → σ* transition will depend on the ease with which n - electrons can be excited. If, in the ground state the n-electrons are stabilized by hydrogen bonding with solvents or by other means, the absorption will be shifted to lower wavelength i.e. a hypsochromic shift will occur.

15.4.2 Olefinic and Other Chromophoric Groups

Let us consider the case of a simple olefin like ethylene. Ethylene consists of one σ - bond and one π–bond. The bond formation in ethylene is represented by the energy diagram in Fig. 15.7.

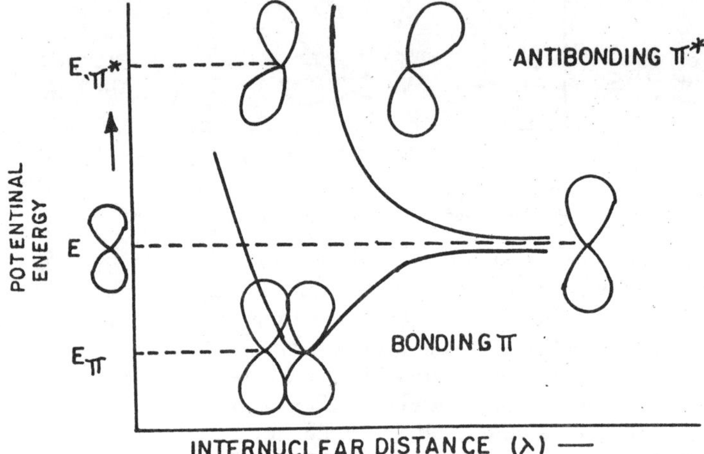

Fig. 15.7. π-Bond in ethylene.

The π bond is weaker than σ bond i.e. π -electrons are at higher energy level than σ electrons. consequently $\pi \longrightarrow \pi^*$ transition takes place at a longer wavelength than $\sigma \longrightarrow \sigma^*$ i.e. $\Delta E_{(\pi \longrightarrow \pi^*)} < \Delta E_{(\sigma \longrightarrow \sigma^*)}$. Thus substances like ethylene, propylene, 1-octene etc which contain *isolated* double bonds undergo $\pi \longrightarrow \pi^*$ transition at 170 – 200 nm. The $\pi \longrightarrow \sigma^*$ transition can also take place but for these transitions $\Delta E_{(\pi \longrightarrow \sigma^*)}$ is >> $\Delta E_{(\pi \longrightarrow \pi^*)}$ and therefore they are observed in far UV regions. Ethylene normally shows two peaks of unequal intensity, a stong peak at λ_{max} = 165 nm (ε_{max} = 10,000) and a weak peak at λ_{max} = 210 nm ($\varepsilon_{max} \cong 1000$). Both these peaks are due to $\pi \longrightarrow \pi^*$ transitions. However, if auxochromes are substituted for the ethylene protons (e.g. NR_2 to vinyl carbon) a bathochromic shift to 250 nm takes place. This shift is due to resonance interaction. Similarly, differences in the absorption spectra of cis and trans isomers of disubstituted olefins occurs. The values for λ_{max} and E_{max} of the trans isomer are generally greater than those of cis isomer e.g. in case of diphenylethylene (Ph(H)C = C(H)Ph) the trans isomer shows a $\pi \longrightarrow \pi^*$ transition at 259 nm (ε_{max} 27,000) while the cis isomer has a lower value at λ_{max} = 280 nm (ε_{max} = 13,500).

Thus we have learnt that transitions occur in molecules which contain isolated auxochromes or π or σ bonds All these transitions take place below 200 nm which is below the region for which commercial instruments are designed for laboratory work.

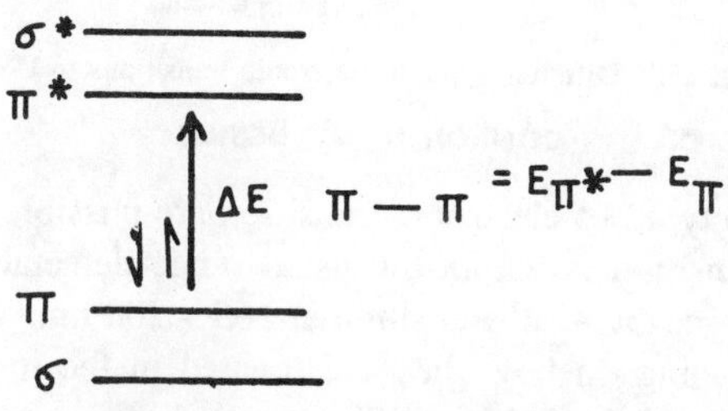

Fig. 15.8. $\pi \longrightarrow \pi^*$ transitions

Now, let us consider chromophoric groups like C = O, C = S, –N = N– in which σ, π and n - electrons are all present. The various types of transitions that can take place in these chemical moieties are : (i) $\sigma \longrightarrow \sigma^*$,(ii) $\sigma \longrightarrow \pi^*$, (iii) n $\longrightarrow \sigma^*$, (iv) $\pi \longrightarrow \pi^*$ (K– band). (v) n $\rightarrow$ p* (R-band) and (vi) $\pi \rightarrow \sigma^*$. These transitions are shown by means of an energy diagram in the Fig. 15.9. Of these various transitions only n $\longrightarrow \pi^*$ takes place in the region above 200 nm (with a low ε) e.g. in the case of acetaldehyde (CH_3—C(H) = O) n $\rightarrow \pi^*$ transitions takes place at 294 nm (log ε = 1.08) and $\pi \rightarrow \pi^*$ transition occurs at 190 nm (log ε = 2.0) So in general, an absorption at 275 – 294 nm region is a positive indication of an aldehyde or ketonic carbonyl function. The n $\longrightarrow \pi^*$ transition is also affected by the solvent and this will depend upon the nature of the chromophore itself, e.g. carbonyl group can be represented by its resonance or hybrid forms as :

$$>C=O \longleftrightarrow C^{+}—O^{-} = C^{\delta+} \cdot O^{\delta-}$$

Here, the degree of contribution to the hybrid by the polar form will depend on the nature of the substitution on the carbonyl carbon e.g. The electron releasing groups will make the hybrid more polar while the electron withdrawing groups will make it less polar. The hybrid will be stabilized by hydrogen bonding or non-bonding interactions of C = O with the solvent if its ground state structure is more polar than its structure in the excited state. Therefore, hypsochromic shift will occur in a polar solvent, e.g.

acetone absorbs at 279 nm due to n $\rightarrow \pi^*$ transition when the absorption is measured in a non-polar solvent like hexane. The value shifts to 264.5 nm when the absorption is measured in a polar solvent like water.

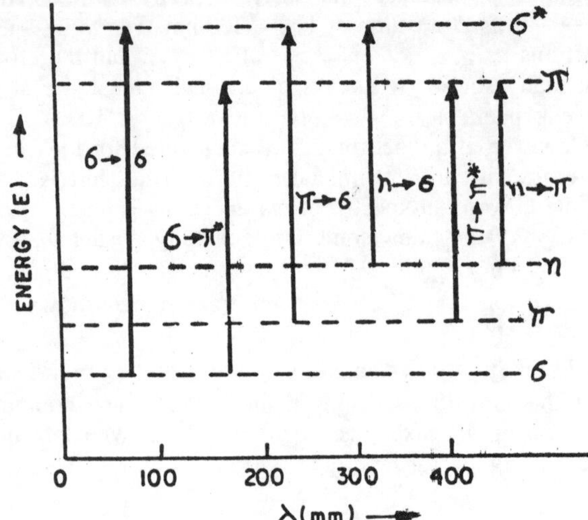

Fig. 15.9. Different type of electronic transitions in UV region.

15.4.3 Effect of Conjugation on the position of UV Bands

We have already learnt that 6 types of electronic transition are possible for various chromophoric groups and out of these n $\rightarrow \pi^*$ transition is within the usual range detectable in the laboratory instruments. Normally simple olefin undergoes $\pi \rightarrow \pi^*$ transition at 165 – 200 nm. When there are two double bonds, absorption will change depending on how they are located in the molecule. If two double bonds are isolated $\pi \rightarrow \pi^*$ transition will still be at 165 – 200 nm, when they are conjugated, absorption will occur at longer wavelength i.e. a bathochromic shift will be produced due to conjugation. It also means that conjugation lowers the energy needed for the excitation of electrons. One of the good examples of a system containing two conjugated double bonds is 1, 3-butadiene having a structure $H_2C = CH - CH = CH_2$. 1, 3-Butadiene is a diolefin and can be represented by its resonance structures as : $H_2C^{\delta+} - CH = CH - C^{\delta-}H_2 \longleftrightarrow H_2C^{\delta-} - CH = CH - C^{\delta+} H_2$. The energy requirement for 1, 3-butadiene can be explained by means of molecular orbital theory. In butadiene, all the 4 carbon atoms are sp^2 hybridzed, and one pure p orbital is associated with each carbon atom. Due to resonance $C_1 = C_4$ and $C_2 = C_3$. All the p orbitals can be treated as forming a molecular orbital (M.O.) covering all the four carbon atoms. The bonds produced are delocalized bonds. The wave equation for butadiene can be written as $C_1\Psi_1 + C_2\Psi_2 + C_3\Psi_3 + C_4\Psi_4$. The molecular energy diagram for ethylene and 1, 3-butadiene is shown in Fig. 15.10.

Thus in butadiene, the easiest $\pi \longrightarrow \pi^*$ transition involves excitation of electron from Ψ_3 to Ψ_3. The energy required is $E_{\Psi_3} - E_{\Psi_2} = \Delta E_2$ which is less than in ethylene. Therefore, π ——> π^* transition in conjugated system is at longer wavelength than in isolated olefin. 1, 3-Butadiene shows absorption at 220 nm in a non-polar solvent.

In an isolated carbonyl (C = O) group the $\pi \rightarrow \pi^*$ transition absorbs at 170 nm and n $\rightarrow \pi^*$ at 290 nm (e.g. acetaldehyde) but in crotonaldehyde which is a conjugated system the $\psi_2 \longrightarrow \psi_3^*$ transition occurs at 218 nm (ε_{max} = 18,000) and n $\longrightarrow \psi_3^*$ transition takes place at 320 nm (ε_{max} = 30 in ethanol) as shown in Fig. 15.11.

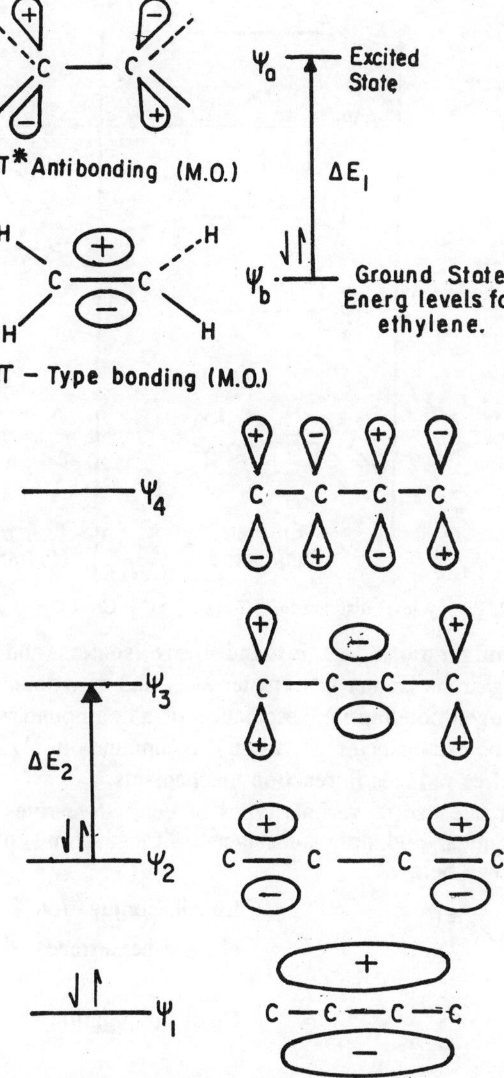

Fig. 15.10. Molecular orbital energy diagram for ethylene and 1, 3-butadiene.

15.5 Applications

The various applications of UV spectrophotometry in chemical and pharmaceutical analysis are enumerated below :

(i) Determination of structure of drug substances by using qualitative rules and comparing them with model compounds.

(ii) Quantitative estimations of drug substances and relating it to structure e.g. assay of alkaloids, antibiotics and other drugs.

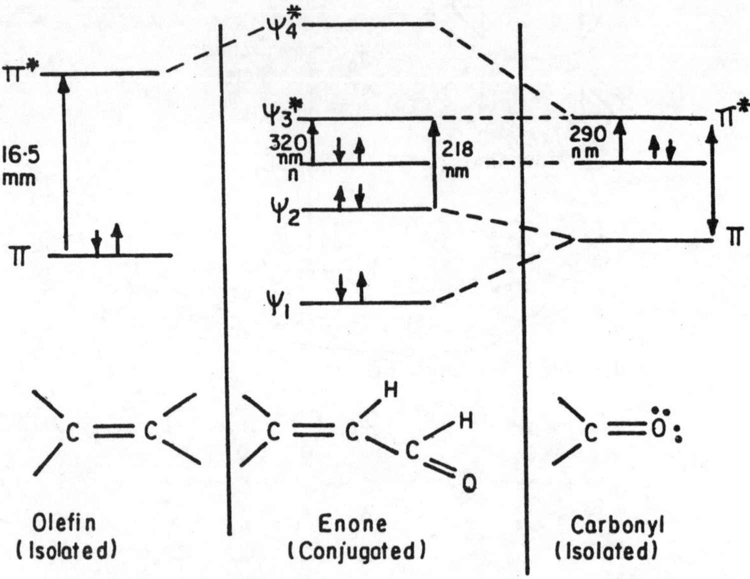

Fig. 15.11. Energy level diagram for C = C , C = C — C = O and C = O.

(iii) Determinations of configurations like *cis* and *trans* isomers and steric interactions between neighbouring atoms e.g. trans isomer has greater λ_{max} and ε_{max} than the cis isomer.

(iv) Determination of hydrogen bonding i.e. association of a compound with the solvent and its effect on the absorption can be established e.g. carbonyl compounds in H_2O.

(v) Detection of ions and free radicals in reaction mechanisms.

In order to be able to make use of various types of qualitative rules for solving the problems of structure elucidation of chemical and drug substances, various forms of chemical systems may be recognised and these are shown below :

(i) >C=C–C=C–C=C — Linear Conjugation (1, 3, 5-hexatriene)

(ii) >C=C(–C=C<)(–C=C<) — Cross conjugation

(iii) Cyclic diene

(iv) Semicyclic diene. (exocyclic double bond)

(v) A B — Homoannular diene (Two double bonds are conjugated

(vi) 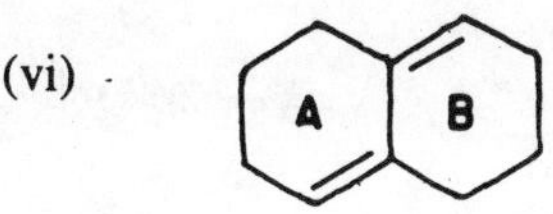

and are in the same ring)
Heteroannular diene
(Two double bonds belong
to two different rings)

Further various types of rules have been framed for calculating the theoretical (expected) values for chromophores incorporating above type of conjugated system and can then be compared with the observed values. These rules are titled as Woodward and Fieser rules for dienes and Nielson's rules for α, β - unsaturated ketones. Practice problems are available in the text books, However, a detailed correlation chart for solving such types of problems is incorporated in this Chapter.

15.6 The Interpretation of Ultraviolet Spectra

Empirical Rules for Calculating the Ultraviolet Absorption Maxima of Aliphatic and Alicyclic Compounds

I. α, β — Unsaturated ketones

Parent system $\;>\underset{\beta}{C}=\underset{\alpha}{\overset{|}{C}}-\underset{\underset{O}{\|}}{C}-R$ $\qquad \lambda_{max} = 215\ m\mu$

Structural variation	increment in λ_{max}
α — alkyl substituent	+ 10 mμ
β — alkyl substituent	+ 12 mμ
exocylic C = C	+ 5 mμ
cyclopentenone system	– 11 mμ
C = C extending conjugation	+ 30 mμ
each γ — or σ —alkyl substituent	+ 18 mμ
presence of a homoannular diene	+ 39 mμ

II. Conjugated Dienes

Parent system $\;>C=\overset{|}{C}-\overset{|}{C}=CR$ $\qquad \lambda_{max} = 214\ m\mu$

structural variation	increment in λ_{max}
alkyl substituent	+ 5
exocyclic C = C	+ 5
presence of homoannular diene	+ 39
C = C extending conjugation	+ 30

III. α, β — Unsaturated Acids and Esters

parent system $\rangle C = \overset{|}{C} - \underset{\underset{O}{\|}}{C} - OR$ λ_{max}— 200 mμ

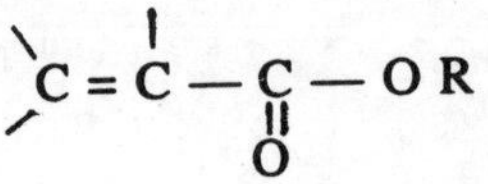

where R = H or alkyl

structural variation	increment in λ_{max}
alkyl substituent	+ 8
exocyclic C — C	+ 5

Empirical Rules for calculating the Ultraviolet Absorption Maxima of Benzene Derivative

Structure	λ_{max}
C_6H_5–$\overset{|}{\underset{|}{C}}$–	250—270 mμ (100—500)
C_6H_5–$\overset{|}{\underset{|}{\ddot{X}}}$– x = atom with at least one unshared electron pair	260–280 mμ (500–2000)
C_6H_5–$\overset{|}{C}$ = X X = C, O or N	240 — 250 mμ (10,000)
C_6H_5–$\overset{|}{C} = \overset{|}{C} - \overset{|}{C}$ = X X = C, O or N	280—290 mμ (10,000 — 30,000)

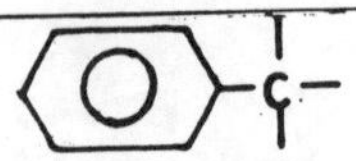

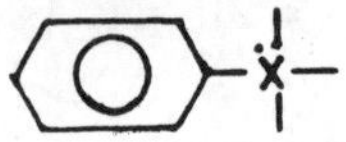

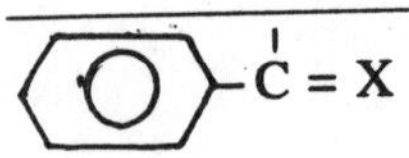

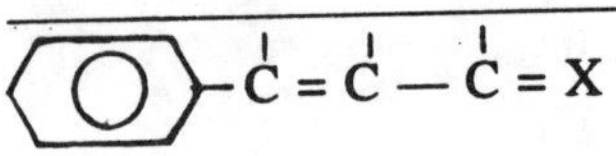

The Ultraviolet Absorption Spectra of Some Representative Compounds

Compounds	λ_{max} (ε)
isolated double bonds	
Acetaldehyde	293 mμ (ε 12)
acetaldehyde	204 mμ (ε 60)
acetone	271 mμ (ε 16)
acetonitrile	160 mμ
ethylene	193 mμ (Σ 10,000)

olefins (R = alkyl)	at 210 mμ (not max)
$RCH = CHR$ or $R_2C = CH_2$	ε 200 — 1000
$R_2C = CHR$ or $R_2C = CHR$	ε 1400 — 5600
$R_2C = CR_2$	ε 4400 — 10500
atiphatic and alicyclic conjugated systems	
butadiene	217 mμ (ε 20,900)
trans—$CH_3CH = CHCOCH_3$	224 mμ (ε 9.750), 314 mμ (ε 38)
cis — $CH_3CH = C(CH_3)COCH_3$	235.5 mμ (ε 4,570)
trans — $CH_3CH = C(CH_3)COCH_3$	230 mμ (ε 12,800)
Benzene derivatives	
aniline	230 mμ (ε 7,000), 280 mμ (ε 1470)
anisole	265 mμ (ε 2300)
benzene	256 mμ (ε 230)
phenol	273 mμ (ε 2050)
toluene	262 mμ (ε 270)
acetophenone	244 mμ (ε 13000), 278 mμ (ε 1100)
benzaldehyde	244 mμ (ε 15800), 280 mu (ε 1500)
benzoic acid	230 mμ (ε 10000), 270 mμ (ε 800)
benzonitrile	230 mμ (ε 12500), 270 mμ (ε 650)
nitrobenzene	252 mμ (ε 10000), 280 mμ (ε 1000) 330 mμ (ε 130)
styrene	244 mμ (ε 12000), 282 mμ (ε 450)
2, 4 — dinitrophenylhydrazones	
benzaldehyde 2, 4 — dinitrophenylhydrazone	378 mμ (ε 29,200)
propionaldehyde 2, 4 — dinitrophenylhydrazone	359 mμ (ε 21,800)
heterocycles	
furan	200 mμ (ε 10,000), 252 mm (ε 1)
pyridine	195 mμ (ε 7,500), 250 mμ (ε 2000)
pyrrole	210 mμ (ε 16,000), 340 mu (ε 300)
thiophene	235 mμ (ε 4.500)
aromatic systems with extended conjugation	
trans — benzalcetone	220 mμ (ε 12,000), 86 mμ (ε 23,500)

cis — benzalacetophenone	250 mμ (ε 13,700), 292 mμ (ε 8,800)
trans — benzalacetophenone	228 mμ (ε 9,800), 308 (ε 24,300)
benzophenone	252 mμ (ε 20,000), 330 mμ (ε 180)
diphenyl	252 mμ (ε 18,000)
naphthalene	220 mμ (ε 110,000), 275 mμ (ε 5,600), 314) mμ (320)
1 — phenylbutadiene	223 mμ (ε 12,000), 280 mμ (ε 28,000)
cis — Stilbene	230 mμ (ε 24,000), 285 (ε 12,000)
trans — stilbene	230 mμ (ε 13,000), 295 mμ (ε 25,000)

EXERCISE 1:

(a) Verification of Beers — Lambert Law with Benzoic acid.

(b) Find the concentration of an unknown solution.

PROCEDURE

(i) Prepare 500 ml of N/1000 benzoic acid as a stock solution.

(ii) From the stock solution, prepare 100 ml each benzoic acid solution of 2, 4, 6, 8 and 10 percent respectively. Determine the absorbance for each solution at 250 nm. Plot a graph between concentration versus absorbance and show that Beers—Lambert Law is obeyed.

(iii) From the stock solution, prepare another solution of unknown concentration. Determine the absorbance of this solution. Find the concentration of the solution from the graph obtained in step ii.

EXERCISE 2 : Determine the λ_{max} for benzene, phenol and aniline, using UV spectrophotometer and explain the shift in λ_{max} for phenol and aniline with respect to benzene. Also determine the λ_{max} for phenol in alkaline medium and aniline in acid medium. What change do you get in λ_{max} and why ?

Substance	λ_{max} E — Band	λ_{max} B — Band	Medium
C_6H_6			Neutral
C_6H_5OH			Neutral
C_6H_5OH			Alkaline (pH = 13)
$C_6H_5NH_2$			Neutral
$C_6H_5NH_2$			Acidic (pH = 3)

EXERCISE 3 : Determine in grammes per litre the quantity of sulphanilamide and sulphathiazole in a given mixture, using UV spectrophotometer.

Theory : When a solution contains several solutes the absorbances are additive, provided that there is no reaction between the components of the mixture.

Thus,

$$A_1 = A_{1,\,a}.\,1.C_a + A_{1,\,b}.1.C_b$$

and

$$A_2 = A_{2,\,a}\,.1.C_a + A_{2,b}.1.C_b$$

where $A_{1,a}$ and $A_{1,b}$ are the optical densities of a and b at λ_1; those at λ_2 are $A_{2,a}$ and $A_{2,b}$; C_a and C_b are the molar concentrations of the components in the solutions. The solution of these simultaneous equations is obtained by the method of determinants or successive approximation.

Apparatus : Spectrophotometer (ultra-violet range); 1.0 cm quartz cells; solutions of sulphanilamide and sulphathiazole in water (4 mg per litre each); mixed solution of sulphanilamide and sulphathiazole containing 3.2 (x) and 0.8 (y) mg per litre of water, respectively.

Procedure : Find the absorption peaks of the pure substance at 25°C. Measure the optical densities of the solutions of the pure components and of the mixed solution at the peaks thus found. Multiply each density by 250, in order to obtain the result in grammes per litre, and set up the two simultaneous equations.

Observation : The absorption curves show peaks at 260 mμ for sulphanilamide and 286 mμ for sulphathiazole. The optical densities found are shown in the table below :

Substance	Optical density	
	260 mu	286 mμ
Sulphanilamide	0.403	0.127
Sulphathiazole	0.272	0.315
Mixture	0.392	0.176

Calculations

$$0.392 = 0.403 \times 250x + 0.272 \times 250y$$

$$0.176 = 0.127 \times 250x + 0.315 \times 250y$$

Hence, x = 0.0033 and y = 0.0009 grammes per litre.

Prepare a similar table for given unknown mixture.

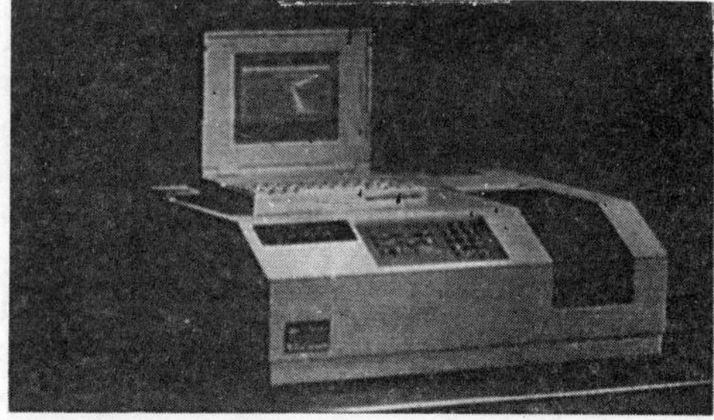

Fig. 15.12 UV-VIS Lambda 12/14 Spectrophotometer (Courtesy of Perkin Elmer)

16

Flame Photometry And Atomic Absorption Spectrophotometry

16.1 General

When an element is heated in a flame or an electric arc a spectrum of light is produced that is characteristic of the element. In flame photometry, a solution of a metal compound is sprayed into a flame, and the radiation emitted is compared to the radiation emitted by a known concentration of the same metal compound. The specific wavelengths emitted by the elements are observed as spectral lines in the visible and u.v. range. As the intensity of the spectral lines is proportional to the concentration of the elements in solution qualitative determinations can be performed by this procedure.

16.2 Theory

We have learnt from atomic structure that atoms exist in certain energy states in which their various electrons are arranged in definite energy levels. under normal conditions the electrons remain in the ground state at their lowest energy levels and do not radiate any energy. But when sufficient amount of external energy are added to an atom one or more electrons will be removed to higher energy levels that are farther removed from the nucleus of the atom.

The result in the formation of the excited state of the atom which is unstable due its short life time and the electrons will tend to return to the ground energy state. This return of electrons may take place in single jumps or a series of jumps and the extra energy imparted to the electrons will be emitted in the form of photons of radiant energy. The wavelength of these photons will be determined by the frequency of the energy difference between the energies of the atom in the ground and the excited state.

As the electrons exist in definite energy levels only certain electronic transitions in an atom are possible, the number of wavelengths or spectral lines emitted by the excited atom will be limited. The collection of spectral lines produced by an excited atom is called its ''emission spectrum'' and will be characteristic of that atom. Generally speaking, the ''line spectra'' are produced due to the excitation of the electrons in the outer most shell of the atom because these electrons are weakly held to the nucleus

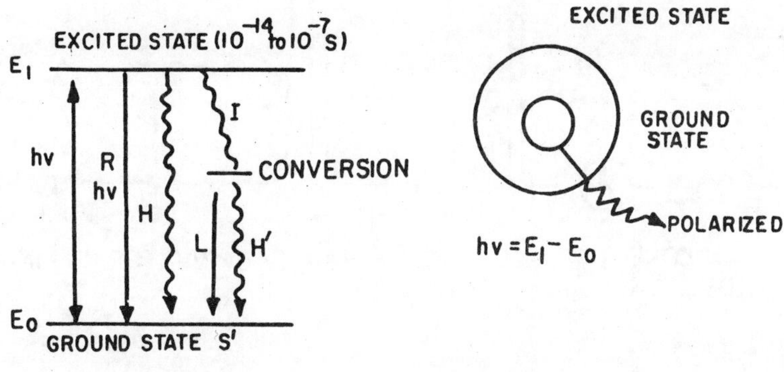

Fig. 16.1. Electronic Excitations.

and can be readily excited than those which are placed deeper in the atom. The intensity of a spectral line is normally related to the number of excited atoms, but is mainly depended upon the frequency of quantum of energy (i.e. photon) released when an electron jumps from one energy level to another.

Emission spectra are of three types, namely : (a) Line (b) Band and (C) continuous. The line spectra consist of sharply defined and often widely and irregularly spaced individual lines of a single wavelength. These spectra are characteristic of the elements and are due to excitation of gaseous atoms or atomic ions. The line spectra are also called as *atomic spectra* and are used for the purpose of analysis.

Band spectra consist of groups of lines, each of a single wavelength that become closely spaced as they approach the end of the band. The band spectra are also called "molecular spectra" since they are radiation emitted by excited molecules.

Continuous spectra are obtained when solids are heated to incandescence. They are characterised by the absence of any sharp lines as a function of wavelength, on the other hand when gases and vapours are heated to high temperature, they yield a series of lines or bands.

16.3 Means Of Excitation

The emission spectra of elements can be produced with aid of an (i) electric arc or (ii) electric spark or by (iii) thermal energy of a flame. In electrical excitation, a direct current or alternating current arc or an electric spark is used as the source. Liquid or powdered samples for analysis are placed upon or incorporated in a carbon electrode. In order to excite the sample, an arc or a series of sparks are then applied which carry the current across the gap between this electrode and a second electrode placed a short distance away (1—20 mm). The intensities of spectral lines obtained with a spark source are more constant and reproducible than those obtained with an arc source. The arc sources provide a higher sensitivity of detection than spark sources.

A common source for producing emission spectra of elements is a hot flame. The temperatures of the flame vary with the gas used for combusion, but they are generally lower than those obtained by

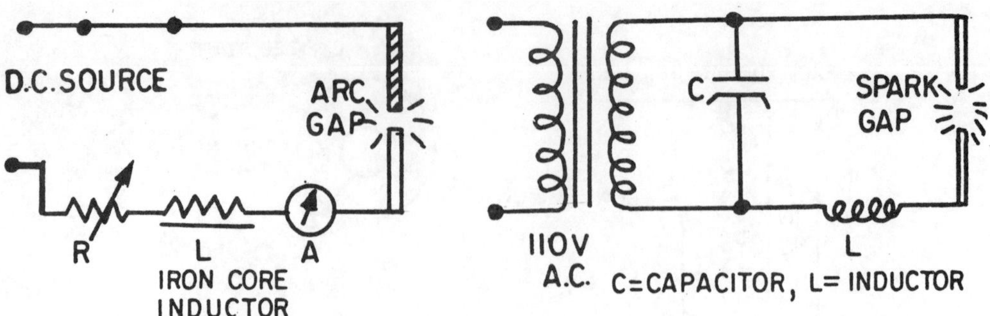

Fig. 16.2. Electric Arc

Fig. 16.3. Electric spark

electrical means. An ordinary natural gas-air flame has sufficient energy to excite the alkali metals like Li, Na, K but for divalent metals like Ca, Mg, Ba etc hotter flames (H_2, acetylene with O_2) are needed.

A flame is used for (i) transforming the sample to be analysed from the solid or liquid state into the gaseous (ii) decomposing the molecular compounds of the sample into simpler molecules or atoms and (iii) exciting the atoms to emission.

The main requirements of a satisfactory flame are (a) proper temperature to carry out the main functions of the flame (b) spectrum of the flame should not interfere with the emission of the material being analysed.

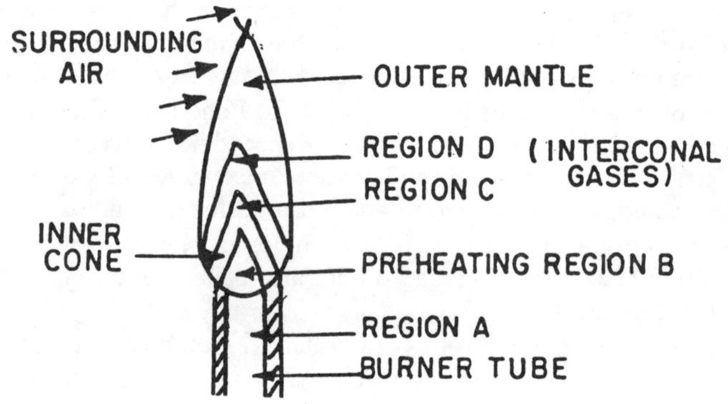

Fig 16.4 Structure of a Flame

The structure of a flame is shown in the Fig. 16.4 the unburnt gas mixture which emerges from the region A of the burner tube passes into a region of pre-heating region B (1 mm thickness) in which it is heated by conduction and radiation from the reaction zone C and by diffusion of radicals into it, which initiate oxidation. No chemical and thermal equilibrium exists in region B. The gases emerging from zone C, consists mainly of CO, CO_2, H_2 and H_2O (and N_2 if air is used as one of the original gases) with smaller amounts of species like H, O and OH, but the actual composition will depend upon the initial mixture. The thermal equilibrium will be completely reached in zone D. In the outermost mantle, flame comes into contact with ambient àir, which causes on one hand cooling effect and on the other hand a gradual supply of fresh O_2 for further combustion of the flame gases.

It is reported that flames excite fewer lines of each element and reproducible conditions of excitation are difficult and consequently accurate quantitative evaluation becomes difficult.

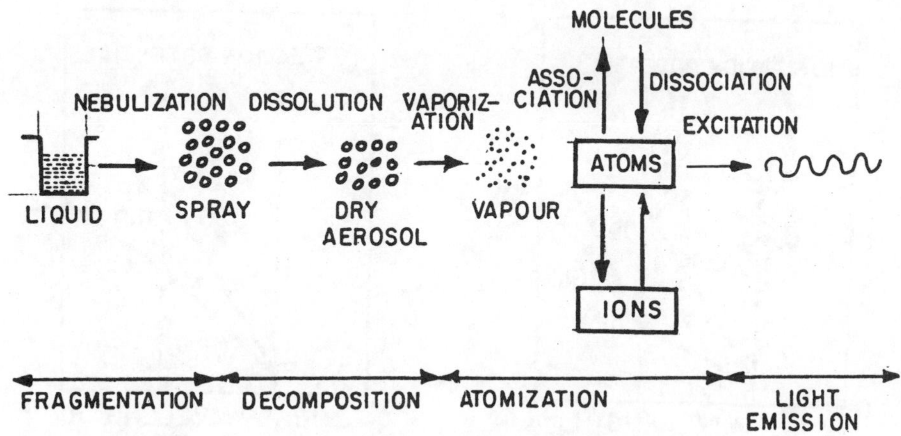

Fig. 16.5 Sequence of events the sample undergoes.

16.4 Emission Spectra

When a solution of a sample in the form of an aerosol is uniformly delivered into a flame, the following changes occur : (i) The water or other solvent is vapourized leaving minute particles of dry salt, (ii) at the high temperature of the flame, the dry salt is vapourized and part or all of the gaseous molecules are progressively dissociated to give neutral atoms which are the potential emitting species (iii) some of the free metal atoms may unite with other radicals or atoms in the flame gases and are introduced into the flame concomitantly with the test element, (iv) the vapours of the neutral atoms or molecules of the test element are then excited by the thermal energy of the flame. Ionization of the neutral atoms may also occur to some extent, (v) the excited atoms or molecules or ions fall back to the ground electronic state, partly by collision with other species and partly by emission of light.

The process which takes place after the formation of the gaseous salt molecules can be explained as follows :

e.g. NaCl + OH (from flame gases) $\rightleftharpoons$ NaOH + O (from flame gases) $\rightleftharpoons$ NaO

Gaseous molecules $\rightleftharpoons$ neutral atoms $\rightleftharpoons$ ionized atoms

NaCl $\qquad$ $Na^o + Cl^o$ $\qquad$ $Na^+ + e^-$

The neutral atoms and ionized atoms of Na, the molecules of NaOH and NaO will be excited and produce their characteristic emission spectra. The equilibrium quantities of various species will depend on variables like (a) flame temperature, (b) gas-phase components, (c) free electron concentration, and (d) other anionic species besides OH radicals and oxygen atoms.

By controlling the temperature of the flame, the number of elements excited and the type of energy level transition can be regulated. The most prominent line in each case is the line resulting from the transition between the lowest excited level and the ground state.

It should be understood that the emission power varies with temperature and is controlled by excitation or Boltzman factor $e^{-Ej/KT}$ which depends exponentially on temperature.

Where K = Boltzman constant.

E_j = excitation energy of the excited state.

Also, for a given emission line, the occupation number of an excited energy level, N_j is related to the number of ground state (not introduced into the flame) N_o.

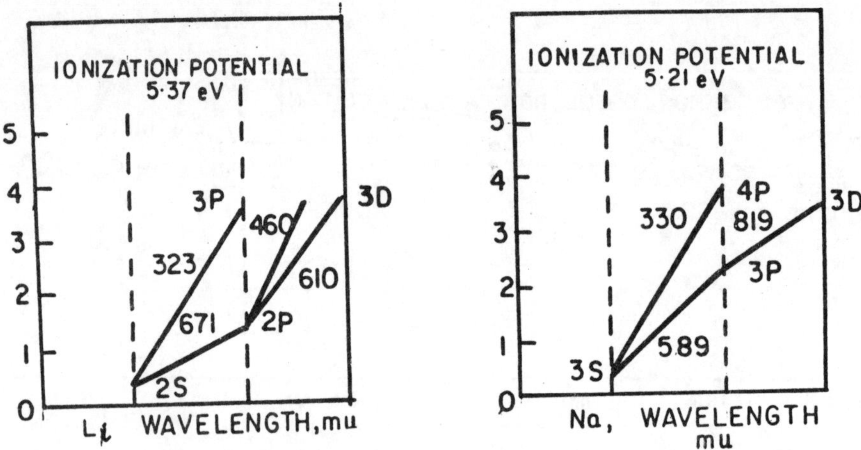

Fig. 16.6. Partial energy level diagram for Li and Na.

$$\therefore \quad N_j = N_o \frac{g_i}{g_o} e^{-E_j/kT}$$

Where g = statistical weights for particular energy level and at values of $\frac{N_J}{N_O}$ for lines for elements calculated at different temperatures.

Usually the fraction of atoms in the first excited level is a small fraction of the total number of atoms introduced into the flame and becomes appreciable only at high temperature. Consequently the ionization reduces the content of neutral metal atoms in the flame and there is decrease in the emissivity of atomic spectral lines. This can be explained by means of equations for example for an element A as given below:

Ionization of A : $A = A^+ + e^-$

$$K_1 = \frac{[A^+[e^-]}{[A]} = \frac{X^2}{(1 - X^2)} P$$

Where X = degree of ionization, P = partial pressure of metal in all forms of burnt gas in atmosphere

The change in degree of ionization with temperature can be obtained by Saha equation stated below:

$$\text{Log } K_1 = \frac{-5050 E_i}{T} + \frac{5}{2} \log T - 6.50 \log \frac{g_A + g_{e-}}{g_A}$$

where E_i is ionization potential in eV, T is absolute temperature and g is statistical weights of ionized atoms.

16.5 Instrumentation Aspects

The light emitted by excited atoms can be examined by means of a spectrophotometer. Each wavelength of the emitted radiation can be adjusted and allowed to pass through slit systems in a spectrophotometer. Then they are made to strike a photomultiplier tube which generates a signal indicating the intensity of the spectral line. In this way routine quantitative analysis of inorganic materials by emission spectroscopy can be achieved by a direct method.

Generally speaking for the quantitative analysis of alkaline earth metals like Li, Na, K and alkaline earth metals like Ca, Mg and Ba, an inexpensive system like a Photoelectric flame photometer is routinely used as it is easy to isolate the required light by means of filters alone. A schematic diagram for a simple flame photometer is represented in the Fig. 16.7.

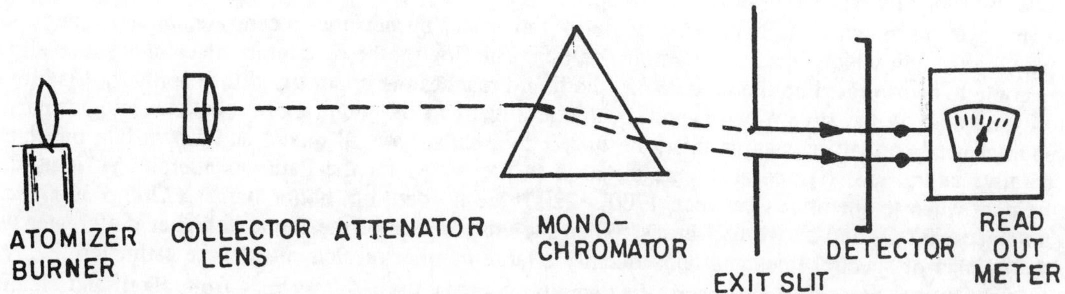

Fig. 16.7 A schematic diagram of a Flame Photometer.

The components of a simple flame photometer consist of (i) an atomizer, (ii) a burner, (iii) an optical system, (iv) a photosensitive detector and (v) a read out meter for indicating the output or the final concentration.

(i) Atomizer and Burner: The most important part of a flame photometer is the atomizer-cum-burner assembly. The function of an atomizer is to produce a fine, uniform spray of the solution containing the sample. The spray is carried to the burner flame by the stream of oxidant (air or O_2) that supports the combusion of fuel gas (methane, propane or butane). The apparatus is also provided with pressure regulators and flow meters to regulate the fuel and the oxidant so that reproducible spray and flame characteristics are maintained during the analysis.

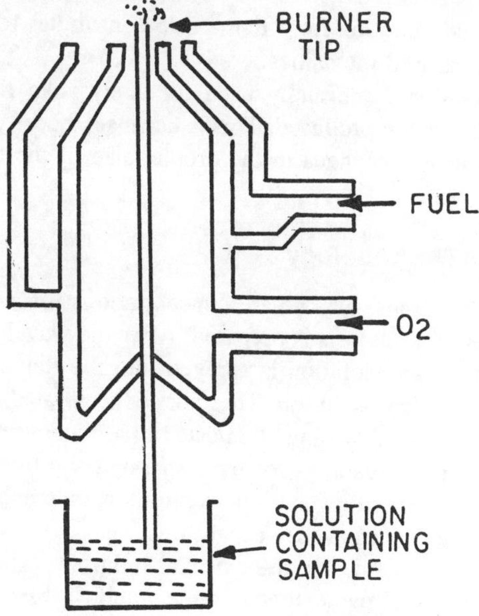

Fig. 16.8. An Atomizer-cum-burner assembly.

The atomizer may be a separate component or may be combined with the burner as a single unit. In an atomizer that is separate from the burner component the stream of oxidant atomizes the sample solution in the atomizer chamber. The larger drops contained in the aerosol collect along the walls of the chamber and are removed through a drain. While the fine droplets are carried in the form of a mist to the burrer flame. Before the sample mist reaches the burner, it gets mixed with fuel gas. An ordinary meeker burner can be used for this type of atomizer.

However, in the case of combined assembly of atomizer-burner unit, a central capillary tube is also attached to the unit which dips in the sample solution. The flow of the oxidant in the capillary tube allows the sample to be aspirated up the tube. When the liquid reaches the upper tip of the capillary, it is broken into a fine mist by the stream of oxygen. In this arrangement the atomizer becomes an integral part of the burner head so that the sample mist, the fuel & the oxidant are all mixed and drawn into the flame. Generally, natural gas, H_2 and acetylene are used as fuel gases for the flame excitation. Air is used as an oxidant when temperatures between 1700 – 2200° are needed, but hotter flames (2700 – 3200°) can be obtained with O_2 and above fuel gases. When the temperature of the flame is higher the greater will be the number of spectral lines and consequently a large number of elements can be estimated.

(ii) Optical System and Detector : In flame photometry the spectral lines from alkali and alkaline earth metals can be obtained with low temperatures and for this purpose an ordinary flame photometer with built in filters is adequate for their determination. The spectral lines thus obtained passes through the filter and falls on the phototube where it is converted into an electric current which can be measured directly or is first amplified and then measured

16.6 Sources of Errors in Flame Photometry

In quantitative flame photometry various types of errors and interferences can crop up due to factors enumerated belows :

(i) An unstable flame and an atomizer that does not deliver the standard and the unknown sample solution at a constant rate or droplet size will lead to an error. Therefore a controlled flow rate of the fuel and the oxidant is required.

(ii) The continuous background radiation from flame also contributes to the error and therefore should be subtracted from the measured intensities.

(iii) Although an aqueous solution is normally used for analysis in flame photometry but when an organic solvent is used, errors are produced. This is because, vicosity and surface tension of organic solvent being different leads to changes in the droplet size of the mist and the rate at which it is delivered to the flame.

16.7 Calibration Curve and Methodology

To begin with a series of solutions of known concentrations of a standard whose composition approximates that of the element for analysis is prepared. After the wavelength for analysis is chosen and the flame is properly adjusted a blank solution is sprayed into the flame. The instrument is adjusted to give a zero meter reading for the blank solution. The most concentrated solution of the standard is then introduced into the flame and the meter reading is adjusted to a maximum value. Thereafter, without any further instrument adjustments, meter readings for the remaining solutions of the standard are taken and a calibration curve of emission intensity versus concentration is prepared. Usually a straight line is obtained, but there can be a deviation from the straight line.

Now, Under the same instrument conditions, the unknown solutions from a sample under investigation are introduced into the flame in the same manner. Meter readings for these unknown solutions are read and their concentrations are obtained from the standard curve. In order to ensure that constant conditions are maintained throughout the analysis period, the standard solutions are usually checked before, during and after the analysis of each series of unknown solutions.

16.8 Atomic Absorption Spectrophotometry

16.8.1 General

Three types of flame methods for the quantitative analysis of inorganic substances (elements) are available. These are stated as ; (i) flame emission, (ii) atomic absorption and (iii) atomic fluorescence. All of them involve a procedure in which a fine spray of the sample solution is introduced into a flame where it is desolvated, vapourized and atomised. The emission spectroscopy and the flame method has already been discussed in detail. In this portion atomic absorption technique will be explained.

16.8.2 Atomic Absorption

In this method, radiation from an external light source emitting the spectral line that corresponds to the energy required for an electronic transition from the ground state to an excited state is passed through the flame. The flame gases are treated as a medium containing free unexcited atoms capable of absorbing radiation from the external source. When the radiation corresponds exactly to the energy required for a transition in a particular inorganic element from the ground electronic state to an upper excited state, unabsorbed radiation then passes through a monochromator. The monochromator isolates the exciting spectral line of the light source. It is then emitted and passed to the detector.The absorption of radiation from the light source depends on the population of the ground state which will be proportional to the concentration of the solution sprayed into the flame. The absorption is determined by the difference in the transmitted signal in the presence and absence of the test element.

In atomic absorption spectroscopy the unexcited atoms are able to absorb radiation from an external source (usually a hollow cathode lamp) at the same characteristic wavelength. The procedure involves in the production of uncombined and unionized atoms in the atomic vapour.

The ratio of the number of atoms which become excited N^* to the number which remain in the ground state N^o is given by Boltzman distribution as explained below :

$$\frac{N^*}{N^\circ} = A \exp - \frac{E}{kT} \quad \text{Also } E = h\nu = h\frac{c}{\lambda}$$

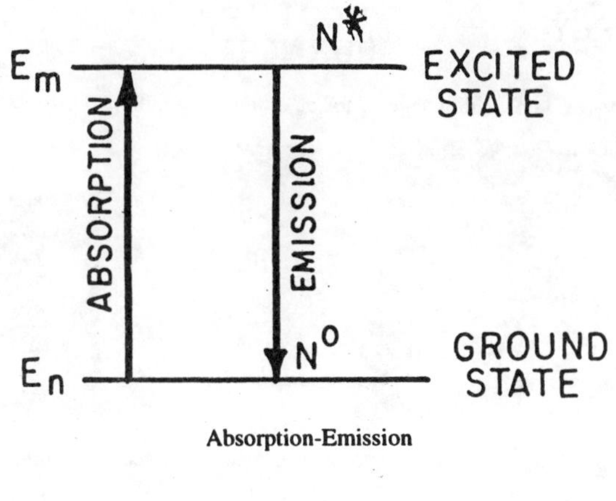

Absorption-Emission

We can also use the equation :

$$\frac{N^*}{N^\circ} = \frac{g_m}{g_n} e^{-\Delta E/kT}$$

where g_m and g_n are statistical weights of the two states.

or we can use :

$$I_V = VA_{nm}\, h\nu N^o \left(\frac{g_m}{g_n}\right) e \left(\frac{-\Delta E}{kT}\right)$$

Where I_V is the intensity of spectral emission V = flame volume, A_{nm} = Einstein transition probability that the excited atom will make the transition E_m - E_n in unit time with emission of a photon.

16.8.3 Atomic Fluorescence

In this mode, the method comprises the irradiation of the atomic vapour of a test element into the flame with a suitable illuminating source placed at right angles to the flame and the optical axis of the spectrometer. The incident radiation will be absorbed at wavelengths corresponding to the atomic absorption and will be then released in the form of fluorescence. The emitted radiation will depend upon the number of fluorescing atoms and therefore on the concentration of the solution sprayed into the flame. The source of illumination is a hollow - cathode lamp and the fluorescence emission is observed at an angle of 45° or 90°.

16.9 Instrumentation Components

A schematic diagram for an atomic absorption spectrophotometer is shown in the Fig. 16.9 The atomic absorption spectrophotometers available in the market can be operated in the emission mode by using the same flame and the atomizer or nebulizer system. Therefore, they can be used for both emission or absorption work and in a routine manner a large number of inorganic elements can be quantitatively estimated.

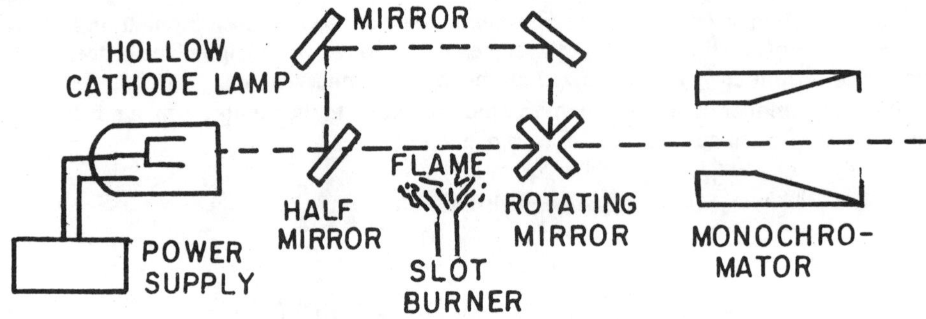

Fig. 16.9a. Schematic Diagram for an atomic absorption spectrophotometer

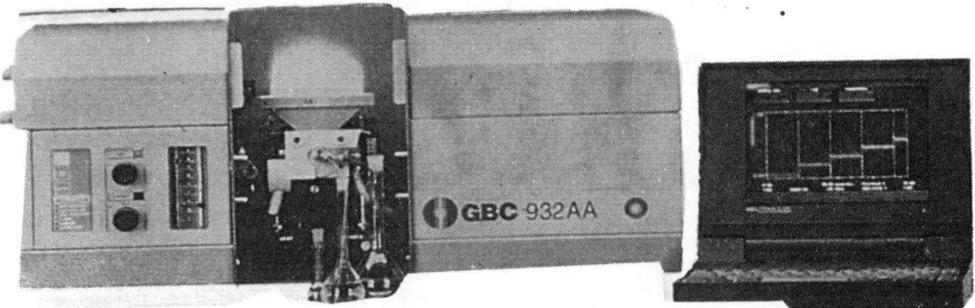

Fig. 16.9b. Model GBC-932 atomic Absorption spectrophotometer

The important components of an atomic absorption spectrophtometer are : (i) pressure regulator and flow meters (for fuel and oxidant) (ii) nebulizer and burner assembly (iii) optical system, (iv) detector, amplifier and read out system, and (v) a suitable light source like hollow cathode lamp.

For reproducibility and error free results, a constant thermal environment in the flame is required, therefore gas pressure and gas flow are held constant. Generally the pressure for fuel is maintained around 10 Psi and 30 Psi for oxidant and a flow range of 1 – 4 litre per minute.

In order to convert the test substance in the sample solution into atomic vapour, a premixed and laminar type of burner shown in Fig. 16.10 is used. In the premixed burner, an aerosol is produced in the mixing chamber. The coarse and fine droplets of the aqueous sample solution are separated whereby the fine droplets are converted into a mist which is delivered into the flame. The flow spoilers inside the expansion chamber ensure adequate mixing and smooth delivery to the flame. The fuel and oxidant are mixed in the body of the burner along with aspirated sample. In the laminar type of burner, the burner head is usually elongated and consists of an array of holes to get a maximum amount of flame. The burner is made up of aluminium or stainless steel and has a 10 cm slot and is of 0.38 – 0.6 mm in width.

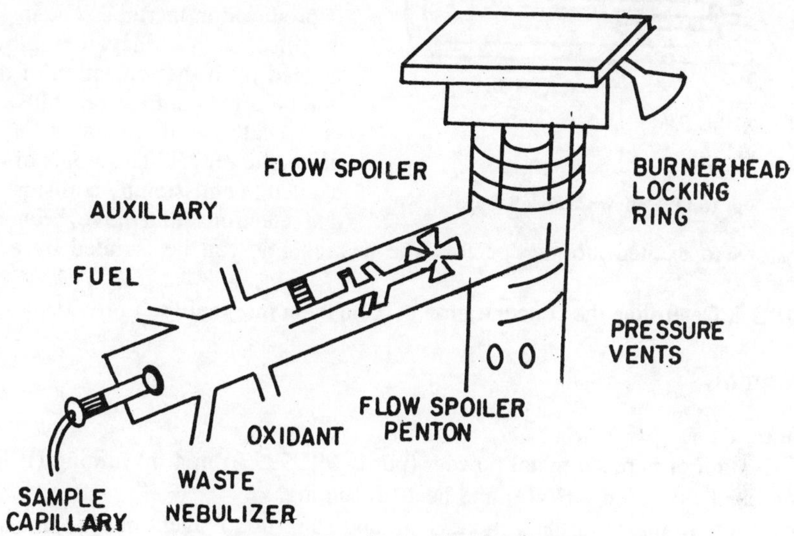

Fig. 16.10. Premixed and Laminar burner

The composition and temperature of the flame is given in table 16.1 below :

Table 16.1

Fuel	*Oxidant*	*Temperature °K*	*Burning Velocity*
1. Natural gas	Air	1700–1900	55cm/sec.
2. Propane (0.3)	" (8)	2000	45 " "
3. Acetylene (1.2)	" (8)	2450	16011
4. Hydrogen (6)	" (8)	2300	320
5. Acetylene (3.5)	Nitrous oxide (10)	3200	220

The most convenient method to measure atomic absorption at the peak is to use a sharp light line

The most convenient method to measure atomic absorption at the peak is to use a sharp light line source of appropriate wavelength i.e. a lamp emitting a sharp atomic spectrum of the element. The first resonance line which corresponds to the transition from the ground to the lowest excited state is normally used. The light of a specific element must not suffer interference from other spectral lines such as from (a) impurity elements, (b) electrode material or (c) carrier gas.

The most common source of excitation or line source used in atomic absorption spectroscopy is a hollow cathode lamp that generates a line characteristic of specific elements. A design of a hollow cathode lamp is described below :

It consists of an anode and a cylinderical cathode enclosed in a glass-tight chamber. The cathode is made up specified element and is cup shaped. The material of which anode is made is not critical. The tube is evacuated and filled with an ultrapure filler (carrier) gas like argon or neon at 1.5 torr. By applying a high potential (100 - 200 V) across the electrodes a low pressure discharge is produced in the tube. The inside of the cathode is filled with a negative glow. Positive ions formed from the ionization of the inert filler gas bombard the cathode on collision with the metal in the cathode, the metal is "*sputtered*" into the discharge region. The atoms of the metal are then excited to emission by collisions with the gas ions and electrons that have been solwed down by previous collisions to excited atomic spectra. The desired line can be isolated by a narrow bad pass monochromater.

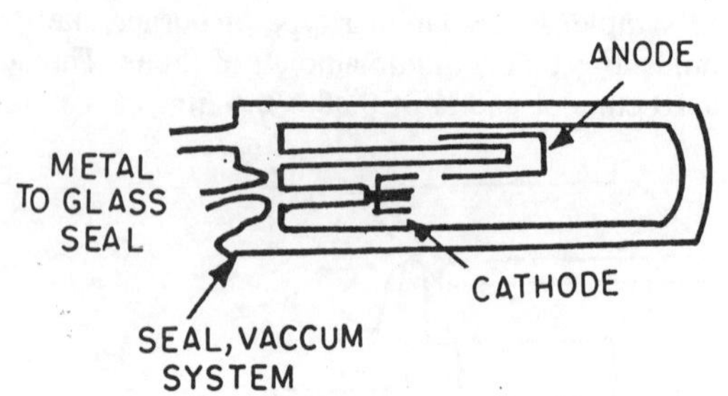

Fig. 16.11. Hollow Cathode Lamp.

EXERCISE 1. Determine the concentration of Zinc in an inorganic salt provided to you using A.A.S.

Standard Solution

(a) Stock Solution

1. Dissolve 0.1 gm of pure Zn metal powder (purity 99.9999%) in 4 ml fuming HCl. and heat to near dryness. Add 1 ml. fuming HNO_3 and heat till fuming.
2. Cool and dilute to make up the volume 1 lit. and store in a reagent bottle. This stock solution has 100 ppm of Zn.

(b) Working Solution

1. Dilute 1 ml. of stock solution with water to make up total volume 50 ml. This will give a working standard solution of λ ppm Zn concentration.

Sample Preparation

1. Weigh 0.1 to 0.2 gm of sample salt and mix in 4 ml of conc. HCl in a 10 ml beaker. Heat the solution near dryness and again add 4 ml of conc. HCl heat again to near dryness. Finally add 1 ml of fuming HNO_3 and heat for sometime.
2. Dilute the sample 100 times with deionized water.

Setting of the Instrument

(Standard condition). Set the followings :

1. λ : 214 nm
2. Hollow cathode Lamp : 15 mA.

3. Slit : 4
4. Function : Absorption
5. Range : UV
6. Fuel Pressure in control Pannel : 8 lb/sq. in.
7. Air Pressure in control Pannel : 30 lb/sq. in.
8. Flow rate fuel air : 9 : 9
9. Flame : reducing (lean blue)

Sample Analysis

Operate the instrument as per instructions given by the instructor or in the manual.

Calculation

$$\text{Conc. of Zn} = \frac{\text{Reading in ppm}}{\text{wt. of sample (in ppm)}} \times \text{dilution factor} \times 10^{-6}$$

Results

μg/g of sample or ppm/ml of solution.

EXERCISE 2. Determine the conc. of Cu in the (bone) material provided to you.

Preparations

1. Standard Solution

Take 1 gm of Cu metal powder or Cu SO_4 equivalent to 1 gm Cu and prepare the standard as given in Experiment 1. HNO_3 and $HClO_4$ in place of HCl and HNO_3.

2. Sample Preparation

(a) Ashing :

1. Weigh about 5 gm of plant material (oven dried and powdered) and place in a Silica crucible.
2. Heat the sample on a hot-plate till charred completely.
3. Place the crucible with charred sample in a muffle-furnace at 500°C for 1 hr.

(b) Acid Digestion :

1. Take out the sample, cool and dissolve all the ash into 4 ml fuming HNO_3. Heat near dryness.
2. Again add 4 ml HNO_3. Heat near dryness and add 1 ml $HClO_4$ till white fumes arise.
3. Dilute the sample with water to make up the total volume 100 ml.

(c) Standard Conditions Of Instrument :

1. λ : 324
2. Hollow cathode lamp : 30 mA
3. Slit : 4
4. Function : Absorption
5. Range : UV
6. Fuel pressure : 8 lb/sq. in.
7. Air pressure : 30 lb/sq. in.
8. Flow rate fuel : Air : 9 : 9
9. Flame : reducing (lean blue)

Sample Analysis

As per instruction supplied by the instructer or as described in the manual.

Calculation

$$\text{Concentration of Cu (ppm)} = \frac{\text{Reading} \times \text{dilution factor} \times 10^{-6}}{\text{wt. of sample}}$$

17

Fluorimetry

17.1 General

In the previous chapters we have learnt that when on atom or a molecule absorbs radiant energy it can produce electronic excitation and ionization in certain cases. If the energy is high enough to allow the electrons to be raised to excited states and then lose the energy by reemission in random directions, the process is called *luminescence.* The luminescent process is of two types. (a) fluorescence and (b) phosphorescence. The two phenomenon can be differentiated from each other in terms of (i) excited electronic state and (ii) the time interval between the absorption and reemission of the radiant energy. The excited and reemitted radiation may normally lie in the visible and U.V. regions of the spectrum.

In order to understand details of fluorimetry and its instrumentation, it is necessary that we clarify our mind on some of the fundamentals such as difference between *electron* orbital and *electronic state* An orbital essentially describes the volume element at a given distance and direction from the nucleus where there is a high probability of finding an electron. Normally, the electrons in a molecule occupy orbitals that are atomic in character. Therefore, we can say that the properties of all electrons in all the orbitals of a molecule are responsible for the electronic state of the molecule i.e. the wave function of an electronic state will be a combination of the wave functions of the electrons in each of the orbitals of a molecule. When an electron is moved from one orbital to another, the state of the molecule is changed, therefore it is necessary to consider the electronic state of the molecule rather than consider only the orbitals involved in such an electronic transition.

Further, we must know that in a molecule three types of electronic states are possible namely ; (i) ground state (ii) transition state and (iii) excited state. The most normal state of the molecule is the ground state i.e. the state of lowest energy. The transition state is considered to be a sort of a vibrationally excited ground state i.e. a state of strained condition. On the contrary, the excited state will be a state much higher than the ground state. It will have a different electron distribution from the ground state. Normally, there can be only one ground state in a molecule where as many different excited states are possible. The exact nature of these excited states depends upon the particular orbitals involved in the molecule.

A majority of organic compounds contain an even number of electrons, hence their electronic states may be either a *singlet state* or a *triplet state*. The ground state of most organic molecules will be a *single state* in which all of the electrons in the molecule will have their spins paired (↑↓). If one set of electron spins in a molecule becomes unpaired ↑↑ or ↓↓ the resulting electronic state is called a *triplet state* .

Since substances which contain delocalized π—electrons are expected to show fluorescence, ethylene molecule may be utilized as a model example for studying such electron excitation. The position with ethylene is that it is in sp^2 hybridized configuration. Each carbon atom forms three sp^2 hybrid orbitals with an angle of 120° to each other and having a p_z orbital perpendicular to the plane of the three sp^2 orbitals. During bond formation each of the carbon atom will utilize two of the sp^2 orbitals to form σ bonds with hydrogen atoms and the third sp^2 orbital can form a low energy *bonding* σ orbital or a higher energy *antibonding* σ* orbital. The two p_z orbitals of the carbon atoms will combine to form *bonding* π orbital and *antibonding* π* molecular orbital. Thus in the ground state, ethylene molecule will have two electron in σ orbital and two electrons in the p orbital while the σ * and π* will remain vacant. This state will be represented by $\sigma^2\pi^2$. The various conditions for electronic states in ethylene are shown in Fig. 17.1.

Ground State	Excited Singlet		Triplet State
π*—	π* ↑	↑↓	π* ↑
π ↓↑	π ↑	*	π ↑
$\sigma^2\pi^2$	$\sigma^2\pi\pi^*$	$\sigma^2\pi^{2*}$	$\sigma^2\pi\pi^*$

Fig. 17.1. Electronic states in ethylene.

As π and π* orbitals are already at higher energy states than σ and σ* orbitals, the former only will be of any significance for any such electron excitations. Thus the exacitation of π electrons will give rise to two possible excited singlet states in ethylene i.e. $\sigma^2\pi\pi^*$ and $\sigma^2\pi^{*2}$. The $\sigma^2\pi\pi^{*2}$ involves raising of one electron from π orbital and placing it in π* orbital and $\sigma^2\pi^{*2}$ singlet state consists in promoting both π electrons to the π* orbital. A third excited state called *triplet state* is also possible and involves raising of a π orbital electron into a π* orbital but with a change in the spin. The above three excited states of ethylene involve only π electrons and result from π → π* transitions.

17.2 Fluorescence

When a molecule is exposed to a photon, it will absorb energy and in the process an electron will be raised into an orbital of higher energy. It the source of energy is removed the excited molecule while coming down to the ground state will reemit the absorbed radiation by a radiationless process. This radiationless or luminescent process will be either fluorescence or phosphorescence depending upon the type of excited state from which luminescence occurs and its relationship to the ground state.

If a molecule at the lowest vibrational level of an excited state returns to the ground state by emission of a photon, the process is called *fluorescence* . As the life time of an excited state is approximately 10^{-8} seconds, therefore the life time of fluorescence will be the intrisic life time of the excited state. Due to the vibrational (thermal) relaxation of the molecule after photon absorption and before photon emission the emitted photon in fluorescence will have lower energy (i.e. longer wavelength) than the excited photon absorbed by the molecule. This shift in the fluorescence spectrum from a shorter wavelength to a longer wavelength is known as *stokes shift*. Thus the phenomenon of fluorescences comprises in the absorption of a photon to go to an excited state, relaxation from higher vibrational levels of that excited state to its lowest vibrational level followed by emission of a photon to the vibrationally excited state of the ground state and again relaxation of the molecule to the lowest vibrational level of the ground state.

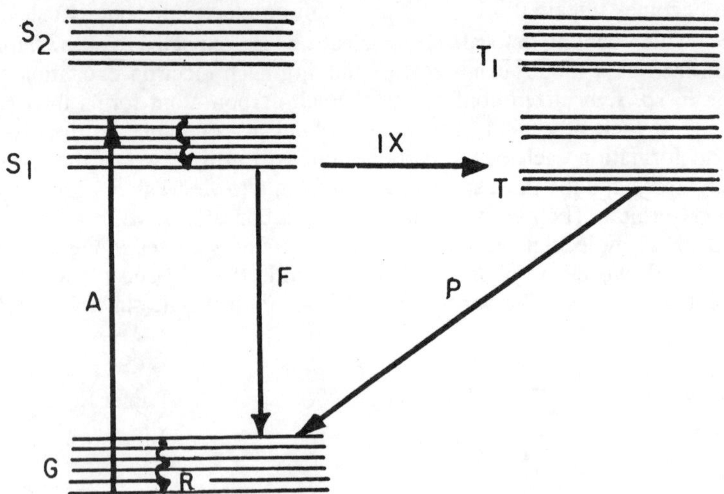

Fig. 17.2. A = photon absorption, F = fluorescence
G = ground state, P = phosphorescence
R = relaxation, S = singlet, T = Triplet
IX = Interstate cross over.

17.3. Phosphorescence

The transition from ground state of a molecule to the lowest triplet state though forbidden is possible and then the emission of light from the lowest triplet state can occur in two different ways. One way is by intersystem crossing of electrons from zeroth vibrational level of the lowest excited state of the molecule by vibrational coupling with the lowest triplet state. This emission is called *phosphorescence.* The life time of the lowest triplet state is 10^{-4} to 10 second which is the life time of phosphorescence. Therefore this phenomenon is characterized by an after glow not observed for fluorescence. A second way of emission of light from the lowest triplet state is by minimizing collisions of electrons in the triplet state by placing the molecule in a rigid medium to remove the vibrational energy in excess of the zeroth vibrational level of the triplet state. Thus phosphorescence involves a triplet — singlet transition.

17.4 Fluorescence and Molecular Structure

Saturated aliphatic compounds do not show fluorescence because they do not strongly absorb in the UV or visible region of the EM spectrum. However, some of the unsubstituted cyclic organic compounds do exhibit fluorescence in these regions. On the otherhand a majority of organic compounds that contain multiple-con-jugated double bonds with a high degree of resonance stability are expected to show fluorescence. It has been observed that the greater the number of rings in an aromatic hydrocarbon the lower is the energy of the emitted photon. Among the aromatic compounds, the nature of the substituent groups greatly affects their degree of fluorescence, e.g. electron donating groups like $-NH_2$, -OH etc increase the degree of fluorescence while electron withdrawing groups like halogens, -COOH, NO_2 etc diminish or destroy fluorescence. Thus it may be noted that cyclohexane is non-fluorescent, benzene shows weak fluorescence while compounds like anthracene, riboflavin, thiamine and epinephrine are strongly fluorescent.

Benzene, when substituted by groups like –F, $-NH_2$, –OH and $-OCH_3$ shows more intense fluorescence than the parent, But, when substituted with groups like, I, Br and Cl does not show any fluorescence, instead gives phosphorescence involving intersystem crossing.

Substances like benzoic acid, nitrobenzene, benzenesulphonamide, benzaldehyde do not show any fluorescence, but benzonitrile shows intense fluorescence due to interaction of $C \equiv N$ group with p electron of benzene. It is interesting to note that cis-stilbene shows less intense fluorescence than the trans isomer. This is due to the geometry of the molecule, the cis isomer is non-planer. Hydrocortisone though is a weak fluorescent substance. shows strong fluorescence in concentrated H_2SO_4 and ethyl alcohol.

The fluorescence is also affected by the ionization is some organic molecules in their excited states. For example β— naphthol shows different acidities in its lowest excited singlet states (ionic, fluoresces) and in its ground state (non-ionic does not fluoresce). Thus, fluorescence intensity is a function of pH of the solution in some organic molecules.

The intensity of fluorescence in organic compounds may be diminished or stopped due to competing quenching processes taking place in excited states. The quenching of fluorescence takes place because of the transfer of energy from the excited molecules to a particle with which at collides.

Ring closure is conductive to fluorescence of aromatic compounds e.g. fluorescein, phenolphthalein. Similarly metal chelation promotes fluorescence.

17.5 Fluorescence and Concentration

The degree of total fluorescence of a solution will depend upon the number of fluorescent molecules in the solution. It is improbable that all of the energy absorbed by a fluorescent molecule will be reemitted as fluorescence because some of the energy is lost through competing quenching process during the fluorescence process. Inorder to calculate fluorescence intensity use of quantum efficiency of fluorescence ϕf is made. It is defined as the number of quanta emitted by the fluorescent process to the number of quanta absorbed in unit time.

Beer's law states that in a solution of an absorbing substance the absorbance is directly proportional to the concentration. Thus we can say that fluorescence intensity will be proportional to the concentration of molecules in the excited state and therefore of the intensity of radiation. The light absorbed by the sample and intensity of the exciting light does not remain constant but decreases as it travels through the sample. In a dilute solution significant absorption will not occur and the decrease in the exciting light will not be significant. In a concentrated solution, the intensity of light might be different in regions of the sample being irradiated.

Thus the fluorescence intensity will be proportional to the amount of light absorbed which can be expressed as :

$$F = k\,\phi_f\,(I_0 - I)$$

where F = intensity of fluorescence

k = proportionality constant

ϕ_f = quantum efficiency

I_0 = Initial light

I = Transmitted light

As per Beer's Law the fraction of light transmitted is :

$$I = I_o e^{-\epsilon bc} \text{ or } \frac{I}{I_o} = e^{-\epsilon bc}$$

where ε = molar absorptivity or molar extinction coefficient

b = path length (cm)

c = concentration in moles/litre.

The coressponding fraction of light absorbed in then :

$$1-\frac{I}{I_o}=(1-e^{-\varepsilon bc})$$

On rearranging the above equation we have

$$I_o - I = I_o(1-e^{-\varepsilon bc})$$

But the total fluorescence intensity will be equal to the rate of light absorption (quanta per unit time) multiplied by the quantum efficiency of fluorescence ϕ_f ,

$$F = k\,\phi_\phi\,I_o(1-e^{-\varepsilon bc})$$

The above equation can be expanded according to the series :

$$e^x = 1 + x + \frac{x^2}{2!} + \cdots + \frac{x^n}{n!}$$

$$\text{Thus } F = k\,\phi\,I_o\,\varepsilon bc\left[1-\frac{\varepsilon bc}{2!}+\frac{(\varepsilon bc)^2}{3!}+\cdots+\frac{(\varepsilon bc)^n}{(n+1)!}\right]$$

It is to be noted that the dectector does not measure total fluorescence intensity but intensity form a segment of the sample.

$$\text{So } S_f = k\,\phi_f\,g\,\Phi\,I_o\,\varepsilon bc\left[1-\frac{\varepsilon bc}{2!}+\frac{(\varepsilon bc)^2}{3!}+\cdots+\frac{(\varepsilon bc)^n}{(n+1)!}\right]$$

where S_f is signal generated by detector.

g = a constant representing sensitivity and amplification of signal

Φ = a constant represent geometry of the system, rather a solid angle of light viewed by detector.

When the concentration is small or the solution is very dilute, only a small fraction of light is absorbed, the term εbc is not greater than 0.05.

$S_f = k\ \phi_f\, g\, \Phi\, I_0\, \varepsilon bc$ then only linear relationship will exist between concentration and fluorescence (Fig. 17.3).

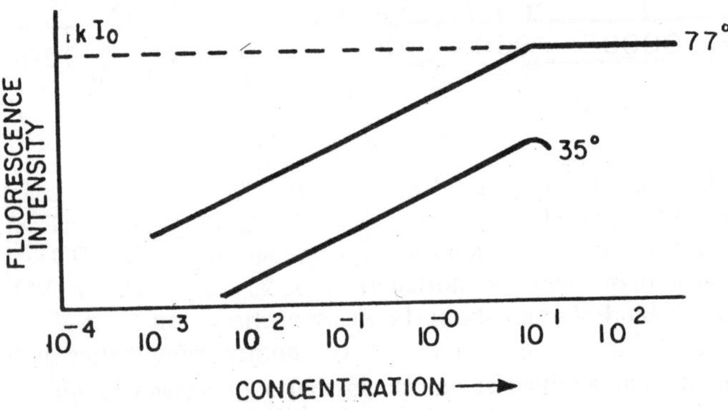

Fig. 17.3. Relation between fluorescence intensity and concentration.

When concentration is large, e^{-ebc} will become zero and the equation $S_f = k\ \phi_f\ g\ \Phi\ I_0$ will be independent of concentration.

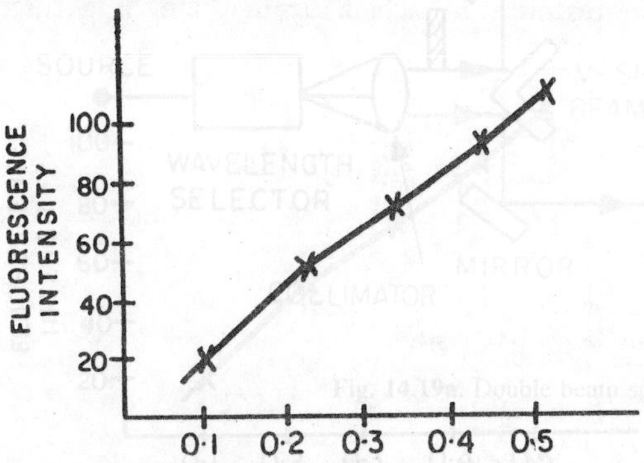

Fig. 17.4. Concentration of Quinine sulphate (mg %)

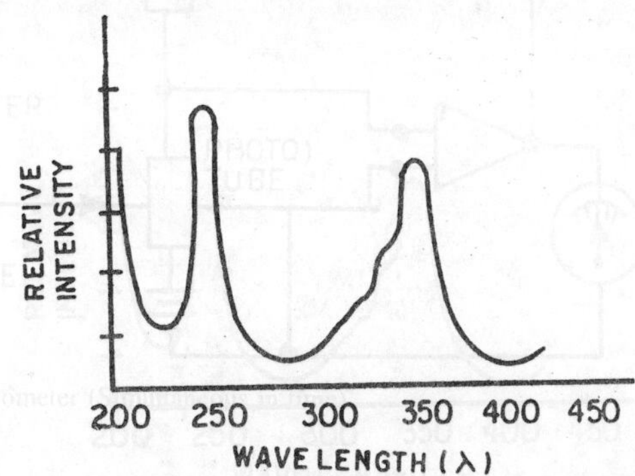

Fig. 17.5. excitation spectra of quinine in 0.05 M H_2SO_4.

17.6 Quenching

As already pointed out fluorescence process is competed by quenching process taking place in the excited states. The quenching can occur in three different ways as explained below.

(i) Collisional Impurity Quenching : The loss of fluorescence can occur by formation of excited complex between the excited sample species and the ground state impurity molecule and then subsequent non-radiative energy losses e.g. dissolved O_2 as impurity quencher.

(ii) Energy Transfer Quenching : This is another type of impurity quenching and will take place when an impurity present whose first excited singlet state is at an energy below that of excited singlet of the sample species. non-radiative energy transfer can occur between the impurity and the sample species.

(iii) Concentration Quenching : This is a kind of self-quenching and take places with increasing concentration. The quenching occurs due to the formation of a collisional complex between one molecule of the sample species that has been excited to singlet state and a second identical unexcited molecule.

The reactions for fluorescence can be represented as shown below :

$$M + h\nu \longrightarrow M^* \text{ (Absorption)}$$
$$M^* \longrightarrow M + h\nu \text{ (Fluorescence)}$$
$$M^* + Q \longrightarrow Q^* + M \text{ (Quenching)}$$
$$Q^* \longrightarrow Q + \text{Energy.}$$

where M is a sample in ground state,
M* is the excited sample,
Q is a quenching agent
hv is the photon of radiant energy

Quenching takes place due to the presence of an anion or ions with loosely bound electrons. Iodide, thiocyanate are powerful quenchers than those with tightly bound electrongs like fluoride and perchlorate. The oxidizing ions like nitrate has a good quenching effect. Organic substances like polyhydroxy phenols, amines as well as antioxidants are efficient quenchers.

During quenching there is no permanent reaction between the fluorescent substance and the quencher. There is usually a reversible oxidation-reduction reaction involved between the quencher and the excited molecule and then the regeneration of the original substance.

17.7 Instrumentation Aspects

The main components of a fluorimeter are (i) a source of radiant energy with which to irradiate the sample (ii) a sample holder and (iii) a detector to measure fluorescence. A schematic diagram of a filter fluoremeter is shown in the Fig. 17.6.

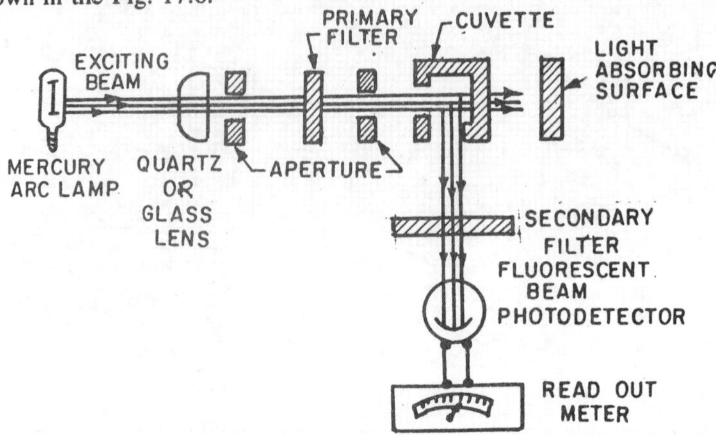

Fig. 17.6 A schematic diagram of a typical fluorimeter.

A mercury vapour lamp with glass or fused silica envelope is a common excitation source from which a suitable activation beam is isolated by means of a filter. The principle lines from mercury discharge lamp are at 366, 405, 436, 546 and 578 nm. The selection of the exciting wavelength is made by inserting a primary filter in the incident beam before the sample. A light source like high-pressure xenon-arc lamp provides a high level of ultraviolet and visible light.

When both excitation and emission spectra are needed two monochromators are necessary, one for the light source and one for fluorescence. For studies in ultraviolet, lenses or cuvettes made of quartz or fused silica are used.

The phototube is placed at right angles to incident beam and with masking slits in position the detector views only the illuminated liquid and not the illuminated cuvette faces. This also minimizes the reflection of any of the intense exciting radiation. A secondary filter is placed in front of the detector to remove the reflected and scattered exciting radiation. The secondary filter should be selected such that they absorb the scattered primary radiation but not the fluorescent light. Although fluorescence is emitted in all directions and can be viewed from any angle. But in practice 90° angle is the most convenient angle selected in designing fluorimeters.

Different models of spectrofluorimeters including those with microprocessor controls are available, which can provide both the fluorescence emission spectrum and the excitation spectrum. Their operation consists in that a suitable wavelength in the emission spectrum is selected, and the second monochromator is set at this point. The excitation spectrum is then plotted by scanning the first monochromator. The optical diagram of a spectrofluorimeter is shown is Fig. 17.7 below.

A 150-w xenon lamp is used as the source and the chopped radiation is allowed to pass through a Czerny—Turner monochromator. It is then focused on to a sample cuvette where it is partially absorbed. The fluorescent emission is analysed by the second monochromator. Further, a beam splitter is inserted to cut away a fixed fraction of incident beam from the main path and monitered by means of an auxillary detector. This helps in correcting the output of the main photomultiplier tube for changes in the luminescence of the xenon lamp as the wavelength is scanned.

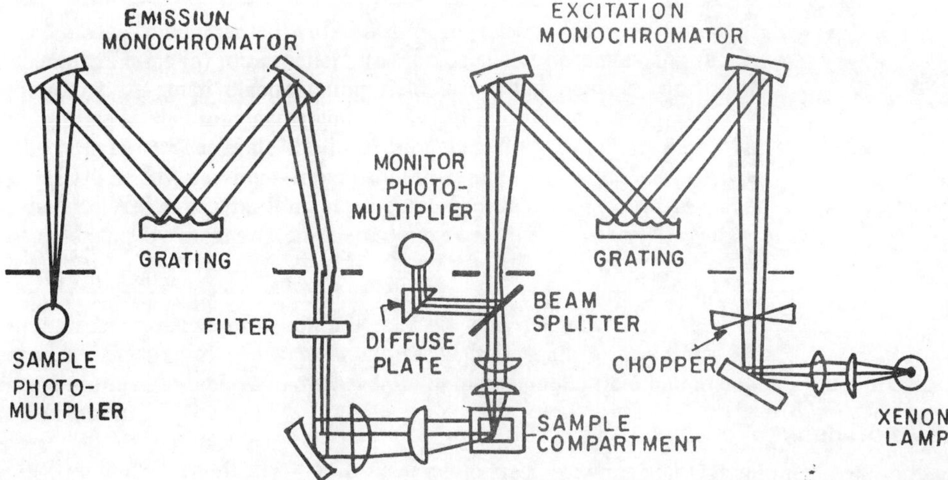

Fig. 17.7 optical diagram of a spectrofluorimeter.

17.8 Applications

Fluorimetry is selective because fewer substance show efficient fluorescence. It is also a very sensitive method because determination in the range of nanogram quantities or below can be measured. A variety of inorganic substances and minerals show fluorescence in the visible region while organic and organometallic compounds absorb in the ultraviolet region. For example selenium is determined by its complexation with 3, 3′— diaminobenzidine. Similarly cadmium is determined by reaction with bis (dimethylaminomethyl) fluorescein after it has been freed from other interfering ions.

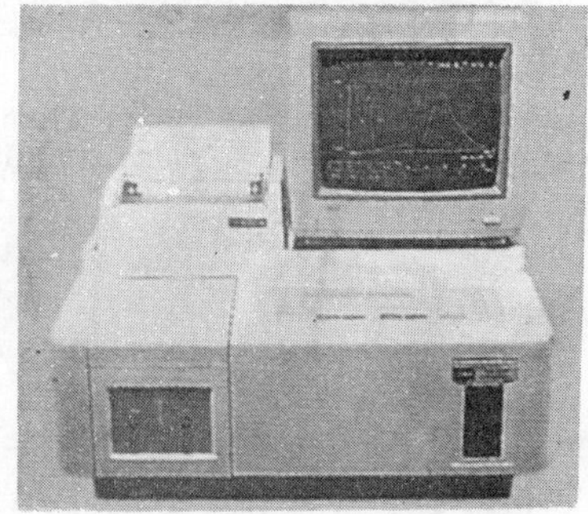

Fig. 17.8 Spectrofluoro-Photometer Model FP-777 JASCO (Courtesy of JASCO)

A large number of pharmaceutical compounds have been assayed by fluorimetric procedure. Some of these compounds are listed in Table 17.1.

Table 17.1. Some pharmaceutical Compounds analysed by fluorimetry

Compound Name	Excitation (nm)	Fluorescence (nm)	Concentration required (µg/ml)
Allylmorphine	285	355	0.1 at pH 1
Amytal	265	410	0.1 at pH 14
Aureomycin	355	445	0.02 at pH 14
Chloroquine	335	400	0.05 at pH 11
Chlorpromazine	350	480	0.1 at pH 11
Cinchonidine	315	445	0.01 at pH 1.
Cinchonine	320	420	0.01 at pH 1.
Epinephrine	295	335	0.07 at pH 1.
Folic Acid	365	450	0.01 at pH 1.
Hydrocortisone	460	520	75% v/v in H_2SO_4 in ethanol

(*Contd.*)

LSD	325	465	0.002 at pH of in CNCL
Nicotinamide	250	430	
Norepinephrine	295	335	0.06 at pH 1.
Oxychloroquine	335	380	0.08 at pH 11.
Pentobarbitone	265	440	0.1 at pH 13.
Procaine	275	345	0.01 at pH 11.
Procainamide	295	385	0.01 at pH 11
Physostigmine	300	360	0.04 at pH 1.
Quinine	250,350	450	0.002 at pH 1.
Reserpine	300	375	0.008 at pH 1.
Terramycin	390	520	0.05 at pH 11.
Riboflavine	270, 370, 445	520	inaqueous buffer at pH 6
Vitamin A	325	470	0.01

17.9 Phosphorimetry

As explained in the beginning of this chapter, phosphorescence differs from fluorescence in (i) its longer decay time i.e. 10^{-1} to 10 seconds (10^{-7} to 10^{-9} seconds for fluorescence) and (ii) by a shift to longer wavelength.

A compound that shows phosphorescence should also possess fluorescence therefore a phosphorimeter should be able to distinguish between the two phenomena. One method of measurement of phosphorescence is to incorporate a rotating shutter called phosphorescope in an instrument. This device incorporates a definite delay between the time intervals during which the sample is irradiated and phosphorescence measured. An alternative method is to use a pulse technique instead of a rotating shutter. The primary source of radiation consists of a flash tube which is triggered by an electronic timing circuit. After a selected time interval, the photomultiphier is activated and phosphorescence measured. Another technique possible in phosphorimetry is time resolution. This technique is useful in the determination of mixtures or multicomponent analysis provided the individual components of the mixture have different decay times.

EXERCISE : 1. To draw the calibration plot for the fluorimetric estimation of quinine sulphate.

Reagents

0.1N Sulphuric Acid : Take about 300 ml distilled water in the 1 litre flask, add 3 ml conc. H_2SO_4 slowly (use 10 ml measuring cylinder). Add distilled water to make the volume upto 1 litre. Mix well.

Quinine Sulphate Solution

Stock Solution A : Weigh 100 mgms quinine sulphate powder. Transfer to a 100 ml volumetric flask, using a small funnel. Add 30-40 ml. 0.1N-H_2SO_4 and dissolve the powder. Make the volume to 100 ml with 0.1N-H_2SO_4. Mix well and label. This contains 1 mgm/ml of quinine sulphate.

Stock Solution B : Pipette 1 ml of stock solution A to another 100 ml volumetric flask. Make the volume to 100 ml using 0.1N-H_2SO_4. Mix well and label. This contains 10 μg/ml of quinine sulphate.

Stock Solution C : Pipette 10 ml of stock solution B to a 100 ml volumetric flask. Make the volume to 100 ml using 0.1N-H_2SO_4. Mix well and label. This contains 1 μg/ml quinine sulphate.

Standard Solution : Using stock solution C. prepare standard solutions of known concentrations, as given below (Use graduated pipettes) :

Test-tube No.	0	1	2	3	4	5
ml. of stock solution C	0.0	1.0	2.0	3.0	4.0	5.0
ml. of 0.1N-H_2SO_4	10.0	9.0	8.0	7.0	6.0	5.0

Procedure

Follow the procedure as given in the instruction manual or as per the instructor. Use standard solution No. 6 (containing 0.5 μg/ml quinine sulphate) for adjusting 100 on the dial scale.

Filters

Primary filter : B Hg - 1 (365 nm)
Secondary filter : N 440 (450 nm) (or B 470)

Observations

S. No.	Concentration (μg/ml)	Fluorescence Intensity (F)
1	0.0	
2	0.1	
3	0.2	
4	0.3	
5	0.4	
6	0.5	

Plot Fluorescence intensity vs. Concentration of quinine sulphate.
This is F_o (blank).

Results

1. The calibration plot for quinine sulphate is attached.
2. The plot is linear/non-linear in the concentration range studied (.................μ.g/ml to μg/ml).
3. The concentration of quinine sulphate in the given sample (concn. unknown) is ....μ.g/ ml.

Sample Calculations

Ex. The following data was obtained for fluorimetric estimation of Penicillin as an aminoacridine derivative :

S.No.	Sample Concentration (μg/10 ml)	Fluorescence Intensity (F)	
1.	0.0 (Blank)	9.1	(F_o)
2.	1.5 (Standard)	32.7	(F_s)
3.	Sample	28.8	(F_u)

What is the concentration of penicillin (in μg/ml) in the sample ?

$$\text{Conc. (unknown)} = \text{Conc. (std)} \times \frac{(F_u - F_o)}{(F_s - F_o)}$$

$$= 1.5 \times \frac{(28.8 - 9.1)}{(32.7 - 9.1)} = 1.5 \times \frac{19.7}{23.6}$$

$$= 1.25 \ \mu g/10 \ ml \text{ or } 0.125 \ \mu g/ml$$

The concentration can also be read directly from the calibration plot.

EXERCISE : 2. To study the pH dependence of the fluorescence of quinine sulphate solutions.

Reagents

Prepare stock solutions of quinine sulphate (stock solution A, B and C) as in experiment No. 1, except that use distilled water instead of 0.1N-H_2SO_4 in all cases.

Prepare 10 ml each of the standard solutions of quinine sulphate as given below :

Test-tube No.	1	2	3	4	5
Volume of stock solution C (in ml.)	1.0	2.0	3.0	4.0	5.0
Distilled water (in ml.)	9.0	8.0	7.0	6.0	5.0

Procedure

Follow the procedure as given in the instruction manual or as per instructor. Use the same settings of control knobs as in Experiment No. 1.

Observations

S. No.	*Concentration (μg/ml)*	*Fluorescence Intensity*
1	0.1	
2	0.2	
3	0.3	
4	0.4	
5	0.5	

Plot Fluorescence intensity vs. Concentration, at the neutral pH.

Result

Compare F vs C plot at neutral pH (as above) with the plot at acidic pH (as in Experiment No. 1)

Record your conclusions regarding the effect of pH on the fluorescence of quinine sulphate solutions.

EXERCISE : 3. To study the "quenching" effect due to the presence of varying concentrations of iodine ion on the florescence of quinine sulphate solution.

Materials

Quinine sulphate solution (Stock solution C,

Potassium iodine

0.1N sulphuric acid

1 volumetric flask (100 ml) for KI solution.

10 ml graduated pipette for KI solution.

20 ml test-tubes.

1 Test-tube stand.

Reagents

1. **Potassium Iodide Solution** : Dissolve 200 mgms. KI solution in 100 ml. of 0.1N-sulphuric acid (contains 2.0 mg/ml KI).
2. **Quinine Sulphate Solution** : Use stock solution C, prepared in Experiment No. 1 (1 μg/ml quinine sulphate). Prepare standard solutions as given below (use graduated pipette) :

Test tube No.	1	2	3	4	5
ml. of stock solution C.	5.0	5.0	5.0	5.0	5.0
ml. of KI solution	0.0	1.0	2.0	3.0	4.0
ml. of 0.1N H_2SO_4	5.0	4.0	3.0	2.0	1.0

Procedure

Follow the procedure as described in the instruction manual or as per the instructor. Use the same settings of control knobs as in Experiment No. 1.

Observations

S. No.	*Concentration KI* (mg/ml)	Fluorescence Intensity
1	0.0	
2	0.2	
3	0.4	
4	0.6	
5	0.8	

Plot Fluorescence intensity vs. Concentration of potassium iodine.

Result

Compare F vs. C plots in presence of iodine ion with the plot obtained in its absence (Exercise No. 1). Record your conclusions.

18

Infrared Spectrophotometry

18.1 General

The region in the electromagnetic radiation spectrum extending from 0.8 to 200 μ is known as infrared. This can be further split into three parts namely : (i) 0.8 to 2.5 μ or 12500 to 4000 cm^{-1} (near IR) (ii) 2.5 μ to 15 or 4000 to 667 cm^{-1} (ordinary IR) and (iii) 15 to 200 μ or 667 to 50 cm^{-1} (far IR). Most of our attention will be focused on the region between 0.8 to 50 μ because this can be explored with the aid of commercial instrumentas and also wherein the spectra arise mainly from the stretching and bending movements of atoms within molecules. The infrared spectra are used for the identification and study of molecular structure of compounds.

18.2 Theory

The normal modes of vibration of a molecule can be described by three coordinates in space. Therefore, the system as a whole will have 3n degrees of freedom of motion. From this, three degrees must be deducted from the whole for translation of a molecule as a rigid unit and three for rotations of the molecule about each principal axis (two if molecule is linear). This leaves a remainder of 3n-6 degrees of freedom for the description of independent modes of vibration of a molecule (3n-5 degrees of freedom for a linear molecule).

There are two kinds of fundamental vibrations :

(a) **Stretching,** in which distance between the two atoms increases or decreases, but atoms remain in the same bond axis, e.g. $A \longleftrightarrow B$ where A and B represent the two atoms and the double arrow as the stretched bond. The stretching is of two types (i) *symmetrical* stretching and (ii) *asymmetrical* stretching. For example, in a three-atom system like H — C — H the symmetrical stretching will have two hydrogen atoms move towards and away from the central atom of carbon in unison, altering the interatomic distance without change in the valince angle (Fig. 18.1).

In asymmetrical stretching one hydrogen atom will approach the carbon while the other will move away from carbon.

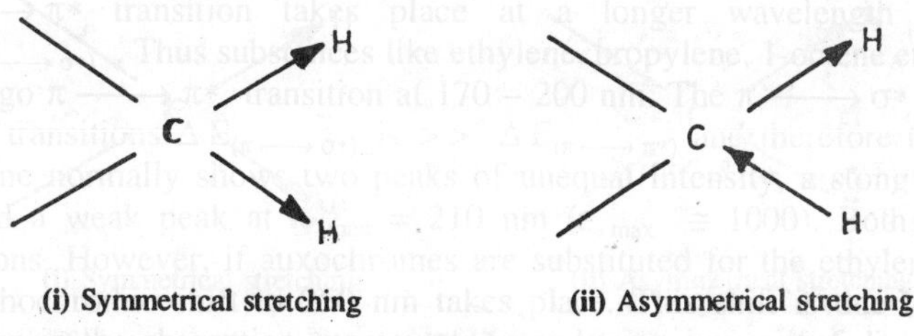

(i) Symmetrical stretching (ii) Asymmetrical stretching

Fig. 18.1.

(b) Bending and deformation, in which the position of the atom changes relative to original bond axis. There are four types of bending vibrations (Fig. 18.2) : namely, (i) wagging (ii) rocking, (iii) twisting and (iv) scissoring.

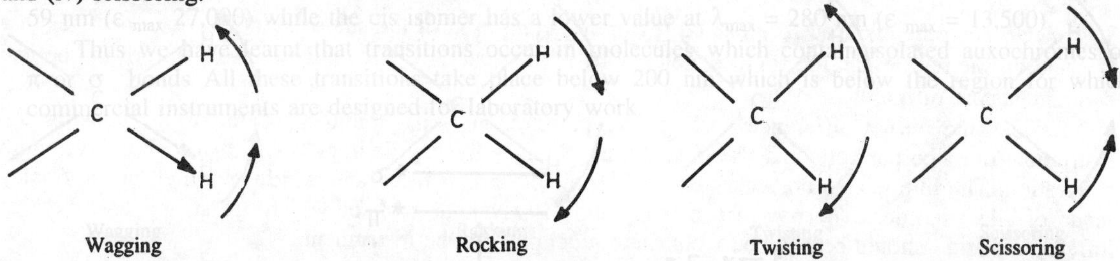

Fig. 18.2.

In *wagging*, the structural unit swings back and forth in the plane of the molecule (in plane bending). In *rocking*, the structural unit swings back and forth out of the plane of the molecule (out of plane bending). In *twisting*, the structural unit rotates about the bond which joins it to the rest of the molecule. In *scissoring*, the two atoms connected to a central atom move towards and away from each other with deformation of valence angle.

In addition to the above described absorption the infrared spectrum made also show *harmonic* and *combination* vibrations. The harmonic vibrations also known as *overtones* possess a frequency which represents approximately integral multiples of fundamental frequency. The intensities are usually about 1/100 those of fundamental bands. On the other hand a combination band is the sum or the difference between, the frequencies of two or more fundamental or harmonic vibrations.

The two most important requirements for a substance to absorb infrared radiation are :

(i) that the natural frequency of vibration of the molecule is same as the frequency of vibration and (ii) that the vibration so produced brings about a change in the *dipole moment* of the molecule. The positions of the centres of gravity of the positive and negative electrical charges between two dissimilar atoms in a molecule will determine its *dipole moment*. If the values of the dipole moment in the extreme positions differ, a periodically changing electrical field will be set around the molecule. As a consequence, absorption of radiant energy at the vibrating frequencies will take place. In this manner a resonance condition will be established. But diatomic molecules like H_2, N_2, O_2 and ethylene do not absorb any infrared radiation. They are homopolar molecules and do not produce a dipole moment due to their symmetry. In a molecule like CO_2, no dipole moment is created in the symmetrical stretching vibration because the centres of gravity coincide in every vibrational position. But in the case of the asymmetrical stretching vibrations, the centres of gravity of the charges do not coincide. A dipole moment is produced and absorption characteristic of this mode is absorbed in the infrared spectrum (Fig. 18.3).

O = C = O	O = C = O	O = C = O
← → v_1	← ← v_2	δ_1 ↓ ↑ ↓
		δ_2 $O^- = C^+ = O^-$
Symmetrical stretching	Asymmetrical stretching	Bending

Fig. 18.3.

The intensity of infrared absorption band is proportional to the square of the rate of change of dipole moment with respect to the displacement of the atoms. Thus when the magnitude of change in dipole moment is small, a weak absorption band will be obtained, e.g. C ≡ N group. If the change in dipole moment is very large, a strong absorption band will be obtained, e.g. C = O group.

18.3 Instrumentation Aspects

The spectrophotometers used for infrared region are composed of the same essential components as in a UV and visible region, but the sources, detectors and the materials used in the construction of the optical components are different.

Besides the above differences, (i) the temperature and (ii) humidity of the room housing the instrument must be controlled. If the temperature changes by few degrees it will affect the wavelength calibration. The humidity more than 50% will spoil the prism faces and windows which are normal y made of alkali halides. The presence of CO_2 and H_2O vapour both of which are strong absorbers of infrared radiation should be avoided from the optical path of the instrument.

In a *single beam* infrared spectrophotometer, first, a blank curve for the spectral energy source and the atmospheric H_2O and CO_2 absorption is recorded. Then, with the sample brought into the beam, same spectrum is scanned again. The absorption bands of the sample are superimposed on the spectrum of the blank and must be obtained from the two curves by forming quotients. However, the single beam infrared spectrophotometers are no more used or manufactured. With the advancement in instrumentation and computer technology, quite a good number of laboratories now possess *Fourier Transform* infrared spectrophotometers inspite of their high prices. However, *ratio recording* double beam infrared spectrophotometers (Fig. 18.4) are commonly used for identification purposes. The original beam of radiation can be separated in space or time. If it is divided into two equal beams by letting it impinge on front surface mirror it is split in space. If the beam is to be separated according to sharing method, splitting is done through insertion of a rotating sector mirror. It alternatively passes the beam from the open sector to one chamel and reflects from the mirror sector to the second channel. Each of them have a pulse of light as bright as the original beam. Each beam traverses the monochromator-detector system on alternating cycles. The sample is placed in one beam while the reference beam is left empty or contains a reference blank or solution. In the optical null balance method, an AC signal results when the two beams are unbalanced. The amplifier is tuned to the chopping frequency of the light beam; signals of the differing frequency are not amplified. The resultant AC signal activates a servo-mechanism which moves an optical wedge or shutter comb that is mounted in the path of the reference beam, thus reducing its energy until both beams are again balanced. The optical attenatuator is linked mechanically to the recorder pen which is moved across the chart paper as the equilibrium position is sought. the record traced on the chart paper is thus the relative transmittance of the sample. The accuracy and the reproducibility of such type of spectra will depend upon the speed and sensitivity of the detector and amplifier.

In the case of *Fourier - Transform* IR spectrophotometer use is made of *interferometer.* Radiation from IR source is collimated by a concave mirror and passed into the *interferometer.* The pulsating beam which leaves the *interferometer* is then directed into an *oscillating mirror* that is positioned alternately

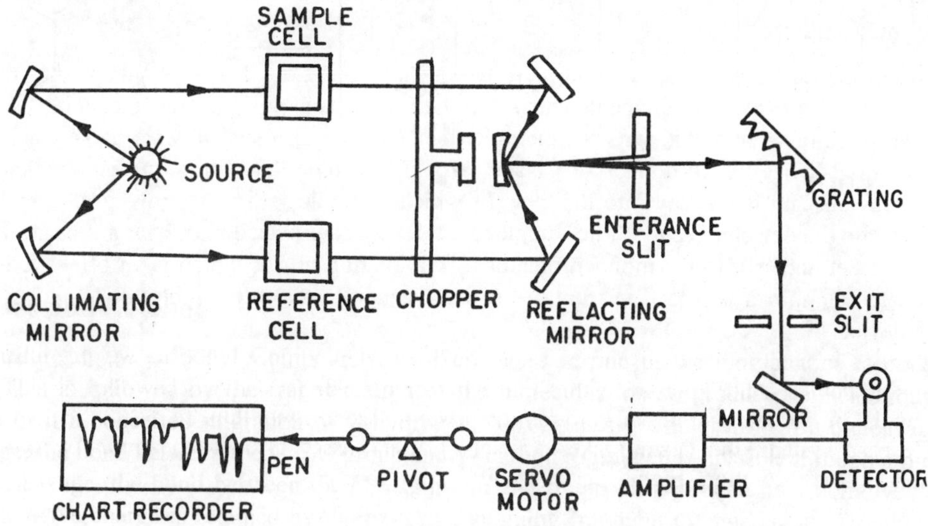

Fig. 18.4. Schematic, automatic, double beam, optical null I.R. spectrophotometer.

to send the beam through the sample cell or through the reference cell. A second *Oscillating mirror* which is synchronized with the first, allows the beams to be focussed on the detector. The *interferogram* cannot be interpreted without a digital computer. The two main important advantages of the Fourier-transform IR spectroscopy are that : (i) it makes use of all frequencies from the source simultaneously rather than sequentially as in a scanning instrument — known as *Fellget advantage* and (ii) the sensitivity of the Fourier-transform method is greater than the dispersive technique because more radiation enters the slitless system — known as *Jacquinot advantage.*

18.3.1 Radiation Sources

The source unit is placed in a separate compartment. The light from the source falls upon a concave spherical mirror which condenses the radiation into an image of the source and then fills the entrance slit of the monochromator. The three common sources which give radiant energy in infrared are (i) Nerst glower (ii) Globar and (iii) Nichrome Wire. These are described below.

(i) Nerst Glower : It consists of a hollow rod 2 mm in diameter and 30 mm in length. It is made from a mixture of zirconium and yttrium oxides. The ends of the rod are fixed to small ceramic tubes with electrical leads for mounting the glower. The leads provide the power connections. The glower is heated to surface temperatures of 1500—2000°C and furnish maximum radiation of about 7100 cm^{-1} (1.4μ). The source must be protected from drafts and provided with ventilation to remove surplus heat and evaporated oxides.

(ii) Globar : It consists of a rod of silicon carbide about 50 mm in length and 4 mm in diameter. It is self-starting and is heated to a temperature of 1300—1700°C furnishing a maximum radiation of about 5200 cm^{-1} (1.9 μ). This source needs water cooling. It is more satisfactory for work at wavelength beyond 650 cm^{-1} (15 μ) because its radiant energy output decreases less rapidly.

(iii) Nichrome Wire : Coils or ribbons of nichrome wire are also used as sources in some of the models of infrared spectrophotometers. The wire is raised to incandescence by resistive heating and heated to surface temperatures of 800—900ºC.

18.3.2 Monochromators

A monochromators is a device for isolating narrow wavelength regions from a source of heterogeneous light. It consists of a dispersing element which may be a prism or a grating together with two narrow slits to serve as entrance and exit parts for the radiation. The entrance slit allows a narrow beam to fall on the dispersing device which deflects the beam through an angle depending on the wavelength. The beam thus fans out and is focused into the exit slit which then allows a narrow band of wavelength to pass through into the detector section. The sample and reference are placed at or near a focus of the beam just before the entrance slit to the monochromator. A collimating mirror which is an off — axis section of a large parabolic mirror is placed in front of the entrance slit to make the light parallel and sent to the dispersing device.

Most of the monochromators in infrared spectrophotometers employ what is called *Littrow design.* The dispersing device is a 30º prism with a plane mirror behind. This allows the dispersed light to be reflected by the mirror and is returned through the prism a second time, thus doubling the dispersion. In the double pass system, the beam makes a total of four passes through the prism with an added improvement in the resolution (Fig. 18.5a & 18.5b).

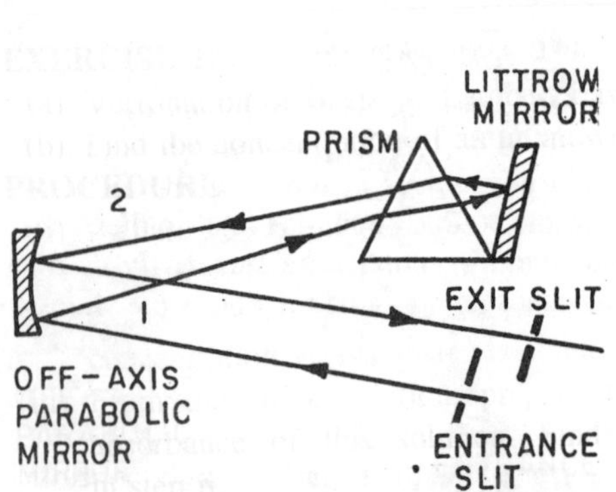

Fig. 18.5a. Single pass monochromator

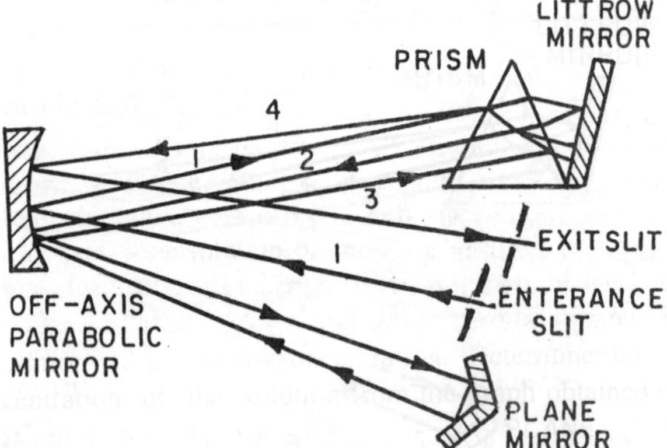

Fig. 18.5b. Double--pass monochromator

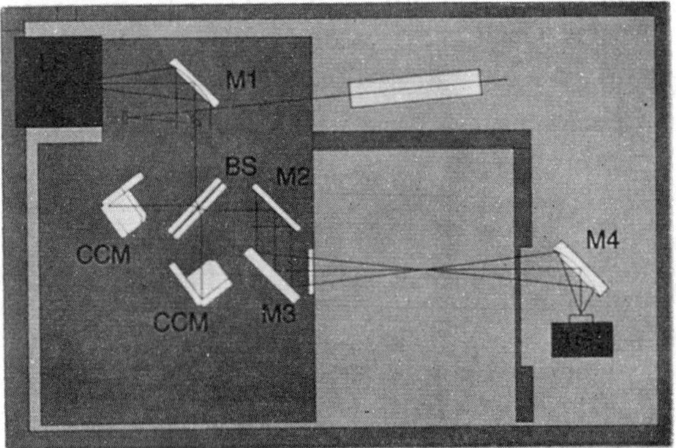

Fig. 18.5c. Optical diagram of a typical FT/IR Spectrometer

18.3.3 Material for Prism Construction

The materials that have been found suitable for the construction of mirrors, windows, prisms etc are following : (i) Glass, (ii) fused silica (iii) fluorides of lithium, calcium and barium (iv) Sodium chloride, (v) potassium bromide and (vi) cesium iodide. Generally, large size crystals of these substances can be grown artificially on a commercial basis and then blanks are cut as per requirements for making prisms, windows, cell surface etc. The long wavelength is fixed by checking the absorption while the short wavelength limit is set by the experimental conditions.

The instruments having a range from 4000—650 cm^{-1} (2.5 — 15.4 μ) make use of sodium chloride (NaCl) prism. With potassium bromide (KBr) prism, the spectrum can be extended to 400 cm^{-1} (25 μ) and with cesium iodide the optics of the spectrum can be extended to 260 cm^{-1} (38 μ).

18.3.4 Detectors

The detectors suitable for infrared spectroscopy are of two types : (i) thermal detectors and (ii) photon detectors. A thermal detector is based on the absorption of energy of a large number of incident photons to produce a response through their heating effects. On the other hand a photon detector is a semiconductor device in which an electron absorbs the energy of a single quantum of infrared radiation and is promoted from valence band to the conduction band producing electrical conductivity. Although photon detectors are faster and more sensitive, but are restricted in wavelength and need cooling. On the other hand thermal detectors can be used over a wider range of wavelength and do not need cooling. However, their response is slow and are less sensitive.

As the thermal detectors give a uniform response for all frequencies they are commonly used in infrared spectrophotometers. Since the radiant power is low for infrared region, so is the detector signal. In order to prevent the faint signals to be lost in the stray and noise signals which are picked up by the wires going away from the detector, a preamplifier is installed as close to the detector as possible.

A thermocouple (Fig. 18.6) is made by welding together at each end two wires made from two different semi-conducting metals of high thermoelectric efficiency. However, these are fabricated with a tiny bit of blackened gold foil as the absorber of radiation. In actual practice, identical junctions between unlike metal wires are welded on to the back surface of the two bits of foil and are mounted in such a way that only the blackened one is subject to radiation to be measured. The cold junction is kept screened and at constant temperature in the receiver housing. The hot junction is exposed to IR radiation which increases the temperature of the junction. The potential difference generated in the wires depends on the temperature difference between the junctions and how much IR radiation falls on the hot junction. As the thermocouples have low impedence, they need to be coupled to a preamplifier through a transformer to be able to respond to the low frequency signals generated by the incident beam of radiation.

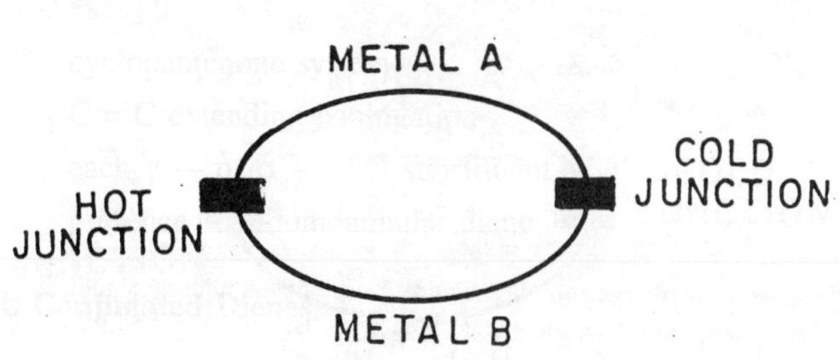

Fig. 18.6. A thermocouple

A second type of thermal detector used in IR spectrophotometers is known as *bolometer*. It is basically a miniature resistance thermometer made either with a small platinum wire or a *thermister* as the sensing element. The thermisters are made of fused mixtures of metal oxides. As their temperature increases, their electrical resistance decreases. This relationship between the temperature and electrical resistance enables them to respond to the IR radiation.

18.5 Sample Handling

The techniques for analysing the samples by IR spectrophotometry differ for solid, liquid and gaseous materials.

For gaseous samples, gas cells equipped with mirrors to allow the radiation to pass through are commercially available. However, sample preparation requires prior removal of water vapour.

For solids or powders, a common or quick way of examining them is convert them into a *mull* or a thick *slurry* . The powdered sample is mixed (10 — 15 mg) with a greasy, liquid medium (A few drops) like paraffin oil, nujol, hexachlorobutaadiene, perfluorokerose etc and made into a paste. The *suspension* thus prepared is then sandwiched between two NaCl plates and mounted on a demountable cell holder. This technique may give difficulties due to scattering of radiation, therefore the liquid medium should possess approximately same refractive index to reduce energy losses.

Another technique adopted for solid samples is by converting them into a *disk* or *pellet* of potassium bromide. A weighed portion pf powdered sample (1.0 mg) is thoroughly mixed in a small ball mill with a weighed quantity of purified and desiccated KBr powder (200 mg). The mixture is placed in a evacuable die and subjected to a pressure of 10 — 15 torr. A highly transparent disk or a pellet is produced which is then placed in a pellet holder and IR scanned. The disk is about 1 cm in diameter and about 0.5 mm thick.

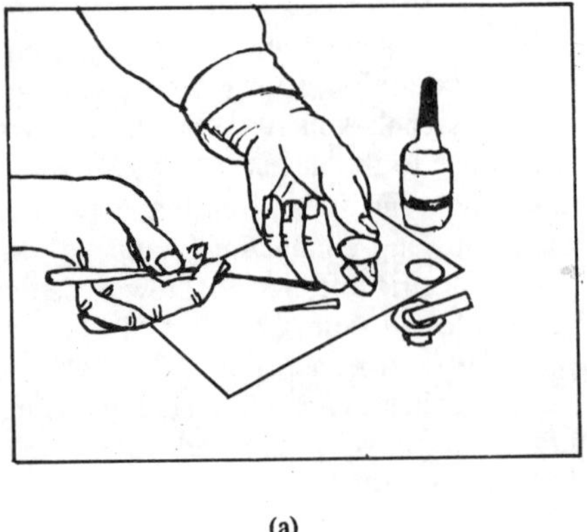

(a)

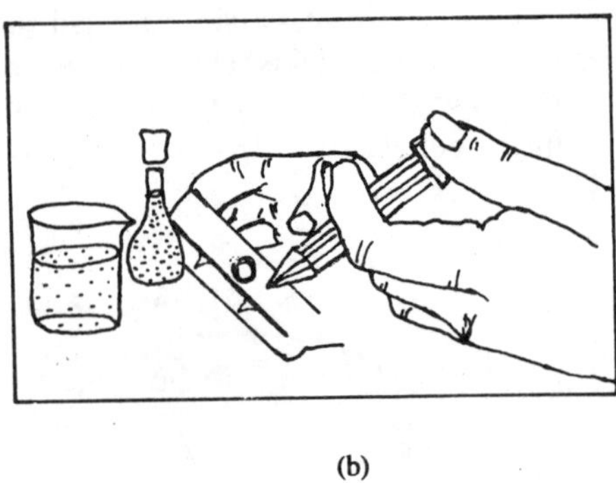

(b)

Fig. 18.7. (a) Preparation of a neat sample for recording the infrared spectrum of a liquid. A drop of the liquid, or mull, is placed between the sodium chloride plates and the plates are secured between the metal retainers of the cell, (b) The filling of a solution cell.

Samples which are liquid at room temperature are generally examined in their pure form. The procedure is called *thin film* technique or *neat form* . A thin layer of the sample is sandwiched between two salt plates and then fixed into a demountable cell holder provided with gaskets. The sample thickness should be such that the transmittance lies between 15 to 70%.

Liquid samples with high viscosity cannot be analysed as such and therefore need to be dissolved in suitable solvents. The solvents should be non-absorbing in the region of interest. Carbon tetrachloride is satisfactory but absorbs between 800 — 740 cm^{-1} (12.5 — 13.5 μ), carbon disulphide absorbs at 2222 cm^{-1} (4.5 μ) and 1540 cm^{-1} (6.5 μ). Solvents chosen should be free from moisture and hydrogen bonding effects. Chloroform, cyclohexane and similar solvents can also be used in a restricted manner.

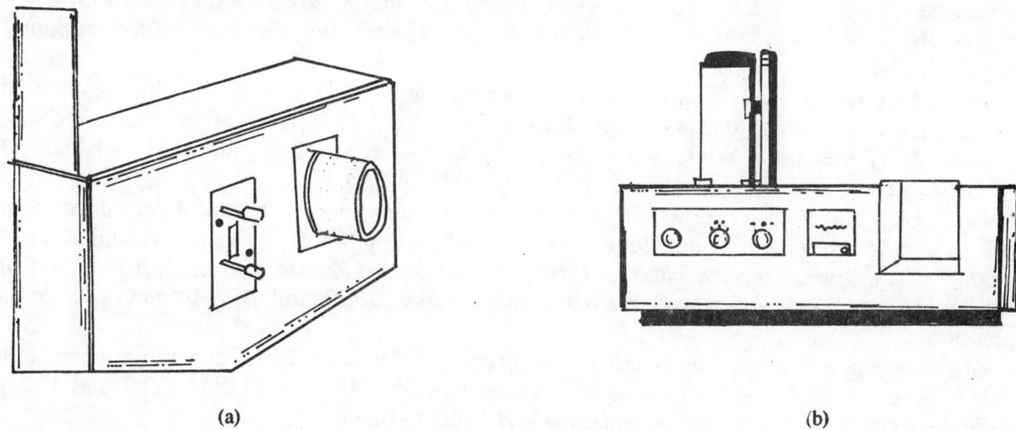

(a) (b)

Fig. 18.8 (a) The cell compartment of a typical infrared spectrophotometer. The left cell is the sample cell and the right cell is a variable thickness cell filled with pure solvent in the reference beam of the instrument. The thickness of the variable thickness cell is adjustable to match exactly the thickness of the sample cell to balance the solvent absorption peak.
(b) A typical infrared spectrophotometer.

The absorption cells available for liquid samples are called *sealed cells* or preassembled cells. It consists of a pair of salt plates separated by a shim or gasket made of a metal or teflon and held together like a sandwich between two metal clamps. Two holes are drilled through the metal frame and to the salt plates for filling and emptying. The cell can be filled and rinsed with the help of a hypodermic syringe. Such cells are demountable type provided with fittings.

18.6 Structural Analysis

The infrared spectrum of a compound gives information on the absorption bands of specific functional groups. The absorption or lack of absorption in specific frequency regions can be co-related with specific vibrational groups and bending motions and in this way one can interpret whether certain functional groups are present or that certain others are absent in a compound.

The fundamental region in the infrared is also called the *rocksalt* region. This region can be divided into the (i) *group frequency* region (400–1300 cm^{-1} or 2.5–8 μ) and (ii) *finger print* region (1300–650 cm^{-1} or 8.0–15.4 μ). In the group frequency region the principle absorption bands are assigned to the vibration units consisting of only two atoms of a molecule i.e. units which are dependent only on functional groups and not on the complete molecular structure.

The absorption in the interval from 4000–2500 cm^{-1} (2.5–4.0 μ) is characteristic of hydrogen stretching vibrations with elements of mass 19 or less. The intermediate frequency 2500–1540 cm^{-1} (4 –6.5 μ) is an indication of unsaturated region. The region from 2500–2000 cm^{-1} (4–5 μ) sshows the presence of a triple bond while the frequency region 2000–1540 cm^{-1} (5–6.5 μ) is an indication of a double bond.

The region 1300–650 cm^{-1} (8.0—15.4 μ) comprises single bond frequencies and bending vibrations of polyatomic systems involving motions of bonds linking a substituent group to the remainder of the molecule. As already pointed out, it is called the ''finger print region''.

The absorption bands which result from overtone and combination bands involving hydrogen atoms show first overtones due –OH and –NH near 9100 cm^{-1} (1.4 μ) and 8500 cm^{-1} (1.5 μ) respectively. On the other hand the combination vibrations obtained from C — H stretching and deformation are found at 4548 cm^{-1} (2.2 μ) and 3850 cm^{-1} (2.6 μ).

On closer study of the exact position of an absorption band one can establish the presence of a particular functional group, e.g. the absorption band at 3000 cm^{-1} (3.3 μ) gives the indication of the presences of C — H stretching. While alkane groups have C — H stretching motion lower than 3000 cm^{-1} (3.3 μ) the alkenes and aromatics have higher than 3000 cm^{-1}.

A band at 1380 cm^{-1} (7.5 μ) shows the presence of a terminal methyl group of on alkane. If this absorption band is in the form of a doublet at 1380 & 1365 cm^{-1} (7.25 & 7.33 μ), it is indicative of a gem-dimethyl group. The absorption band at 1460 cm^{-1} (6.85 μ) is due to the scissoring motion of a methylene group. The presence of groups in a linear chain absorb at 720 cm^{-1} (13.9 μ) and is due to their rocking motion.

The substitution in a benzene ring is usually indicated by a series of weak absorption bands in the region 2000 — 1670 cm^{-1} (5 — 6 μ) along with strong bands at 900 — 650 cm^{-1} (11.1 and 15.4 μ). These absorption bands are due to out of plane C — H bending motions.

The position of free or unassociated –OH group is observed at 3600 cm^{-1} (2.78 μ) in the form of a weak band. It hydrogen bonding is involved, its intensity will be increased & also will be shifted to lower frequencies. When the hydrogen bonding is strong, the band is broadened. The ethers usually show a strong absorption band at 1100 cm^{-1} (9.09 μ) due to the presence of —C—O—C— linkage.

The position of the carbonyl (C = O) group depends upon its surroundings, namely aldehydes and ketones show absorption between 1725 and 1690 cm^{-1} (5.80 — 5.90 μ); carboxylic acid group absorbs at 1700 — 1670 cm^{-1} (5.9 — 6.0 μ); The amide carbonyl is at 1690 — 1600 cm^{-1} ; the ester carbonyl is at 1750 — 1725 cm^{-1} (5.72 — 5.80 μ). The anhydrides show double absorption bands, one band is at 1850 — 1800 cm^{-1} (5.40 & 5.55 μ) and the second band is at 1800 — 1750 cm^{-1} (5.55 & 5.72 μ).

The N — H stretching vibrations are positioned around 3300 cm^{-1} (3.0 μ) in the form of a doublet for a primary amine. The N — H in-plane scissoring motion is found at 1610 cm^{-1} (6.2 μ) where as the out of plane bending is located at 830 cm^{-1} (12.0 μ). The latter is in the form of a broad for primary amines. On the other hand secondary amine shows a single absorption band at 3350 cm^{-1} (2.98 μ). The amine salts are found to absorb at lower frequencies, usually with a weak band at 3140 and 2500 cm^{-1} (3.5 & 4.0 μ). The absorption band at 2040 cm^{-1} (4.9 μ) is due to $N^{+}H_3$ group.

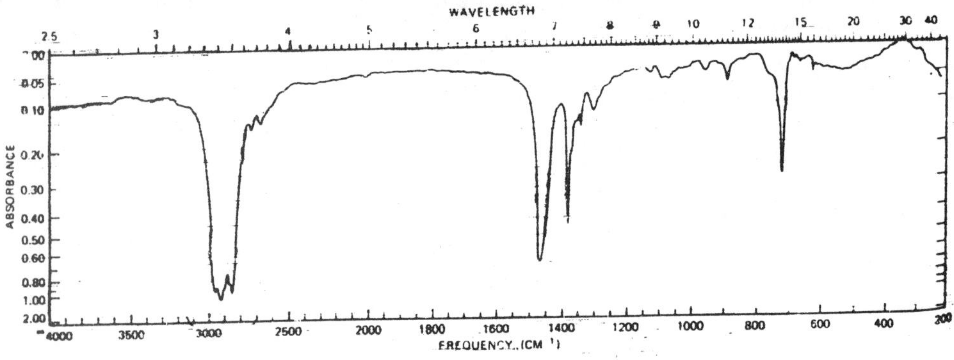

Ir Spectrum No. 1 Dodecane, Neat liquid film.

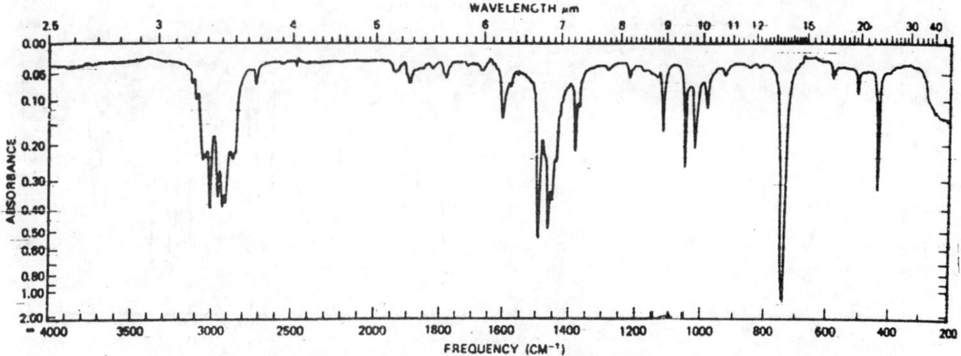

Ir Spectrum No. 2. O-xylene, Thin Film, Neat

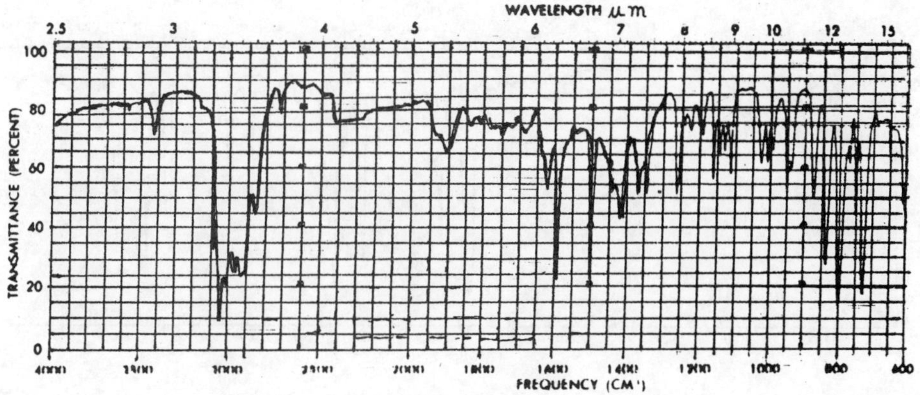

Ir Spectrum No. 3, 2-Methylnaphthalene (melt, NaCl)

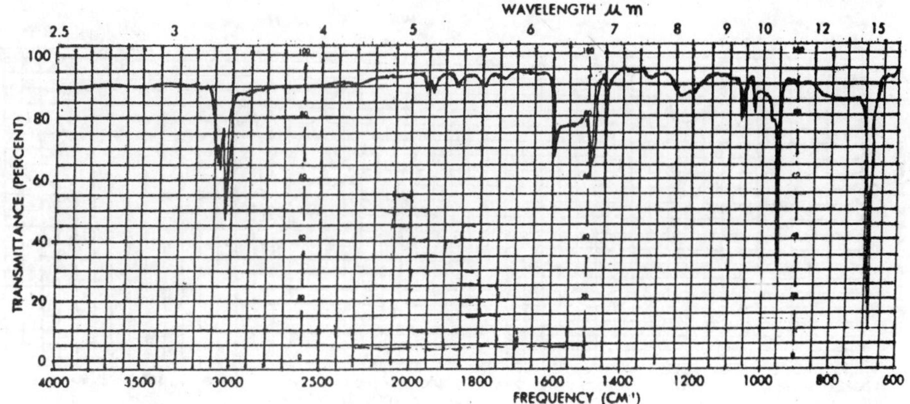

Ir Spectrum No. 4. Trans Stilbene, CCl_4 Solution, NaCl

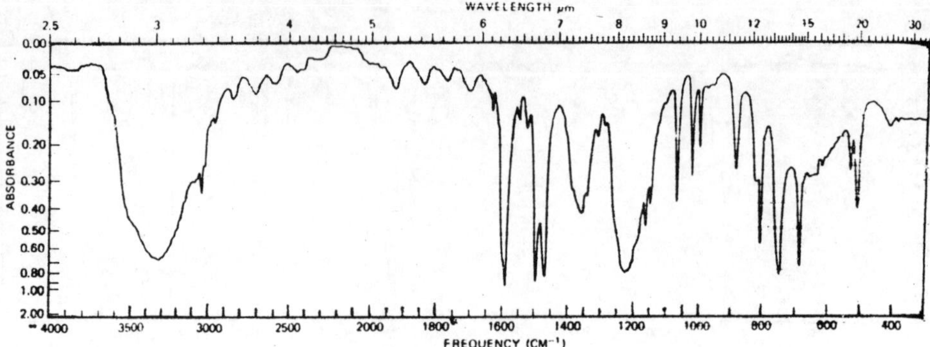

Ir Spectrum No. 5. Phenol, Capillary Cell, Neat

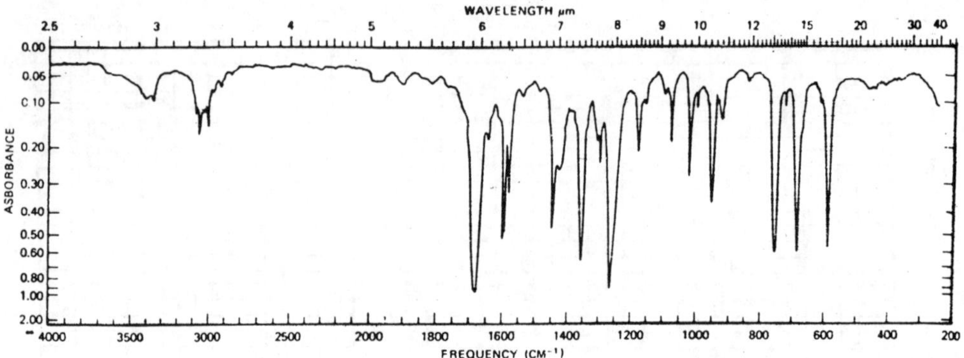

Ir Spectrum No. 6. Acetophenone, Capillary Cell, Neat

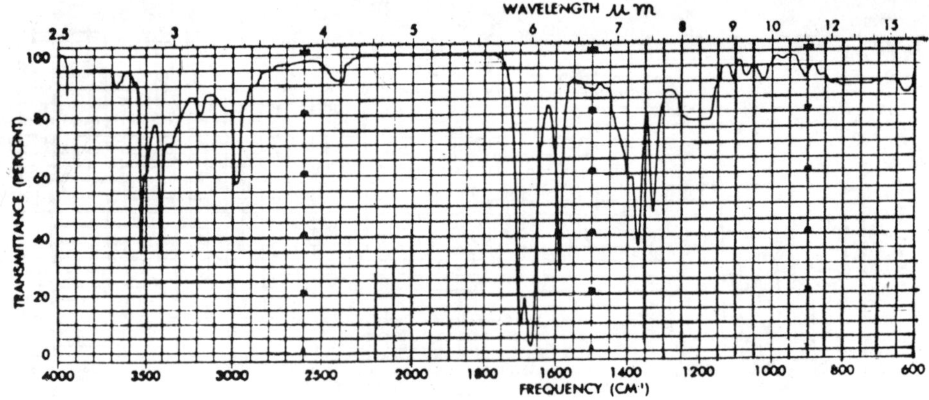

Ir Spectrum No. 7. Acetamide in $CHCl_3$ Solution

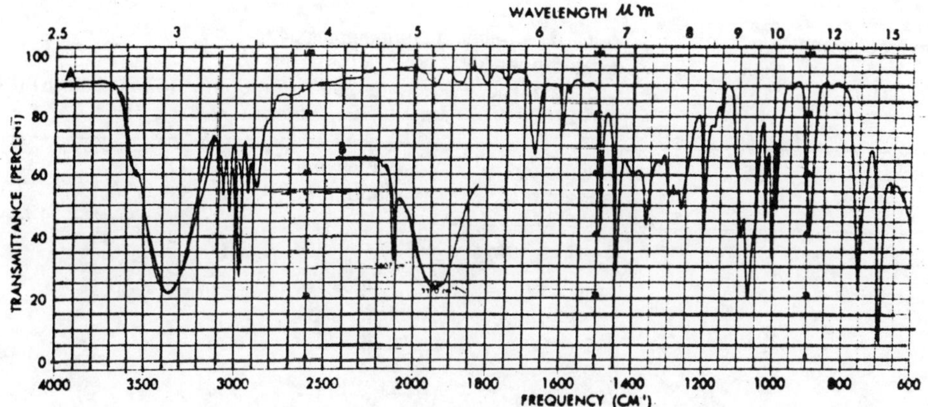

Ir Spectrum No. 8. 1-Phenylethanol, Neat liquid film

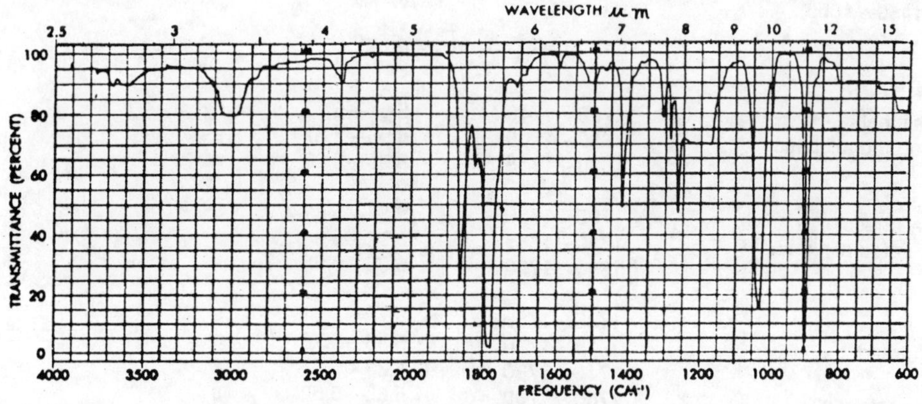

Ir Spectrum No. 9. Succinic anhydride in $CHCl_3$ Solution

The asymmetric and symmetric stretching motions of a nitro group (NO_2) are shown in the form of two strong bands at 1560 and 1350 cm^{-1} (6.41 & 7.40 μ). The stretching frequencies of SO_2 are found at 1400 — 1310 and 1230 — 1120 cm^{-1} (7.14 — 7.63 and 8.13 — 8.93 μ). S = O absorbs at 1200 — 1040 cm^{-1} (8.33 — 9.62 μ) and S — O around 900 — 700 (11.11 — 14.28 μ). For practice purpose some representative infrared spectras have been in corpornted below.

EXERCISE 1. Take the ir of benzoic acid by mull and pellet methods and identify the major peaks.

EXERCISE 2. Take ir of 5% solution of isopropyl alcohol (use solvent CCl_4 for range above 1333 cm^{-1} and CS_2 and below 1333 cm^{-1}) and identify the major peaks.

Table 18.1 Principal Absorption Bands of Selected Functional Groups

	C—H Stretching
Alkanes Alkenes Alkynes Aromatic hydrocarbons	Located in the 2850—3300 cm^{-1} (3.51—3.03 μ) region. Intensity[a] m to s.
	C≡C—H stretching characteristically located near 3300 cm^{-1} (3.03 μ) (s)
Aldehyde C—H	Characteristic. Two bands 2800—2900 cm^{-1} (3.57—3.45 μ) (W) and 2700—2780 cm^{-1} (3.70—3.60 μ) (W)

	Frequency range cm^{-1}	Wavelength range, μ	Intensity
	C—H bending		
Alkanes	1340—1480	7.46—6.75	m—s
Alkenes	1300—1420	7.70—7.04	s
	800—1000	12.5—10.0	s
Alkynes	630	15.9	s
Aromatic[b]	700—900	14.3—11.1	v
	C—C double and triple bond stretching		
Alkenes	1620—1680	6.17—5.95	W—M
Alkynes[c]	2100—2300	4.76—4.35	W—M
Aromatic[d] 1450—1600	6.90—6.25	W—M	
	Carbonyl C=O stretching		
Aldehydes[e]			
Saturated aliphatic	1720—1740	5.81—5.75	s
α, β-Unsaturated aliphatic	1680—1705	5.95—5.87	s
Aryl	1680—1715	5.95—5.83	s
Ketones			
Saturated aliphatic	1705—1750	5.87—5.71	s
α, β-Unsaturated aliphatic	1660—1685	6.02—5.94	s
Aryl	1680—1700	5.95—5.88	s
Esters			
Saturated	1735—1750	5.76—5.71	s
α, β-Unsaturated	1715—1730	5.83—5.78	s
Aryl	1715—1730	5.83—5.78	s
Saturated γ-lactones	1760—1780	5.68—5.62	s
Esters			
Saturated β-lactones	~ 1820	~ 5.50	s
α, β-Unsaturated γ--lactones	1740—1760	5.75—5.70	s
β, γ-Unsaturated γ-lactones	1800	~ 5.56	s
-ketoesters	~ 1650	~ 6.06	
Carboxylic acids[f]			
Saturated	1700—1725	5.88—5.80	s
α, β-Unsaturated	1690—1715	5.92—5.83	s
Aryl	1680—1700	5.95—5.88	s
Carboxylate ion			
—C(=O)(—O) (resonance, O‒‒C‒‒O)	1550—1610	6.45—6.21	s
	1300—1400	7.69—7.15	s

	Frequency range cm^{-1}	Wavelength range, μ	Intensity
Amides[g]			
Solid or concentrated solution	1630—1680	6.14—5.95	s
Dilute solution	1670—1700	5.99—5.88	s
Lactams	1680—1780	5.95—5.62	s
Ureas	1660—1730	6.02—5.78	s
Imides (two bands)	1670—1700	5.99—5.88	s
	1700—1730		s
	Alcohols and phenols		
O—H stretching			
Free OH	3590—3650	2.79—2.74	Sharp bands (v)
Hydrogen-bonded OH	3450—3570	2.90—2.80	Sharp bands (v)
	Intramolecular-no change on diluting solution; Intermolecular-change on diluting solution.		
Chelate compounds	2500—3200	4.00—3.10	Broad peak (v)
O—H bending and C—O stretching			
1° and 2° alcohols	1050—1100	9.50—9.10	s
	1310—1410	7.60—7.10	s
N—H stretching			
1° (two bands)	~ 3400	~ 2.94	Sharp (m)
2°	~ 3500	~ 2.86	Sharp (m)
	3300—3150	3.03—2.86	m
3°	—	—	
Amine salts	3000—3150	3.33—3.18	m
N—H bending			
1° and 2°	1550—1650	6.45—6.06	m—s
Salts (two bands)	1570—1600	6.37—6.25	s
	~ 1500	~ 6.67	s
C—N stretching			
Aliphatic (two bands)	1000—1200	10.0—8.30	w
	1400	7.14	w
Aromatic	1250—1350	8.00—7.41	s
	Nitrites and Isocyanides		
C ≡ N stretching			
Nitriles	2220—2280	4.50—4.38	m
Isocyanides	2050—2220	4.87—4.50	m
	Nitro compounds		
N—O stretching			
Aromatic, asymmetric	1500—1570	6.67—6.37	s
Aromatic, symmetric	1300—1370	7.70—7.30	s
Aliphatic, asymmetric	1500—1570	6.45—6.37	s
Aliphatic, symmetric	1370—1380	7.30—7.25	s
C—N stretching			
Aromatic	~ 860	~ 11.6	m
Aliphatic	usually ~ 915	~ 10.9	m

	Frequency range cm^{-1}	Wavelength range, μ	Intensity
	Halogen Compounds		
... stretching	1000—1400	10.0—7.10	s
C – Cl stretching	600—800	16.6—12.5	s
C – Br stretching	500—650	20.0—16.6	s
C – I stretching	500—600	20.0—16.6	s
	Sulfur compounds		
Thiols; S—H stretching	2550—2600	3.92—3.85	w
Thiocarbonyl compounds ; C=S stretching	1050—1200	9.58—8.33	
Sulfones, including sulfonamides S=O stretching (two bands)	1140—1180	8.77—8.48	s
	1300—1350	7.69—7.41	s

a Intensity; S, strong; m, medium; w, weak; v, variable.
b Position varies with number of adjacent hydrogen atoms.
c If —C ≡ C — H, characteristic C — H stretching also.
d Usually four bands.
e Also display characteristic C — H stretching.
f O — H stretching also—several bands 2500—2700 cm^{-1} (4.00—3.70m) (w).
g Position of band varies appreciably depending spectrum is of the solid, of a concentrated solution, or of a dilute solution. Also seen is NH_2 and NH stretching, similar that of amines.
h These bands are strong, but very variable in position.

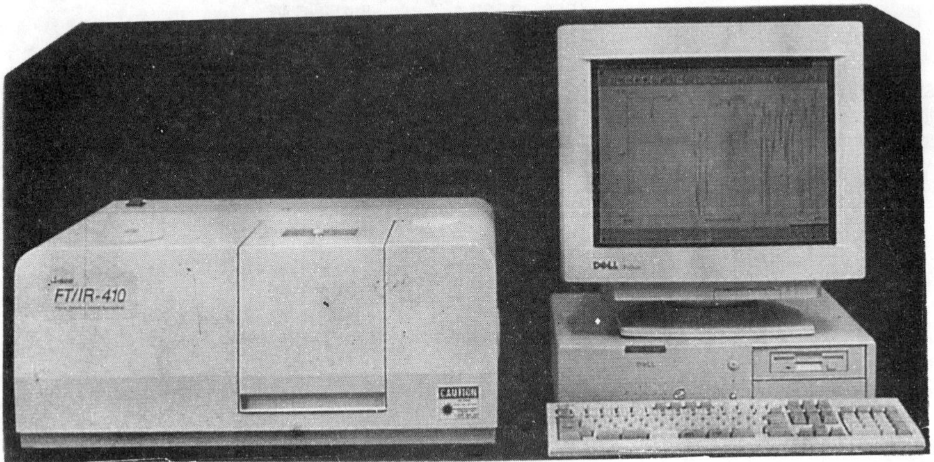

Fig. 18.9 FT Infrared Spectrophotometer Model–410 JASCO (Courtesy of Jasco)

19

Nuclear Magnetic Resonance Spectroscopy

19.1 General

In the previous chapters we have learnt that molecules absorb UV-visible radiation at a wavelength of 200-800 nm and infrared radiation at a wavelength of 2 to 16 μ. Also, while the shorter and more energetic waves in the UV-Vis region affect the energy levels of the electrons, the longer and less energetic IR waves produce only vibration, deformation and rotations in the molecules. However, in the nuclear magnetic resonance spectroscopy, radiation of very long wavelength and extremely low energy, $\lambda = 10^7$ to 10^8 μ or 100 to 10,000 cm in radiofrequency region are used. These waves are not energetic enough to affect the electronic, vibrational or rotational levels of molecules, but will interact with the nuclei of certain atoms that are exposed to a strong magnetic field, therefore the term nuclear magnetic resonance (NMR) spectroscopy has been coined.

19.2 Magnetic and Non-Magnetic Nuclei

We are familiar with the atomic structure and know that atomic nuclei contain nucleonic particles like protons and neutrons. The protons are positively charged which also means that the nuclei are positively charged. The protons, like electrons spin on their own axis. They possess a quantized spin angular quantum number or spin quantum number which is given by $h/2\pi\sqrt{S(S+1)}$. The individual protons and neutrons have spin quantum numbers of $+\frac{1}{2}$ and $-\frac{1}{2}$ only. The total spin quantum number I is a constant for a nucleus. This constant depends on the number of nucleons and the symmetry of charge distribution. In order to calculate the total nuclear spin the following rules are followed :

(i) Nuclei which have an odd mass number i.e. an odd number of nucleons, will have ‹*integral* spin

e.g. $\frac{1}{2}, \frac{3}{2}, \frac{5}{2}$ . . . . etc.

(ii) Nuclei which have odd number of protons and neutrons i.e. even mass number, will have *integral* spin number e.g. 1, 2, 3,---- etc.

(iii) Nuclei which have an even number of protons and neutrons i.e. even mass number, will have *zero* spin. This is because there will be a pairing of opposite spins in the respective nucleons and will cancel each other. All this is depicted in Table 19.1.

Table 19.1

Element	No. of Protons	No. of Neutrons n	Mass number z + n = A	Spin I
H	1	0	1 (odd)	1/2
Deutrium H_2	1	1	2 (even)	1
Tritium, H_3	1	2	3 (odd)	1/2
Boron, B	5	5	10 (even)	3
Boron, B	5	6	11 (odd)	3/2
Carbon, C	6	6	12 (even)	0
Carbon, C	6	7	13 (odd)	1/2
Oxygen, O	8	8	16 (even)	0
Nitrogen N_2	7	7	14 (even)	1
Fluorine, F	9	10	19 (odd)	1/2
Phosphorus, P	15	16	31 (odd)	1/2
Sulphur, S	16	16	32 (even)	0

Further, we should know that the spinning of the positively charged nucleus allows the distributive positive charge to rotate giving rise to the equivalent of a current flowing in a circular path. This in turn produces a magnetic field, with a magnetic moment μ directed along the axis of the spin as shown in Fig. 19.1.

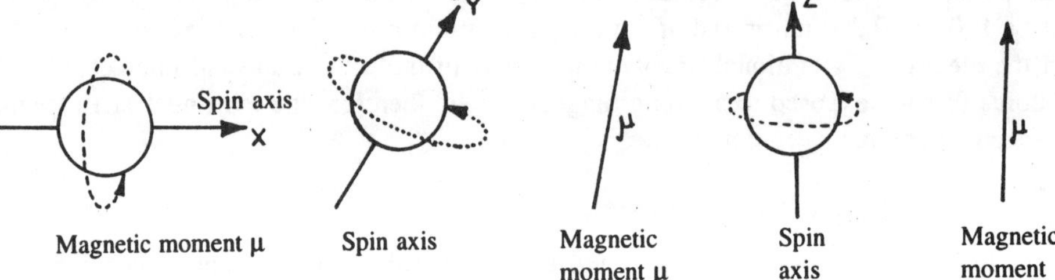

Fig. 19.1. Spining proton

From the Table 19.1, we observe that nucleuses of P^{31}, H^1 and F^{19} have same angular momentum although their masses are different whereas that of S^{32}, O^{16} and C^{12} have zero spin and no angular momentum. Also, nuclie like P^{31}, H^1 and F^{19} having spin quantum number I > O behave like tiny bar magnet i.e. are magnetic, while S^{32}, O^{16} and C^{12} having spin quantum number I = O are non-magnetic in behaviour. Thus a bar magnet (i.e. a magnetic dipole) will change the orientation of another magnetic dipole placed in its neighbourhood and consequently will give rise to a magnetic force. The region of place in which a magnetic force exists is called a magnetic field.

19.3 Nuclear Precession

It is a known fact that when a magnet is placed in a magnetic field, it tries to align itself with the field and comes to rest. If it is disturbed, it will olcillate. The frequency of this ascillation will depend on the strength of the magnetic field. In a similar manner a nucleus will behave like a small bar magnet and when placed in an external field will align with that field and ascillate- when disturbed.

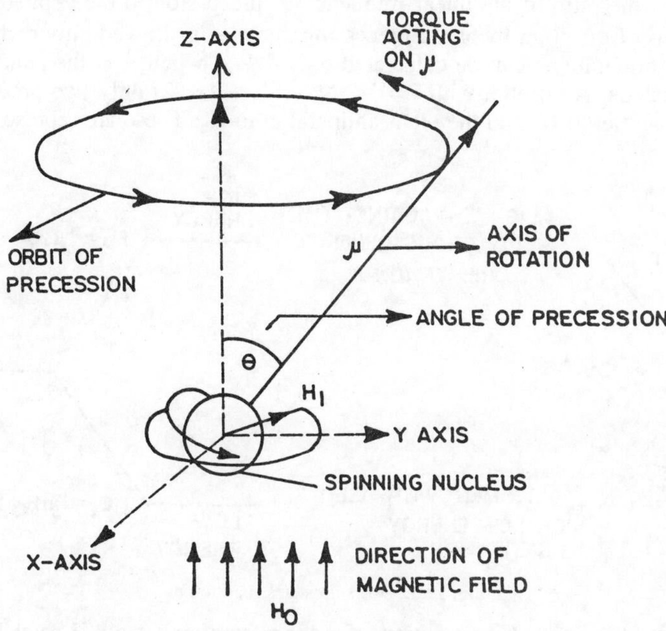

Fig. 19.2. Nuclear precession.

In the Fig 19.2 is shown a nucleus spining on x axis and producing a magnetic moment μ. If a powerful external field H_o is placed along z axis the nucleus will make an angle Θ with it. The external field will exert a force at right angle to the magnetic moment on the nucleus (i.e. torque) in such a way that the nucleus starts *precessing* along the direction of the external field. The angular frequency (ω_L) of this precession (called Larmor precession frequency) will depend on the strength of the applied magnetic field and the nature of the nuclear magnetic. This can be written as :

$$\omega_L = H_o \cdot \gamma \qquad \text{---------1}$$

Where ω_L is Larmor angular frequency. H_o is the applied magnetic field γ is the nature of the nucleus.

Actually, γ is a ratio of the magnetic moment μ of the nucleus to the angular momentum of the nucleus and is called gyromagnetic ratio.

The magnitude of the angular frequency ω_L of a motion can be converted to that of its linear frequency as follows:

Angular frequency = $2\pi \times$ linear frequency

$$\omega_L = 2\pi V_L$$

But $\omega_L = H_o\gamma$

$$\text{or} \qquad 2\pi V_L = H_o \gamma$$

$$V_L = \frac{H_o \gamma}{2\pi}$$

$$\text{and} \qquad \gamma = \frac{2\pi V_L}{H_o} \qquad \text{.............. 2}$$

i.e. γ is a function the ratio of the linear frequency of precession to the applied magnetic field.

However, in terms of quantum theory, a precessing nucleus is allowed only certain orientations with respect to H_O. These orientations can be calculated by 2 I + 1, where I is the spin quantum number of the nucleus. For a nucleus like proton with I = 1/2 (2 × 1/2 + 1 = 2) only two precessional orientations are possible i.e. one parallel to H_o and the other antiparallel to H_o. These are represented in the Fig. 19.3.

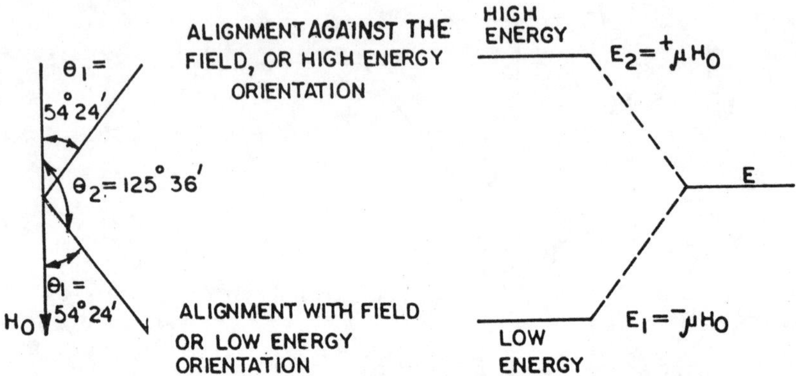

Fig. 19.3. Two spin states for Proton.

Δ E is the energy difference for transition of proton from spin state E_1 and F_2 (i.e. between two states) and can be represented by : Δ E = 2 μ H_o. (For a nucleus with spin quantum number I, this difference in energy is given by : $\Delta E = \frac{\mu H_o}{I}$) Now, if energy equal to 2 μ H_o is supplied to such a system, a hydrogen nucleus will undergo a transition from one spin state to another. The energy for this transition can be supplied by electro-magnetic radiation in the radiofrequency range. If the magnetic field (H_1) of the radiation is oscillating in a plane at right angles to the applied field (H_o) if the frequency of radiation (v) is the same as the Larmor frequency of precession (V_L) of the nucleus, transfer of energy from the radiation to the nucleus can occur. This phenomenon of transfer of energy is called *resonance.*

The energy of radio waves is given by planck equation E = hV and when resonance takes place this energy is absorbed to bring about nuclear transition. But, the energy to bring about transition ΔE for a nucleus of spin quantum number I is given by E = μ H_o/I. At resonance the energy of radiation will be equal to transition energy. This can be written as :

$$E = hv$$

$$E = \frac{\mu H_o}{I}$$

$$\therefore \; hv = \frac{\mu H_o}{I} \quad \text{or} \quad v = \frac{\mu H_o}{Ih}$$

Thus in summery, we can place a nucleus in a powerful magnetic field H_o so that it precesses and then expose it to radio waves whose frequency (V) can be varied with the precessing frequency (V_L) of the nucleus. When the two frequencies (i.e. V_L & V) match, there will be an exchange of energy between the rotating field and the precessing nucleus. This results in the magnetic moment of the nucleus to be reoriented opposite to the direction of external field (H_o).

19.4 Instrumentation Aspects

The chief components of a nuclear magnetic resonance spectrophotometer consist of (i) a magnet (ii) or radionave transmitter and sweep generator (iii) a radiowave receiver or detector and (iv) a recorder as

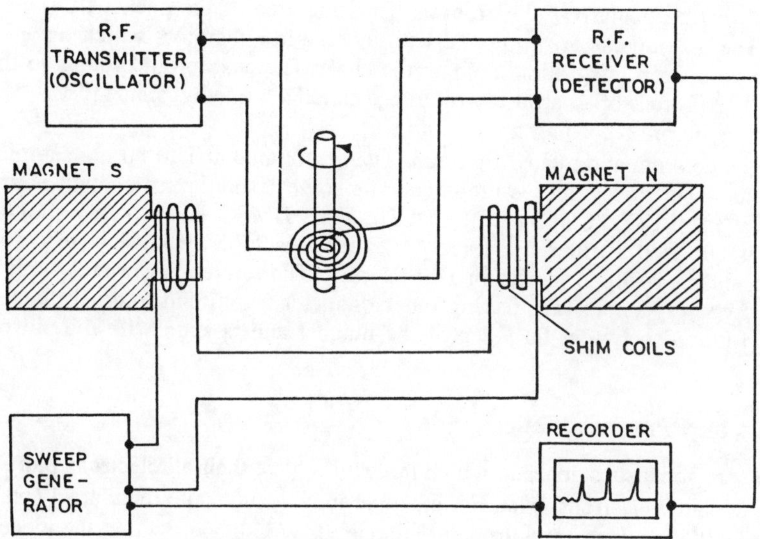

Fig. 19.4 A schematic diagram of a NMR spectrometer

shown in Fig 19.4.

Magnet : A powerful magnet is required to provide a stable and a homogeneous field. The field must remain constant for a long period of time. Magnets of large size, (e.g. 15" in diameter, 23,500 gaus & or 100 MH_z) which are capable of strong fields are used. These magnets contain small air gaps (1.5-2.0") between their poles so that the sample tubes can be spun between the poles. By spinning the solution of sample tubes along their verticle axis between the poles, the inhomogeneity of the field perpendicular to the direction of spinning can be averaged out.

Radio frequency Transmitter and Sweep generator : The radio frequency (r.f.) transmitter coil is placed perpendicular to the magnetic field and can transmit radio waves of some fixed frequency depending upon the size of the magnet e.g. 60, 100, 220, 400 MH_z.

As the magnet and the radio-frequency transmitter both produce fixed fields, (also fixed frequency) sweep generator is also installed to supply a variable dc current to a secondary smaller magnet. By this kind of arrangement the total applied magnetic field can be varied or swept over a small range so that the precession frequency changes with that of the radio frequency field (R.F.) The rate a which the field is swept is in the range of 5-10 milligauss per minute. Thus, for an instrument with a magnet of 60 MH_z (14,000 gauss) this rate will be about 11-12 H_z. When the field is swept at a very rapid rate a ringing pattern or a wiggle is observed on the spectrum.

Radio frequency Detector : The radio-frequency (r.f.) detector or receiver coil is fixed perpendicular to both magnetic field and the transmitter coil and is tuned to the same frequency as the transmitter. By this arrangement the overloading of the receiver is minimized which otherwise would cause the direct coupling of the transmitter and receiver coils. When the precession frequency is matched with radio frequency, the nuclei contained in the sample induces an electromagnetic field (emf) in the detector coil due to the change in the magnetic flux caused by the nuclear transition. This signal is amplified and passed on to the recorder.

Recorder : In practice, R.F. oscillator frequency is held constant and R.F. receiver signal is measured as a function of magnetic field strength. The plot or spectrum consists of signal strength on Y-axis against magnetic field on X-axis. The strength of the resonance signal is directly proportional to the number of nuclei resonating at that particularly field strength. Thus the area of the peak will gives the number of resonating nuclei. The instruments are equipped with automatic integrators which record the peak areas in the form of a superimposed integration trace on the chart. The position of protons in the spectrum are measured relative to 12 protons of an arbitrary reference called tetramethyl silane [TMS, $(CH_3)_4$ Si] which is added to the sample before recording a spectrum.

Sample : For the determination of NMR of an organic compound 1 to 30 mg sample is required. A 2 to 10% dilute solution of the sample is prepared. The solvent should not contain H atom of its own. The solvents generally are CCl_4, $CDCl_3$, CD_3 $COCD_3$, D_2O, DMSO etc. i.e. they should be deuterated compounds. TMS is not used as reference for D_2O, as it is insoluble in D_2O, instead sodium salt of 2, 2- dimethyl-2- silapentane-5-sulphoric acid or DSS is used. The reference is mixed with the sample and placed in a special type of sample tube having outer diameter 5 mm and internal diameter 4 mm. The sample tube is then placed between the poles of the magnet and is spun with the aid of an air driven turbine.

19.5 Diamagnetic and Paramagnetic Fields

We know that there are some substances in which molecules have their all electrons paired whereas there are some in which unpaired electrons exist. For example in NO_2 molecule there are 17 valence electrons, out of which 16 are paired and one on nitrogen is unpaired. We also know that the electrons while they are spinning on their axis, they are also moving in orbits around the nuclei. The two motions due to spinning and orbital of charged electrons generate magnetic moments. On the contrary, in atoms or molecules in which all the electrons are paired, the magnetic moments produced by oppositely spinning electrons balance one another out and consequently no net magnetic moment is produced. Such substances, if they are placed in an external magnetic field will generate a magnetic moment which will oppose the applied magnetic field. As a result of this opposition, these substances are repelled from the applied magnetic field. Such substances are called *diamagnetic substances* and the induced field in opposition to the applied field is called a *diamagnetic field.* However, on the other hand substances (e.g. NO_2, Cu, Mn etc) which contain one or more unpaired electrons possess a permanent magnetic moment because the spin and the angular moments of the unpaired electrons are not balanced out. If these substances are placed in an external magnetic field, their permanent magnetic moments will align with the field and thus will reinforse the external field. These substances as they contain one or more unpaired electrons are called *paramagnetic substances* and their permanent magnetic moments which aligns with the external magnetic field is called the *paramagnetic field.*

Let us consider we have a diamagnetic substance and is placed in an external magnetic field. The induced electronic circulations will produce a diamagnetic field. Therefore the net field actually experienced by the nuclei will be less. This protection of the nuclei from the external field is called *diamagnetic shielding.* The extent of this shielding will depend on the density of electrons surrounding the nuclei contained in the sample and is represented by the expression :

$$H = H_o (1 - \sigma)$$

Where H is the actual field felt, H_o is the external magnetic field.

Thus different protons in a compound will be shielded differently by the electron clouds depending upon the structure of the molecule. For example ethyl alcohol (CH_3—CH_2—OH) contains three different types of protons, namely methyl, methylene and hydroxyl. Proton attached to cabon is covered by a denser cloud than proton attached to oxygen. Oxygen pulls away electrons from C_1 than C_2 and there is decrease in electron density at C_1 and C_2, consequently proton at C_1 and C_2 are less shielded. So when ethyl alcohol is placed in an external magnetic field, the field experienced by OH proton is stronger (less shielding) than that of CH_3 or CH_2 protons. Thus as the external field is slowly increased by means of sweep generator, the less shielded OH protons will resonate at a less strong field. Three groups of signals will appear in the NMR spectrum of ethyl alcohol and the peak areas will be in the ratio of 1 : 2 : 3. (Fig. 19.5)

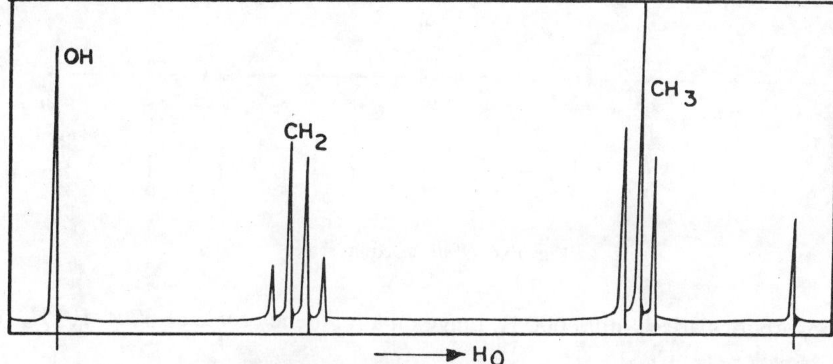

Fi.g 19.5. NMR spectrum of ethanol.

19.6 NMR spectrum and scales of Measurement

For recording the NMR spectrum of a sample when sweep is started the recorder pen moves from left side of the chart paper the right side as the magnetic field increases gradually. The left side of the spectrum is the less strong field or down field and on this side less shielded or deshielded protons or nuclei appear. The right side is the strong field or up field and more shielded protons or nuclei appear on this side.

The NMR spectrum of a compound is a plot of signal strength versus magnetic field. Since it is difficult to measure a magnetic field, therefore, the value of absorption frequencies of the protons is determined with respect to some reference compound though the most suitable standard would have been a bare proton without any shielding electrons, but in reality such is not feasible. A commonly used standard for NMR work is tetramethyl silane (TMS) and is added into the sample solution. The important properties of TMS are that; (i) it is a symmetrical molecule and gives one sharp peak of 12 equal protons, (ii) it is unreactive and does not associate with the sample, (iii) it is volatile and allows recovery of the sample, (iv) the molecule absorbs at high field as it is very much shielded. The difference between the resonance frequencies of protons in the sample (υ sample) and the resonance frequency of the protons in the standard (υ standard) is called *chemical shift*

$$\delta = \frac{H_o - H_{ref}}{H_{ref}} \times 10^6 \text{ ppm}$$

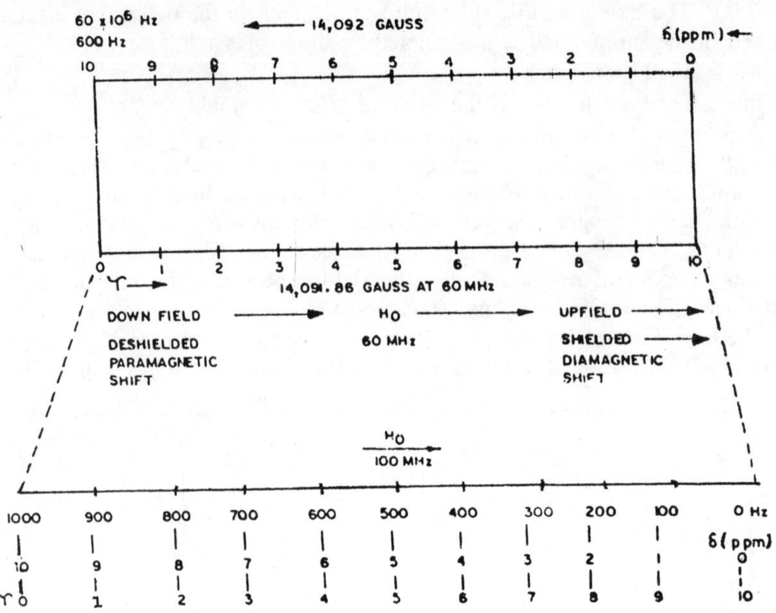

Fig. 19.6. NMR spectrum scale.

The proton absorptions arise within 600 H_z range on a frequency scale of 60×10^6 H_z (i.e. 60 MH_z). Thus 1H_z = 1 cycle/sec. (CPS)

$\therefore$ the value of 120 H_z at 60 MH_z is ≡ 120 CPS at 60 MH_z.

The frequency at which absorption peaks occur are also measured in units called ppm (parts per million). The ppm is obtained by dividing chemical shift by oscillator frequency (H_z) and then multiplying by 10^6 as shown below :

$$\text{PPM} = \frac{\text{Chemical shift } (H_z)}{\text{Oscillator frequency } (H_z)} \times 10^6$$

A chemical shift of 80 H_z downfield TMS measured on a 40 MH_z instrument will become 120 H_z when measured on 60 MH_z instruments as :

$$\frac{60}{40} \times 80 = 120 \ H_z$$

Similarly, when measured with a 100 MH_z instrument it will become 200 H_z as :

$$\frac{100}{40} \times 80 = 200 \ H_z$$

Thus an instrument of 100 MH_z will have a higher resolving power and will give better line separation.

The system δ (delta) scale is criticized by some in the sense that values increase from right to left while the magnetic field increases from left to right. It is dimensionless and is independent of the applied frequency. Thus a peak at 60 H_z (υ 60) from TMS at applied frequency of 60 MH_z would be at δ 1.00 or 1.00 PPM:

$$\delta \text{ or PPM} = \frac{60 \ H_z}{60 \times 10^6 \ H_z} \times 10^6 = 1.00$$

The other system is (tau) scale in which the value of τ is parallel to the increasing value of applied magnetic field. The value of TMS absorption in τ scale is 10 (τ = 10.00-δ) and consequently higher τ value will indicate greater shielding.

The same peak at an applied frequency of 100 MH_z would be at υ 100 but still would be at δ 1.00:

$$\delta \text{ or PPM} = \frac{100 H_z}{100 \times 10^6 H_z} \times 10^6 = 1.00$$

The chemical shift is proportional to the strength of the applied field H_o and therefore to the applied frequency because of the diamagnetic shielding induced by H_o.

19.7 Factors Affecting Chemical Shifts

Earliar, while quoting the example of ethyl alcohol, we indicated that its three different types of protons would be shielded differently by the electron clouds.

The two main types of factors which affect chemical shifts depending upon the structure of molecules are as follows :

(a) Local deshielding caused by paramagnetic currents about the nuclei.

(b) Shielding and deshielding caused by currents in the neighbouring atoms and groups.

(a) The deshielding caused by local paramagnetic currents depends on the existance of low lying excited states of magnetic nuclei. In the case of protons there are no such states, therefore the local paramagnetic effects are negligible in their PMR spector.

(b) In order to understand the effects of shielding and deshielding we will consider representative compounds like (i) ethane, (ii) ethylene (iii) acetylene and (iv) benzene. Normally, on the basis of diamagnetic shielding, we should expect the values of chemical shifts to follow the order of electronegativity of carbon compounds $sp > sp^2 > sp^3$. But, in actual practice we find that acetylene proton has chemical shift intermediate to that of methyl protons on the strong field side and ethylene protons on the weaker field side. In the same way, we may expect the benzene protons to resonate at a frequency similar to those in ethylene because they are in SP^2 state. But we find benzene protons are less shielded than ethylenic protons and appear on the lower field side.

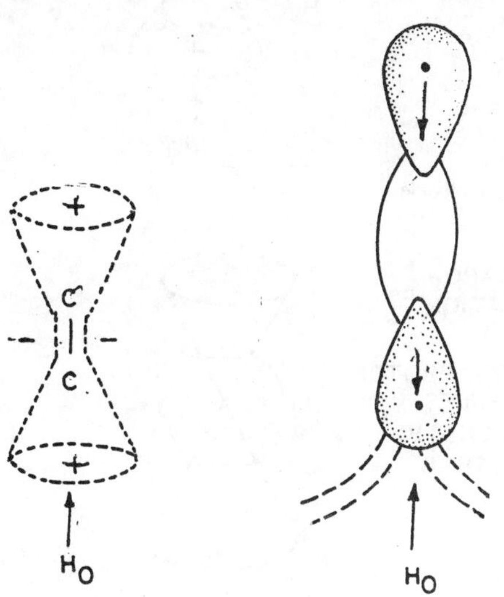

Fig. 19.7. Acetylene molecle.

The position with acetylene is that it is a linear molecule and the π orbitals of the triple bond are symmetrical about the molecular axis as shown in the Fig. 19.7. When acetylene or acetylenic compound is placed in an external magnetic field, the preferred orientation of the molecule is such that its axis is parallel to the applied field. The electron currents flow in a direction perpendicular to the applied field and circulate within the axially symmetrical axis. Thus the degree of shielding experienced by these protons will be higher inspite the sp carbon tend to reduce the electron density around these protons. Similar will be case with groups like C ≡ N.

In the case of ethylenic protons the situation is different because of the side-wise overslap of p-orbitals the π cloud is concentrated to the left and right of the bond axis in a plane perpendicular to that of the paper. When such a molecule is placed in an external applied field π electrons circulate within the π orbital but perpendicular to the applied field and therefore these protons experience a paramagnetic shielding. They have a chemical shift lower than acetylene. Similar is the case with groups like C = O, C = N, C = S etc.

In benzene and aromatic compounds, π electrons being delocalized circulate over a number of atomic centres and thus produce what is called 'ring currents'. These ring currents produce strong deshielding effect than that observed in ethylenic protons therefore, the aromatic protons resonate at lower or weaker field. However, those protons which do not come within the influence of ring currents will not be deshielded.

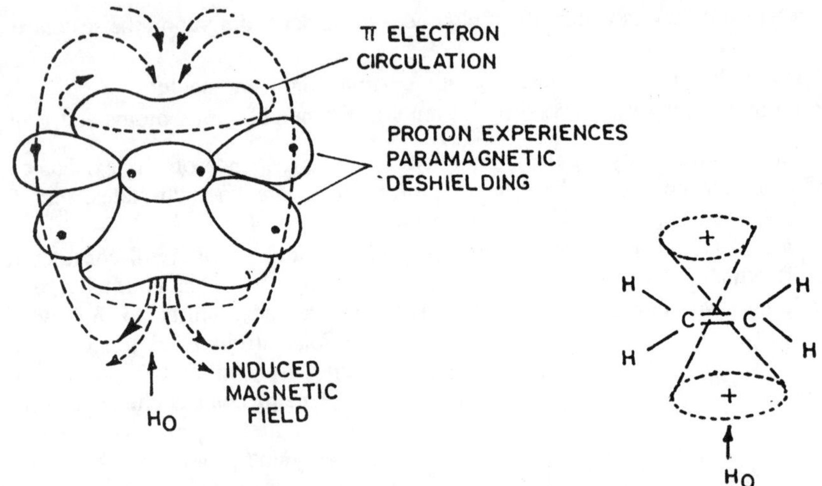

Fig. 19.8. Ethylene molecule.

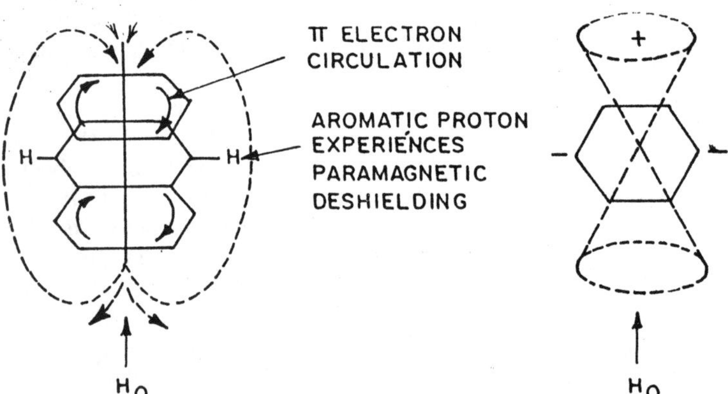

Fig. 19.9. Ring currents in benzene.

19.8 Spin-Spin Interactions

Let us consider the example of ethyl acetate and study its NMR spectrum (Fig. 19.10). Ethyl acetate has the structure HC_3 — CO — O — CH_2CH_3 and contains three different types of protons namely; (i) CH_3 — CO —, (ii) — O — CH_2 and (iii) — C — CH_3. The NMR spectrum will show three groups of peaks representing the three types of protons in the ratio of 3 : 2 : 3. The equivalent protons i.e. protons having identical electronic and magnetic environment will have similar chemical shifts. Accordingly the peak for

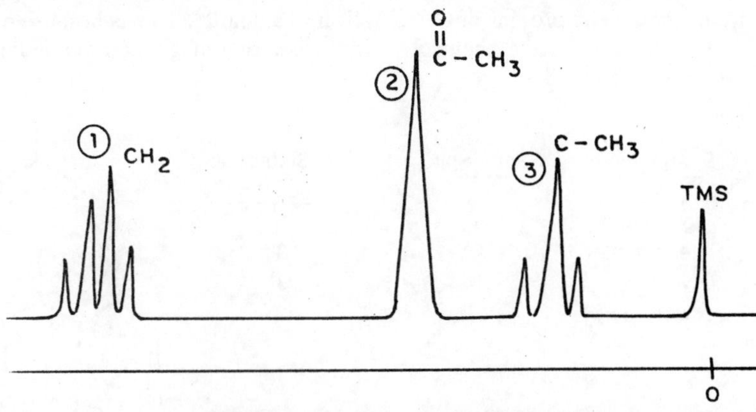

Fig. 19.10. NMR Spectrum of ethyl acetate.

CH_3 CO will show a single peak whereas methylene and methyl peaks will be in the form of multiplets. Further, we know that protons orient their spins with or against the applied field. These orientations will influence the spin of the nearest bonding electron which in turn will affect the spin of the other bonding electron in the orbital and then to the next proton. Thus the information concerning the spin states is transmitted to the neighbouring nuclei by means of the intervening bonding electrons. This effect is called *Spin - spin coupling* and since it causes splitting in the peaks in a spectrum, it is also known as ***spin-spin splitting***. The separation of the two peaks of a doublet depends on the effectiveness of the coupling and is denoted by a *coupling constant* J (in H_z or CPS). It is independent of the applied magnetic field and is not affected by a solvent. There is very little effective coupling between nuclei which are separated by more than three covalent bonds, except in the case of aromatic and conjugated alkenes where electrons are delocalized.

As already indicated ethyl acetate shows three groups of peaks in the ratio of 2: 3: 3. The acetyl,

	Energy Level	Total Spin	Statistical Count
↑↑	High energy Level	+1	1
↑↓ ↓↑	Intermediate Energy	0	2
↓↓	Low Energy Level	−1	1

Parallel and anti-parllel to magnetic field

1 : 2 : 1

Fig. 19.11. Energy level diagram for methylene protons.

$COCH_3$ protons have no neighbouring protons to couple with and thus appear as a singlet. The 3 proton peak of — CCH_3 at high field is split into a triplet. It is because methylene protons orient themselves in the external magnetic field and combinations can be grouped into three energy levels as shown in the diagram (Fig. 19.11).

The peak intensities of the triplet are in the ratio of 1 : 2 : 1. This can also be explained by the following rule. The – OCH_2 has two protons, so we can take n = 2. Thus the multiplicity will be n + 1 = 3. Intensity ratio of 3 sub-peaks will be given by the coefficient in the expansion of $(n+1)^n$ or $(n+2)^2$ = $1n^2 + 2n + 1$ i.e. 1 : 2 : 1.

On the other hand the methylene protons of OCH_2 split into a quartet. This is because of the influence of three protons of C-CH_3 which will orient themselves in the external magnetic field and can be grouped into 4 energy levels as shown in Fig. 19.12.

	Energy Level	Total Spin	Statistical count
↑↑↑	High energy	+ 3/2	1
↑↑↓ ↑↓↑ ↓↑↑	Intermediate	+ 1/2	3
↑↓↓ ↓↑↓ ↓↓↑	Level	– 1/2	3
↓↓↓	Lower energy	– 3/2	1

Parallel and antiparallel to magnetic field.

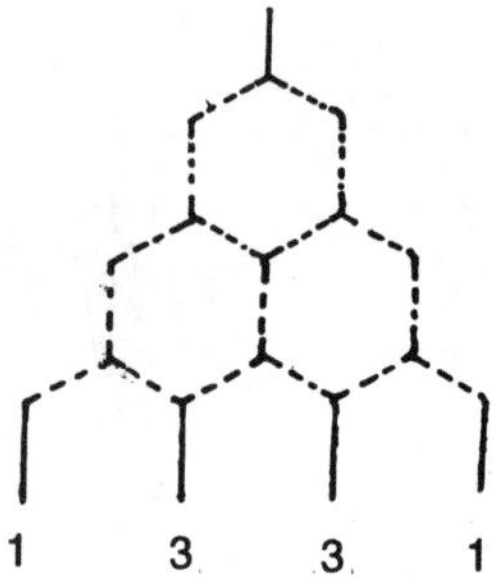

1 3 3 1

Fig. 19.12. Energy level diagram for methyl protons

This can also be explained as : n = 3, the multiplicity will be n + 1 = 4 and a quartet will be obtained. The intensity ratio of this quartet will be given by $(n + 1)^n$

or $(n + 1)^3 = 1n^3 + 3n^2 + 3n + 1$ i.e. 1 : 3 : 3 : 1.

The positions of multiplets i.e. J values are functions of the separations of the energy levels and the relative intensities of multiplets correspond to the orientation probabilities of the neighbouring protons. The multiplicity depends on the number of protons on the adjacent atom. If n is the number of equivalent protons, multiplicity of a group is n + 1. Thus ratio can be 1 : 1, 1 : 2 : 1, 1 : 3 : 3 : 1, 1 : 4 : 6 : 4 : 1, 1 : 5 : 10 : 10 : 5 : 1 in the expansion of $(n + 1)^n$. The integration of the multiplet will be equal to the number of protons responsible for the signal.

In the case of NH_3, multiplicity of equivalent protons is 3 and consequently it gives a 3 proton peak as a triplet having a peak ratio of 1 : 2 : 1.

In substances like HCl, HBr, HI and halogens electric quadrapole causes spin decoupling and therefore no proton-halogen or halogen-halogen (except F) splitting are observed.

After recording the NMR Spectrum for a given sample under a given set of conditions, the number of protons associated with a particular resonance has to be estimated. For this purpose most of the instruments are equipped with automatic integrators which can record peak areas in the form of a superimposed integration trace on the chart. The integration is carried out immediately after the determination of the spectrum and takes a few minutes. This is clearly shown in the nmr spectrum for ethyl chloride in Fig. 19.13.

19.9 Classification for proton Coupling

Various types of non-equivalent protons in organic molecules can be recognized and these are classified into various systems as described below:

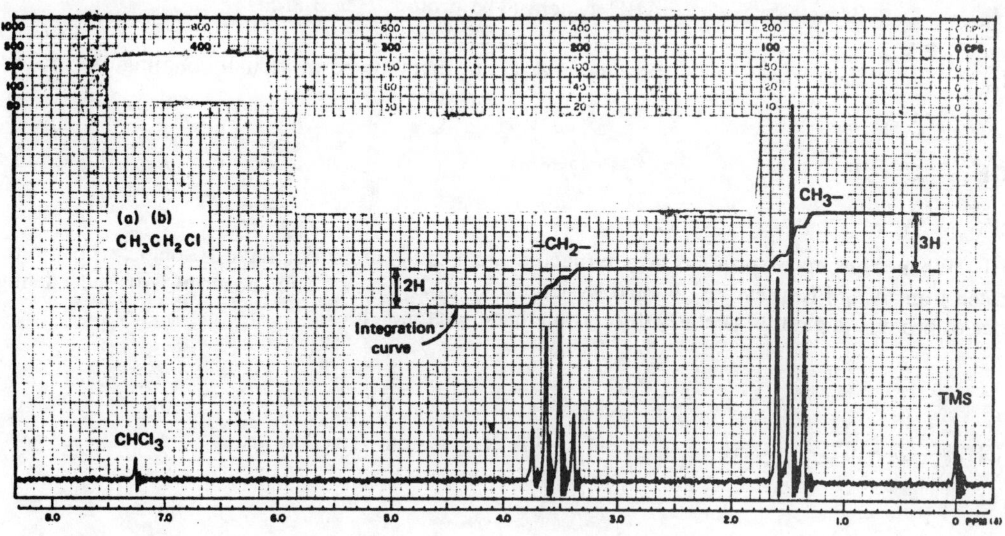

Fig. 19.13. Ethyl chloride in $CDCl_3$ at 60 MHz.

(i) When all the protons in a molecule are electrically and magnetically equivalent there is no coupling involved in molecule, the system is represented by e.g. methane, dichloro ethylene.

H—C(H)(H)—C A_4 system

$Cl_2C=CH_2$ A_6 system

The number of protons is denoted by the sub-script.

(ii) When a group of protons in a molecule have chemical shift comparable to spin-spin coupling, they are represented by letters A, B, C -------------- in the order of increasing shielding. Here the chemical shift difference is small. Examples are ethyl bromide, n-butyl bromide, vinyl bromide. In this case mutually coupled protons A & B are not coupled to any other protons.

$H_3C—CH_2—Br$ A_2 B_3 system

$CH_3 - CH_2 - CH_2 - CH_2 - Br$ A_2 B_3 system

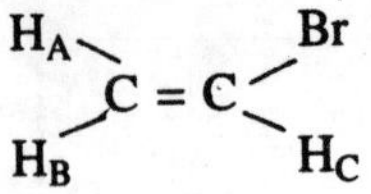

H_A, H_B C = C Br, H_C ABC system (The proton A & B are involved in geminal coupling while protons B & C are involvolved in vicinal coupling.

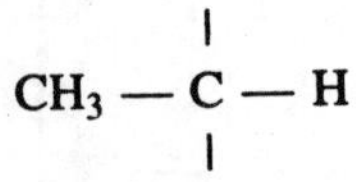

$CH_3 - C - H$ A_3 B system

(iii) When a group of protons in a molecule are nearly equal but have resonance positions well separated from A and B, they are denoted by letters X, Y, Z . . . . . . The subscript is used to denote the number of protons, e.g. ethyl ącetate, difluoromethane, styrene etc.

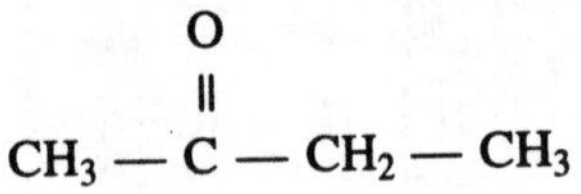

$CH_3 - C(=O) - CH_2 - CH_3$ A_2X_3 system for ethyl group.

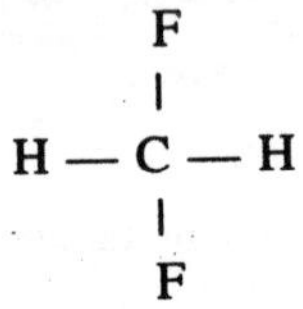

$H - C(F)(F) - H$ A_2X_2 system

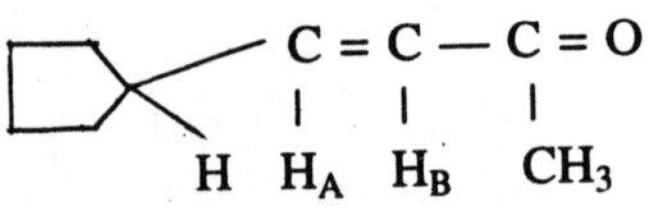

C = C — C = O, H H_A H_B CH_3

ABX System

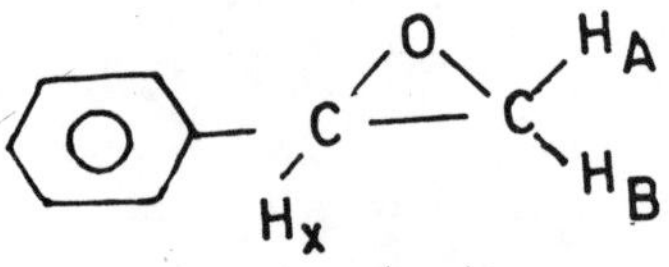

O, C, C, H_A, H_B, H_x

ABX System

C_6H_5, C = C, H_A, H_X, H_B

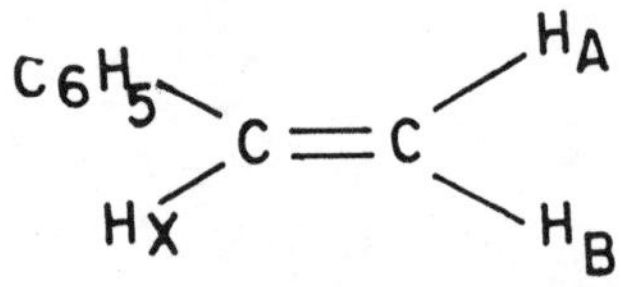

ABX System

The other possible system are described below:

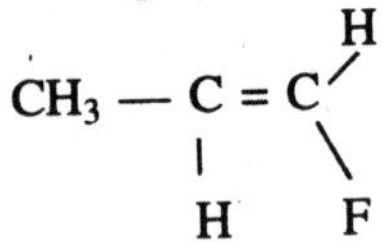

$CH_3 - C(H) = C(H)(F)$ A_3 MNx system

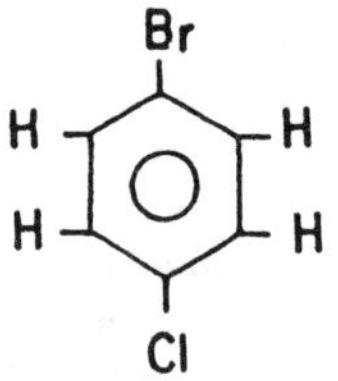

Br, H, H, H, H, Cl

AA′ xx′ system

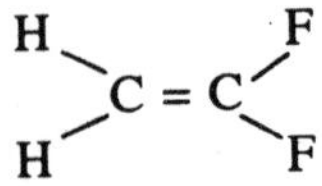

H, H, C = C, F, F AA′ xx′ system

NO_2, H, H, H, H, Cl

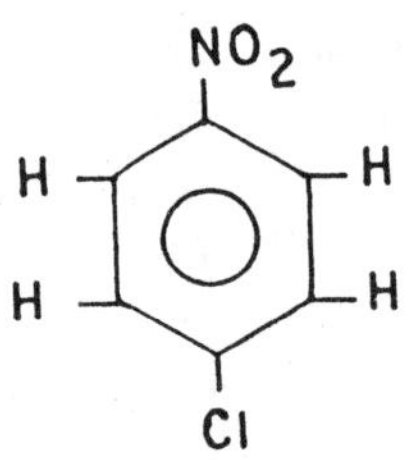

AA′ xx′ system

The values of coupling constants for various types of interacting protons with variety of structural and stereochemical features are described below : These value are useful in assigning structures for such molecules.

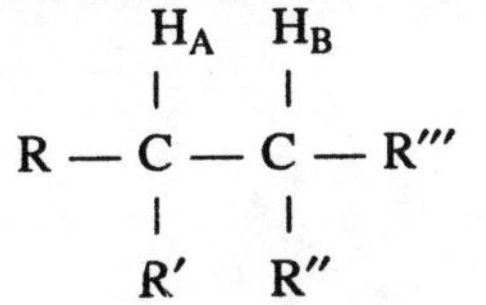

$R-C(H_A)(R')-C(H_B)(R'')-R'''$ J_{AB} (Vic) = 5–8Hz

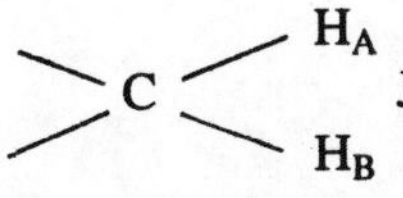

$>C<^{H_A}_{H_B}$ $J_{AB(gem)}$ = 12-15 Hz

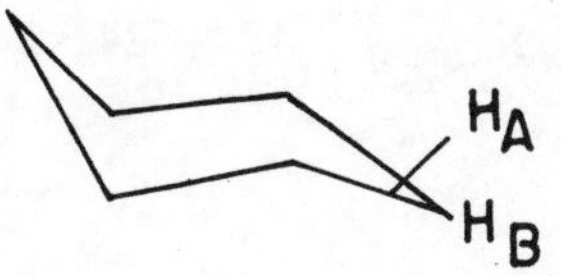

AB(gem) = 12.6 Hz

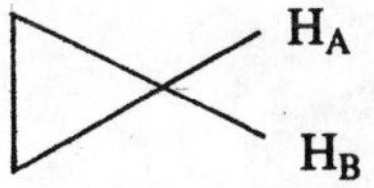

$J_{AB(Gem)}$ = 3.9–8.8 Hz

For a system like A_2, the two nuclei are equivalent, interaction is not observed and a single peak is obtained. If-CH_2– is part of a chain on adjacent C-atoms, they will be treated as equivalent protons. If –CH_2 – is part of a ring, they will be treated as non-equivalent protons, thus it will be like AB geminal coupling having two doublets with J = 12-15 Hz

A system like Ax will show a pair of doublets with equal intensity. If Δ J/J ratio is large, the system will conform to Ax system, if it is small, it will be AB like.

The geminal protons show J values as per the angle Θ.

J_{AB} = 20Hz when θ = 105°
J_{AB} = OHz when θ = 125°

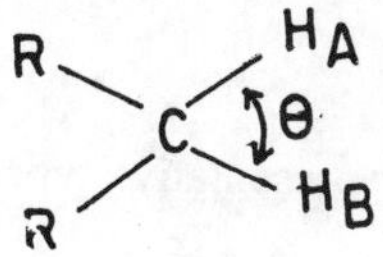

The vicinal protons show J values as per the dihedral angle θ .

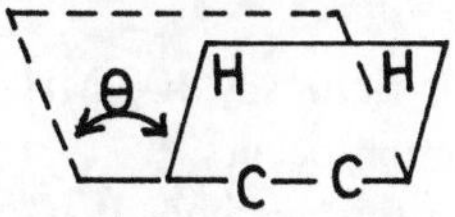

J_{AB} ≈ 10Hz if θ = 180°
minimum if θ = 90°

8Hz if θ = 0°

For compounds containing π electrons coupling occurs over greater distance e.g. trans > cis > geminal.

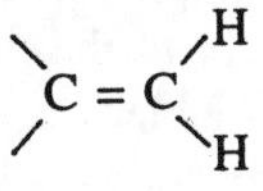

$J_{AB\ (gem)}$ 0–3.5Hz

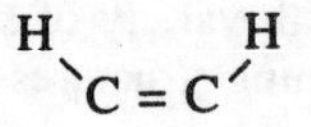

H H \C = C/ $J_{AB\ (cis)}$ 6–14 Hz

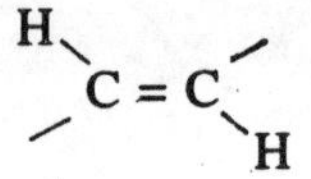

H\C = C/ / \H $J_{AB\ (trans)}$ 11–18 Hz

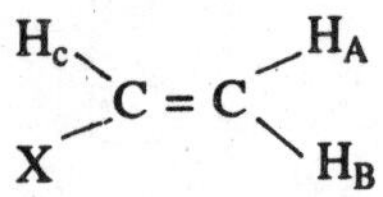

H_C\C = C/H_A X/ \H_B $J_{AB\ (cis)}$ 4.6–19.3 Hz

X = Cl, Br, F, CH_3 $J_{BC(trans)}$ 12.7 – 24.0 Hz

COOH, C_6H_5, H, CN

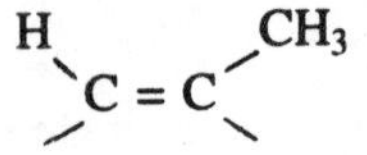

H\C = C/CH_3 $J_{A_3X} \approx 1$ Hz H_A — C ≡ C — H_B J_{AB} = 9.5–9.8 Hz

The aromatic system like benzene shows ortho, meta and para coupling in the range ortho > meta > para.

ortho J = 8Hz
meta J = 2–3Hz
para J = 0–1Hz

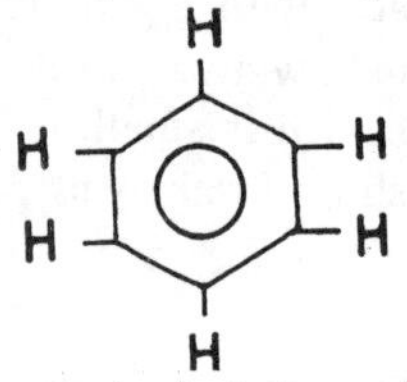

Some representative types of nmr spectras have been attached at the end of this chapter.

19.10 Spin-Spin Decoupling or Double resonance

Normally, spin-spin coupling is of immense help in identifying resonances, but in case of complex molecules it may complicate the spectrum to the point where the spectrum cannot be elucidated. In such cases simplification may be achieved in following ways.

(i) By using an instrument with more powerful homogeneous magnetic field, say 100 MHz instrument than a 60 MHz. Because of higher resolution, a greater line separation occurs.

(ii) By a spin-spin decoupling technique. A *spin decoupler* is used in this method. It is an auxillary oscillator that produces a signal at a selectable frequency and then imposes this field on the sample with great intensity. Say for example, if during an NMR experiment on a simple AX system, the X is irradiated with a second radio frequency signal of frequency (V_X) equal to the precessional frequency of X, then the X-nuclei will undergo rapid changes of spin state. Nucleus A is aware of only one equivalent spin state of X and therefore its resonance signal appears not as a doublet, but as a sharp singlet. Irra-diation of X effectively decouples the signal from A. Similarly, if A is

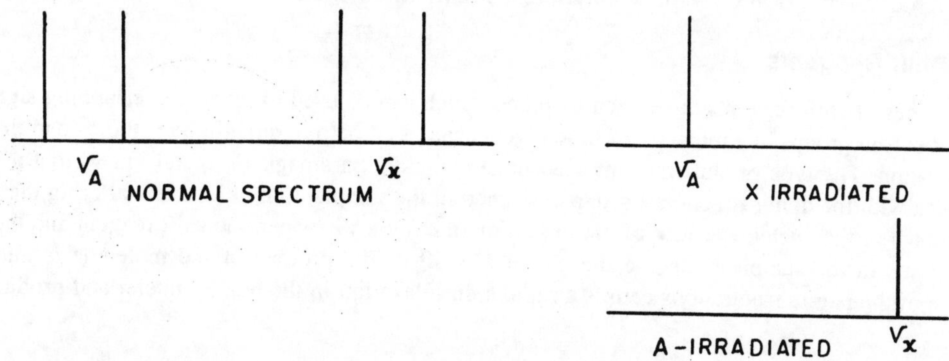

Fig. 19.14 A Double irradiation experiment

irradiated with a second radiofrequency to its own resonance frequency (V_A), then the signal from X will collapse to a singlet. All this is shown in the Fig. 19.14 and 19.15.

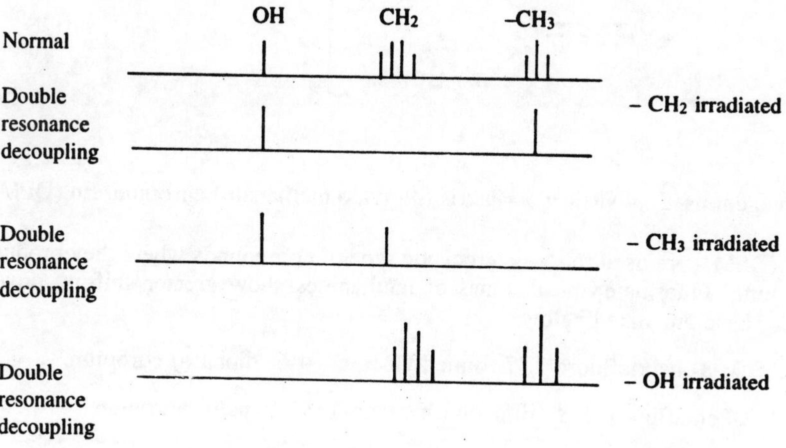

Fig. 19.15 Decoupling experiment on ethanol

The decoupling of different isotopes like ^1H and ^{19}F where the difference in resonance frequencies is large can also be performed.

19.11 Nuclear Overhauser Effect

Another procedure for decoupling is known as *nuclear Overhauser effect* (NOE). The procedure involves the disruption of normal relaxation processes of nuclei from the excited states. The NOE experiment comprises in saturating one signal and observing the intensities of the other signals. Thus if one of the interacting nuclei is saturated by radiation from an auxiliary oscillator, it becomes more difficult for the other nucleus to lose its excess energy and this results in a larger NMR signal. If the nuclei are both protons, the enhancement of signal can be as much as 1.5 times. Hence it is possible to pin point which peaks are due to nuclei in close proximity to each other in the molecule.

19.12 Shift Reagents

Certain types of shift reagents have been invented which can be used to resolve overlapping signals from different proton groups in a molecule. These regents can be of help in quantitative studies and in structure determination. The type of shift reagent used must contain a paramagnetic metal ion so that it can form a complex with the donor functional group contained in the sample, thus selectively altering the magnetic environment of the nuclei. Because of the formation of complex between the shift reagent and the suitable donor atoms in the sample molecule the chemical shift of the protons of the molecule is altered. The presence of the paramagnetic ions causes a rapid spin-relaxation in the nearby nuclei and produces a line broadening of the NMR signal.

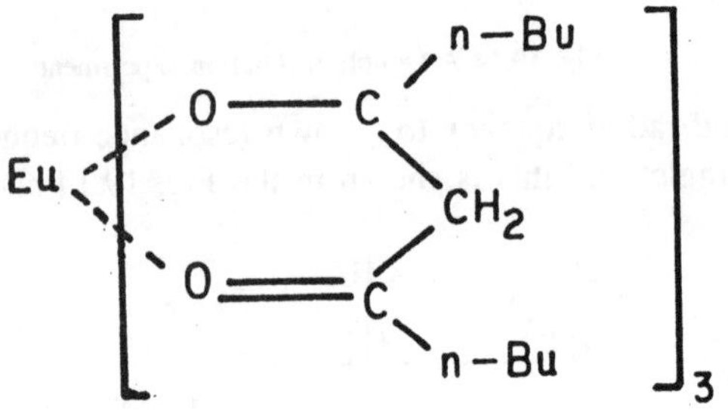

The most common shift reagent used in NMR work is tris (dipivalo methanato) europiun, Eu $(DPM)_3$ show below.

Ytterbium complexes, $Yb(DPM)_3$ are used for N-heterocyclic type of compounds where they produce moderate type of line broadening. Fluorinated β-diketones of lanthanides show greater shifting power than non-fluorinated reagents. These are stated below.

EU $(FOD)_3$ Tris (1, 1, 2, 2, 3, 3- hepttafluoro 7, 7- dimethyloctan - 4 6- dionato) europiun.

EU $(PFD)_3$ Tris 1, 1, 1, 2, 2-Pentafluoro -6, 6- dimethyl heptane-3, 5- dionato) europiun.

EU $(FHD)_3$ Tris (1, 1, 1- trifluoro-5, 5- dimethyl hexane - 2, 4-dionato) europiun.

In the actual practice known amounts of the shift reagent are added successively to the sample which is dissolved in a non-polar solvent. The chemical shift of each proton in the sample molecule changes with each addition of the reagent and the extent of the induced shift is determined. Thereafter a plot of the induced shift against the ratio of the shift reagent to substrate is drawn. From the plots for each proton, structural information may be derived.

19.13 Carbon-13 Nuclear Magnetic spectroscopy

The only stable isotope of carbon is C-13 with a spin quantum number I = 1/2. It has a natural abundance of 1.1% compared to 99.9% abundance for proton nuclei. The C-13 gyromagnetic ratio, which is a proportionality constant between resonance frequency and field strength is smaller than ^1H nuclei by a factor of 0.25. The relative sensitivity for detecting equal numbers of nuclei at a constant field strength is proportional to the cube of the gyromagnetic ratio and therefore the sensitivity of C–13 is 0.016 relative to ^{1}H = 1.00. All the above factors bring down the intensity of C-13 signal by about 600 fold over that of proton nuclei. Lastly, the relaxation time (T_1) of C-13 is relatively long. It is because of the reasons stated above that the use of C-13 NMR spectroscopy has been slow than that of proton NMR spectroscopy.

The C-13 chemical shift range extends over 200 ppm compared to about 10 ppm for protons. Thus, it gives rise to first order spectra and the use of higher frequency instruments is not necessary. It must be noted that as carbon atoms are imbedded within a molecule where intramolecular effects are more important than inter-molecular effects.

A number of techniques are available to observe the C-13 NMR signal. The first improved method of obtaing C-13 spectra were by using larger NMR (10-15 mm) sample spinning tubes which yielded better field homogenity and proton decoupling techniques.

The introduction of Fourier transform technique has also lead to the enhancement of application of NMR spectroscopy in general. This innovation along with a digital computer or time-averaging device has allowed large improvements in signal-to-noise (S/N) ratios to be achieved. The Fourier-transform technique comprises in the application to the sample of a short intense radio frequency pulse that excites the entire range of precision frequencies of the chosen nuclear species, and measurement as a function of time of the resulting free induction signals from the nuclear spins in the sample. This procedure gives a high resolution spectrum. The advantage of this technique in comparison to continuous-wave spectroscopy is that the free induction signal is obtained rapidly so that in a given observation time it is possible to apply the pulse repetitively and store the free induction signals in a time-averaging device.

Earliar, all C-13 chemical shift data were made relative to external carbon disulphide (CS_2) but now they are reported with respect to tetramethylsilane (TMS). Thus, this system is consistant with δ– scale used for protons and has also the advantage that only one compound is used as a reference standard for three nuclei, ^{1}H, ^{13}C and ^{29}Si.

A large amount of data on the position of absorptions in C–13 NMR spectra are available in the literature. This information is of valuable help in solving problems on structure determination. A vast majority of absorptions fall between the carbonyl absorptions at low field and the methyl absorptions at high field. The positions of absorptions of some of the important organic compounds and groups are shown in the Table 19.1.

It has been observed that hybridization has a significant effect on the chemical shift of organic molecules. Thus sp^3 hybridized carbon absorb at high field (0.60 p.p.m), Sp^2 - carbon at low field (80-200 p. p.m.) and Sp- carbon at intermediate value. Further, the exact position of absorption of a specific atom is determined by the electronic effects of any substituents.

Because C–13 has a spin of 1/2 the same as that of a proton, the spin multiplets in the decoupled spectra have similar appearance and interpretation as that of proton multiplet signals.

In the C–13 NMR spectra direct C–13 to C–13 splittings will not be observed, but the spectrum will comprise of a series signals: one of each carbon position, which are split only by the attached adjacent hydrogen or other magnetic nuclei. Further, the C–13 to proton coupling constants are large (O—300 Hz) compared to proton-proton (O—20Hz)

Table 19.2. Chemical shifts of some C–13 Resonances (relative to internal TMS)

Compound Name and groups	PPM
Alkane and alkyl groups	0 — 40
Mono olefines (terminal)	

(Contd.)

	$= CH_2$	110 — 120	
	= C	150	
	= CH	135 — 140	
Mono olefins (internal)			
Diene	= C —	140 — 150	
	= C —	130 — 140	
	$= CH_2$	110 — 120	
Alkynes	≡ C —	80 — 90	
	≡ C—H	70-80	
Carbonyl	C = O	200–220	
	— CO_2	155 — 190	
C ≡ N groups	C = N	130 — 155	
	— C ≡ N	100 — 125	
	—C—N	42 — 62	
Cyclohexane˙			
4 - t - Bu - C_6H_{10} - OR			
R	axial	equatorial	Δ δ
H	67.6	72.5	4.9
Ac	70.4	74.4	4.0
Me	76.5	81.4	4.9
For unsaturated functions			
	— C ≡ N	121	
	C = NOH	161	
	CN^-	178	
Olefines	$= CH_2$ α	106 — 107	
	—CH = (CH_2) β	138 — 150	
	—C = (CH_2) β	144 — 153	
	= CH — (otherwise, in chain)	119 — 144	
	= C— (otherwise, in chain)	124 — 144	
Allenes			
	$= CH_2$	74	
	= CH —	86	
	= CH =	207 — 211	

(*Contd.*)

Dienes (Conjugated & unconjugated)		
	= CH_2	112 — 118
	= CH —	139
	= C	146
Acetylene		
	—C ≡ C –	82
	—C ≡ C (α)	70 — 79
	—C ≡ C (β)	80 — 90
Aromatics		
	= CH — benzene	129
	= CH — alkyl benzene	127 — 132
	= C alkyl benzene	133 — 138
	= CH (naphthalene)	128.1
	= C (naphthalene)	137.4

Monosubstituted benzenes

Substituent	1-c	0-c	m-c	p-c
NO_2	19.6	-5.3	0.8	0.6
$COCH_3$	9.3	0.2	0.2	4.2
CHO	9.0	1.2	1.2	6.2
CO_2 CH_3	2.2	0.4	0.4	4.4
Ph	10	0.4	0.4	0.4
CH_3	9.1	0.3	0.3	2.8
F	35.1	-14.3	0.9	-4.4
Br	-5.4	3.3	2.2	-1.0
I	-32.3	9.9	2.6	-0.4
OCH_3	30.2	-14.7	0.9	-8.4
OH	27.6	-11.8	2.8	-6.1
NH_2	19.2	-12.4	1.3	-9.5
NCH_3	22.4	-15.7	0.8	-11.8

HETEROAROMATIC COMPOUNDS

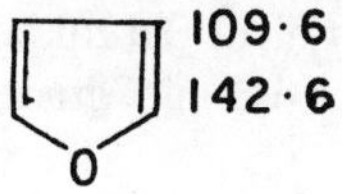

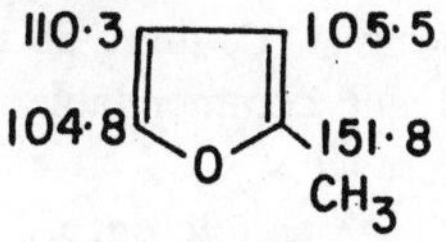

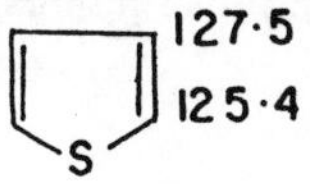

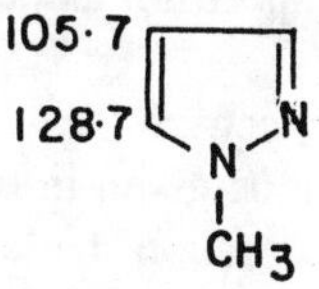

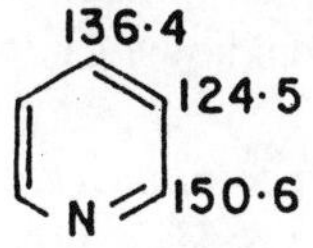

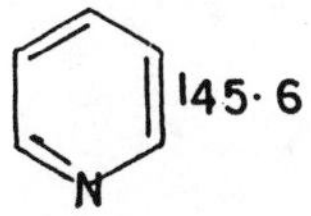

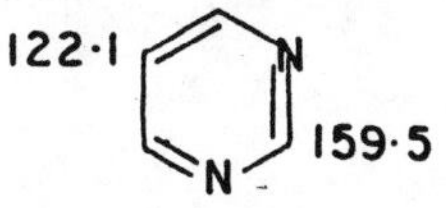

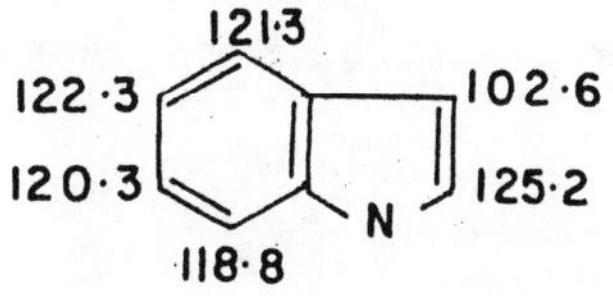

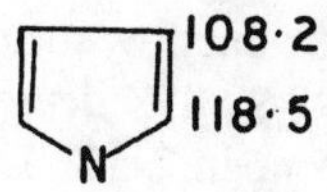

Furan (O): 109·6, 142·6

2-Methylfuran (O, CH_3): 110·3, 105·5, 104·8, 151·8

Pyrrole (N): 108·2, 118·5

Thiophene (S): 127·5, 125·4

N-Methylpyrazole (N, N–CH_3): 105·7, 128·7

Pyridine (N): 136·4, 124·5, 150·6

Pyridine (N): 145·6

Pyrimidine (N, N): 122·1, 159·5

Indole (N): 121·3, 122·3, 120·3, 118·8, 102·6, 125·2

19.14 Applications of NMR Spectroscopy

1. Structure Elucidation : Proton magnetic resonance spectra give information on the number of protons and the pattern of the interacting groups. In conjunction with infrared, ultraviolet and mass spectra, they are extremely helpful in structure determination.

2. Hydrogen Bonding : Proton magnetic resonance spectra can help in identifying hydrogen bonding due to the possibility of rapid exchange of –OH proton.

3.Keto-enol Tautomerism : Nuclear magnetic resonance spectrosiopy is a powerful analytical method for studying quantitatively keto-enol equilibria in organic molecules.

4. Determination of Optical purity : Nuclear magnetic resonance spectroscopy can be used in the determination of finding the ratio of enantiomorphs in a mixture on to assess the optical purity of a compound with having to physically separate the enantiomers.

5. Conformational Analysis : Nuclear magnetic resonance spectroscopy can record signals due to each conformation in a molecule.

6. Quantitative Analysis : One of the important application of nuclear magnetic resonance spectroscopy can be a rapid quantitative means of determining the ratio of compounds in a mixture.

EXERCISE 1. A Case Study On An Unknown Organic Sample By Nmr Spectrometer.

Before running an nmr spectrum of an unknown compound, follow the steps given below :

(a) Adjust the nmr spectrometer by inserting ^{1}H 'HOMO ADJUST'sample (Follow operating instructions of your instrument).

(b) Remove the HOMO ADJUST sample and insert ^{1}H REFERENCE sample for obtaining TMS LOCK (''for obtaining TMS LOCK'' follow operating instructions of your instrument).

(c) Now prepare your unknown sample in 5 mm O.D. tube. 20 mg material in 0.5 ml solvent is recommended. 99-99.8% deuterated solvent commendable (or spectroscopic grade CCl_4). Solvent should contain 2-5% TMS as reference.

(d) In case of liquid, take it neat with 2-5% TMS as reference.

(e) Now insert your unknown sample and take the spectrum as per operating instructions of your instrument.

(f) After taking the spectrum, integrate the whole spectrum.

(g) Take out the chart paper and complete the columns given in the chart.

(h) Analyse the spectrum and complete the observation table. For example, the following observation table has been completed after analysing the spectrum of ethyl benzene.

Observation and Calculation

Table - 19.3

Proton Type	Chemical Shift (ppm)	Splitting	Coupling Constant J (Hz)	Integra-Tion Height Ratio	Proton Ratio	$\frac{\Delta \nu ab}{J}$
a	δ 1.21 (γ 8.79)	triplet	$7H_z$	40	3	$\frac{120}{7} = 17.14$
b	δ 2.62 (γ 7.38)	quartet	$7H_z$	27	2	
c	δ 7.14 (γ 2.86)	singlet	–	68	5	

Interpretation

The interpretation of an unknown structure of a molecule by an nmr spectrum alone is seldom possible. It is only is the case of a simple specturm, sometimes it is possible to get the complete structural information. For a complex nmr spectrum we only get some partial informations which in conjuction with other spectra like, ir, uv and mass, help us in the elucidation of unknown structure.

The spectrum which we have cited in the fore-going example is a simple one and, therefore, structural determination is possible.

From the spectrum we note the following aspects :

1) Proton ratio = 3:2:5
2) Singlet is at downfield, δ 7.14 and triplet at upfield, δ 1.21.
3) Order of splitting is first order since, Δ γ/J is greater than 7.
4) Coupling constant for the triplet as well as for the quartet is $7H_Z$.

We find from the spectrum that a peak appears around δ 7.14, which indicates the presence of an aromatic compound. This is further confirmed from the calculation of proton ratio. We also get an indication that the compound is mono substituted aromatic compound since the singlet at the down field of the aromatic compound contains only five protons. The reason of downfield shift of the singlet is due to the deshielding effect of the aromatic ring.

The triplet and quartet show the same coupling constant hence, the protons under triplet and protons under quartet appear to be coupling each other. Moreover, the compound is of the type A_2X_3 type since, Δ v/J is greater than 7. Further, it is observed that the quartet protons are more downfield than the triplet protons. Hence, the probable structure of the compound, consistant with the nmr spectrum, is :

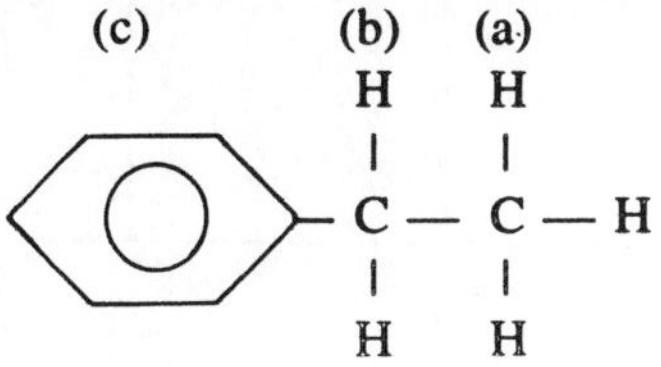

```
 (c)      (b)  (a)
           H    H
           |    |
 C6H5  —   C —  C — H
           |    |
           H    H
```

EXERCISE 2. Take an nmr spectrum of isobutyl alcohol and account for all the peaks.

Proton Type	Chemical Shift (ppm)	Splitting	Coupling Constant Hz	Integration Height Ratio	Proton Ratio	Δ γ / J

EXERCISE 3. Take an nmr spectrum of an unknown compound given by the instructor and establish the structure..

Proton Type	Chemical Shift (ppm)	Splitting	Coupling Constant Hz	Integration Height Ratio	Proton Ratio	Δ γ / J

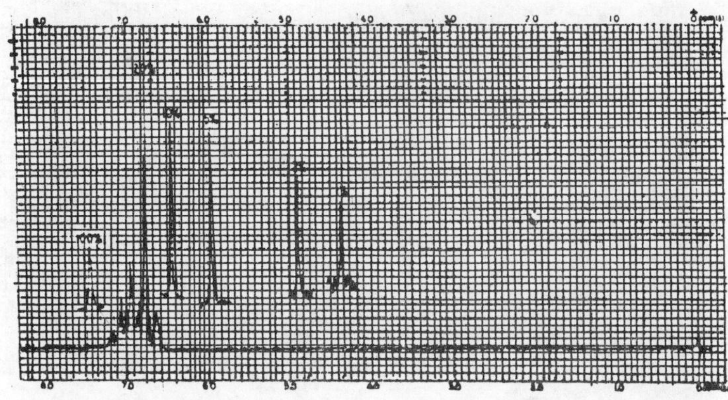

NMR Spectrum No.1. Phenol, 20% (w/v) in carbon tetrachloride, 500 cps sweep width.

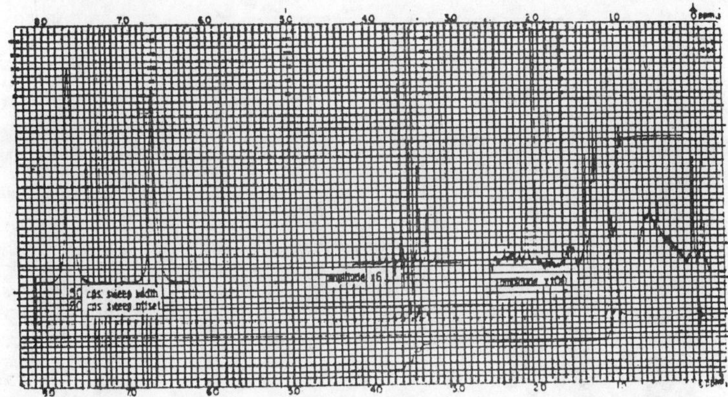

NMR Specturm No.2. Isopropyl ether, pure liquid, 500 cps sweep width.

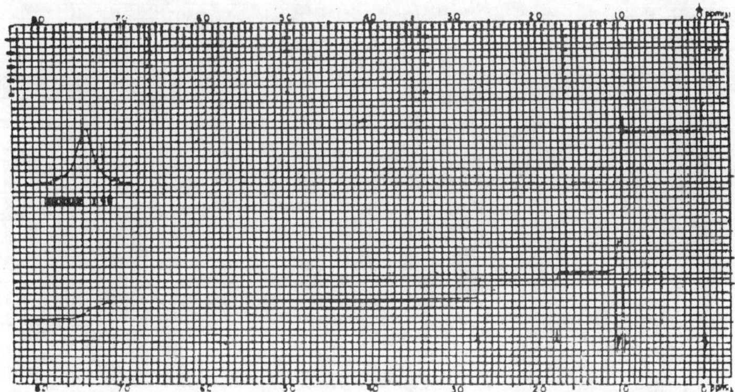

NMR Specturm No.3. Acetylacetone, pure lliquid, 1000 cps sweep width.

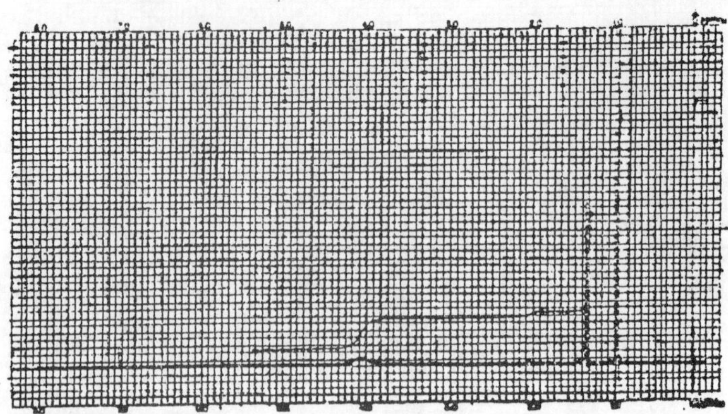

NMR Spectrum No. 4. N-Methylacetamide, 15% (w/v) in carbon tetrachloride, 1000 cps sweep width.

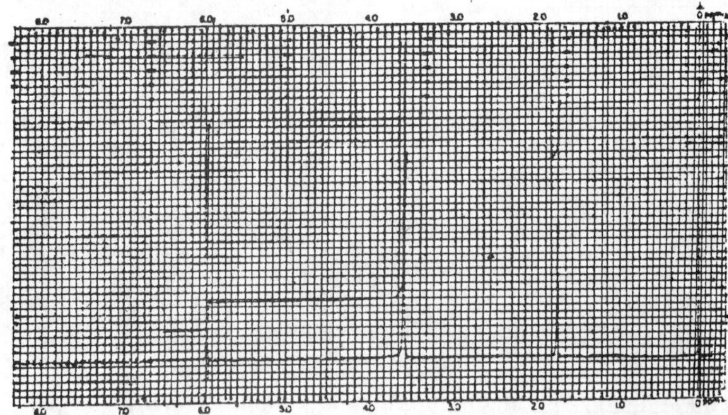

NMR Specturm No. 5. Phenylacetic acid, 15% (w/v) in carbon tetrachloride, 1000 cps sweep width.

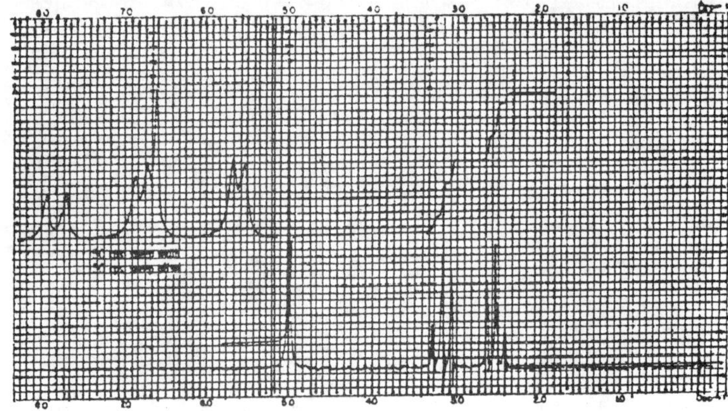

NMR Specturm No. 6. β-Alanine, 15% (w/v) in deuterium oxide, 500 cps sweep width.

FUNCTIONAL GROUP CORRELATION CHART FOR PROTON NMR CHEMICAL SHIFTS

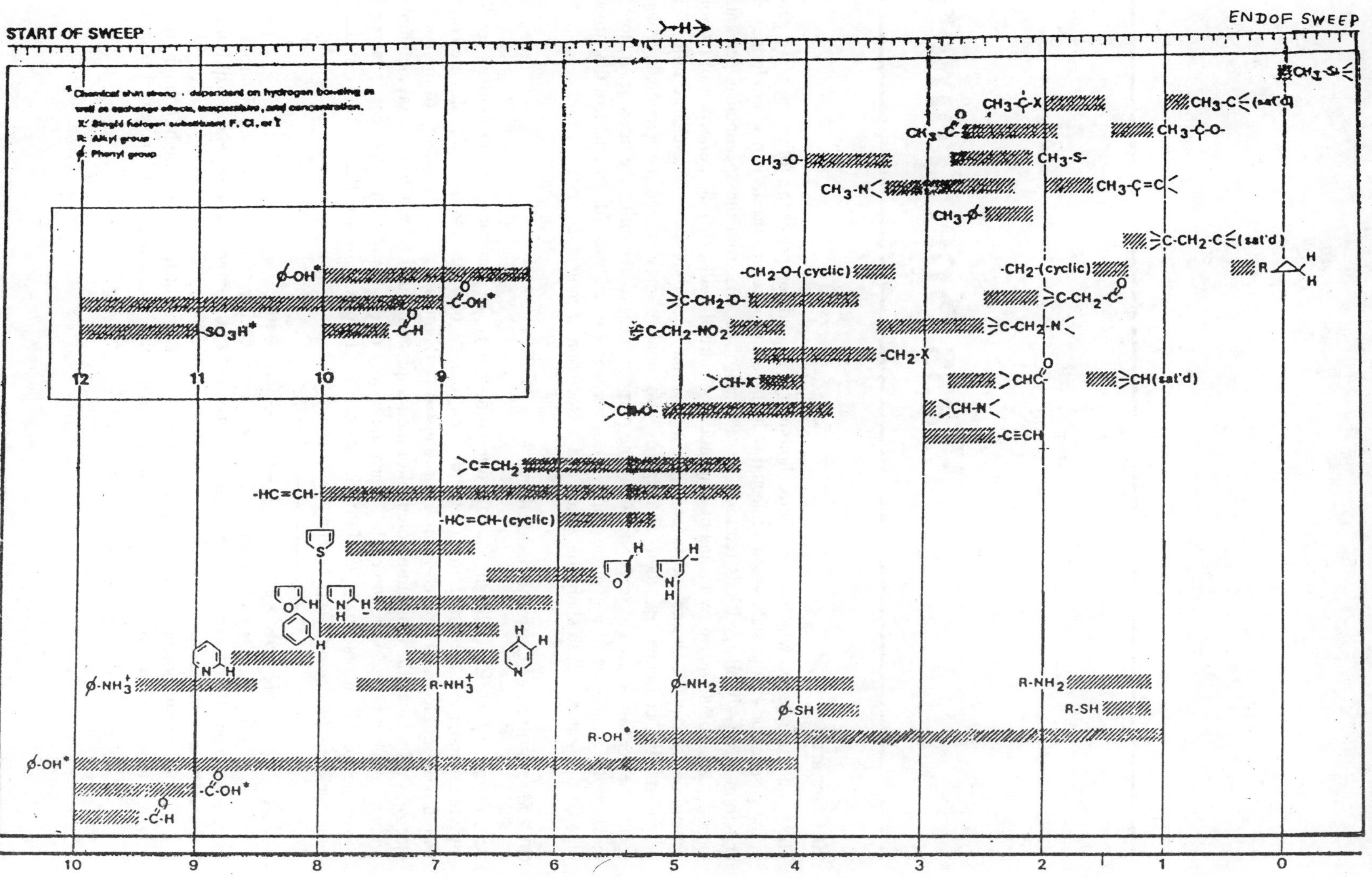

20

Mass Spectrometry

20.1 General

The basic principles on which mass spectrophotometry is based comprises the following : (i) a substance in the gaseous or vapour state when subjected to high voltage electric current is made to loose electrons and form positively charged ions (cations) i.e. a beam of cations from the specimen is generated, (ii) these ions can be deflected by means of magnetic or electrical fields, (iii) the deflection of the ions will depend on their mass, charge and velocity i.e. a spectrum according to mass-to-charge ratio of ions is produced, (iv) consequently, their abundances and relative masses can be recorded. Thus mass spectrometers can be used to serve the following purposes : (a) to determine the mass of an atom, (b) to measure the abundance of a given isotope, (c) to perform gas analysis, (d) to establish the structure of organic compounds, (e) to study ionization and dissociation of molecules.

30.2 Mechanism of Cation Production

An *electron impact* (EI) technigue is utilized to produce ions. The sample in the vapourized condition is introduced under low pressure into a tube called ion source where the entering molecules are bombarded with a beam of electrons emitted from a hot tungsten or rhenium wire. If the energy of the bombarding electrons is less than the ionization potential of the sample molecules (about 10 ev in organic molecules) no change takes place in the molecules. when the energy of the bombarding electrons is increased just above the ionization potential, possibility increases that there will be a collusion between the sample molecules and an electron. This can be shown as :

$$M + e^- \longrightarrow M^{\dot{+}} + 2e^-$$

e.g. $$CH_3—OH + e^- \longrightarrow CH_3 — OH^{\dot{+}} + 2e^-$$

The ion produced is a radical cation. However, it the energy of the bombarding electrons is further increased, some of their excess energy will be transferred to the molecular ions which will bring further fragmentation of the sample molecules.

The electrical potential of the bombarding electrons which is just high enough to initiate fragmentation is called *appearance potential.* The magnitude of the appearance potential is equal to or greater than the sum of the dissociation energy of the fragmented bond and the ionization. When the bombarding electrons have a very high energy, more than one bond in the molecule can be broken.

In actual practice, a voltage of 70 ev is used to accelrate the electrons so that there is enough energy to break any bond in the sample molecules. For example if we introduce methyl alcohol (CH_3OH) vapour into an ion source and then bombard it with a 70 ev beam, it will fragment in the following sequence:

$$CH_3\text{—}OH + e^- \longrightarrow \begin{matrix} & & H & & & & \\ & & | & & & & \\ H & — & C & — & O^{\cdot +} & — & H \\ & & | & & & & \\ & & H & & & & \end{matrix} + 2e^- \quad m/e = 32$$

$$\begin{matrix} & & H & & & & \\ & & | & & & & \\ H & — & C & — & O & — & \overset{\cdot +}{H} \\ & & | & & & & \\ & & H & & & & \end{matrix} \longrightarrow H — C = O^+ — H + H \quad m/e = 31$$

$$\begin{matrix} & & H & & & & \\ & & | & & & & \\ H & — & C & — & O^{\dot{+}} & — & H \\ & & | & & & & \\ & & H & & & & \end{matrix} \longrightarrow C^+H_3 + \dot{O}H$$

$$\begin{matrix} & & H & & & & \\ & & | & & & & \\ H & — & C & = & O^+ & — & H \end{matrix} \rightarrow H — C — O^+ + H_2 \quad m/c = 29$$

It is to be understood here that only one ion can be formed from the decomposition of a singly charged ion as per rules of conservation of charge.

20.3 Instrumentation Aspects

The essential components of a mass spectrophotometer consists of (i) inlet system (ii) the ion source (iii) the electrostatic accelerating system (iv) ion collector (v) amplifier and (vi) a read out system.

There are three different methods of introducing the sample into the ion source, namely : (a) molecular leak (b) direct insertion (c) chromatographic eluent insertion. The choice depends on the volatility of the sample material.

(i) Inlet system : (a) The commonly used method for the gaseous samples is the "molecular leak method". For gaseous sample, the method involves the transfer of a gas from a bulb to the inlet sample reservoir via a sensitive metering device. The gas is held in the reservoir at 10^{-1} — 10^{-2} torr from which it slowly leaks through an opening into the ion source where the pressure is kept around $10^{-5} - 10^{-7}$ torr (1 torr = 1 mm Hg).

For the case of solids and liquids, samples must be vapourized before they reach the reservoir. In order to ensure that such samples are vapourised, the sample handling systems is heated, Liquid samples can be introduced by means of a micropipette syringe through a silicone rubber septum directly connected to the vacuum system. If solid samples are not volatile, they have to be converted to acetates, esters and trimethyl silyl ethers. The sample size varies from 0.1 mg to several milligrams.

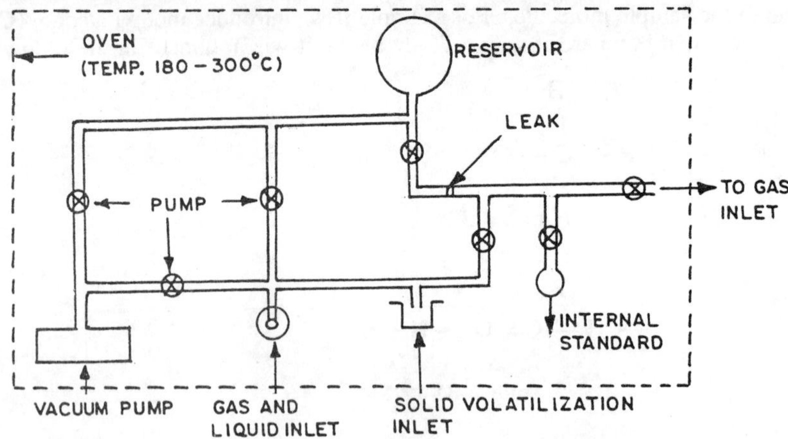

Fig. 20.1. Inlet system for a mass spectrometer.

(b) Direct Insertion : This type of technique is suitable for solids and many liquid organic substances. The sample is placed into a small effusion (knudsen) cell at the end of evacuated ion source through a vacuum lock system. The sample is then evaporated either by heating the probe or by heating the entire ion source.

(c) Chromatographic Eluent Insertion : The procedure here involves a direct attachment of a gas liquid chromatograph with the ion source. The sub-microgram quantities of the separated and purified sample components eluting from the GLC are passed through specially designed separators to remove the carrier gas and the enriched eluent is inserted into the ion source through a vacuum lock system.

(ii) Ion Source : As already explained an electron impact (EI) technique is used for the production of cations. The vapourized sample is introduced under low pressure into the ion source tube and the

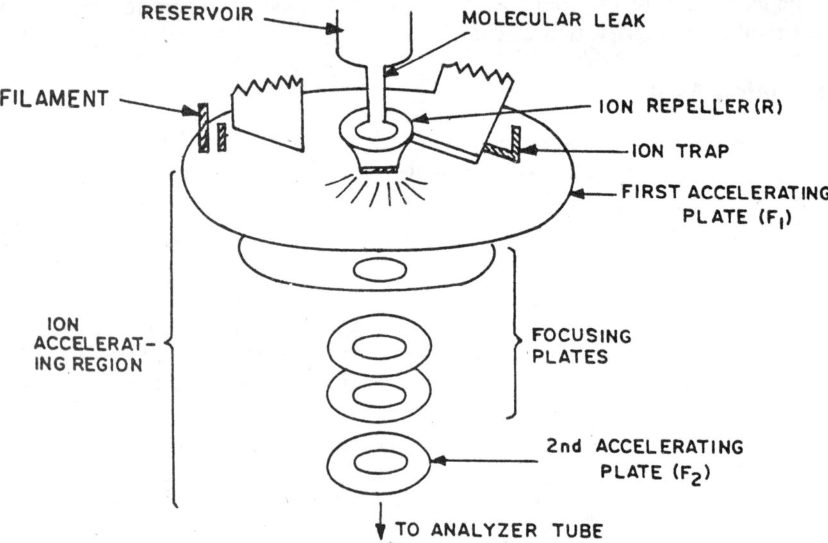

Fig. 20.2. Components of ion source.

sample molecules are bombarded with a beam of electrons emitted from a hot tungston or rhenium wire. An ion source contains (a) ion repellers, (b) ion acceleration plates and (c) ion focusing plates as shown in the Fig. 20.2. A small electrostating field is applied between the repeller electrode and the first accelerating plate so that ions generated are forced into the ion generating region. A potential of 1000—2000 Volts is used to accelerate the ions through a slit system so that a narrow beam of fast moving ions is formed. The fast moving—ionic beam thereafter leaves the ion source and enters into the analyzer tube. In the analyzer tube, the ions are then subjected to a uniform magnetic field (500—1000 gauss) which is generated by means of an electromagnetic placed perpendicular to the direction of the ionic beam.

In single focusing type of instruments there is only one analyzer sector and the dispersed ions arrive at the ion collector through a fine slit system at the end of the analyzer tube. As the accelerating potential experienced by the ions depends where in the source it is formed there is lack of uniforming of ion energies and a spread in their radii of curvature in the magnetic field and therefore there is peak broadening and low resolution.

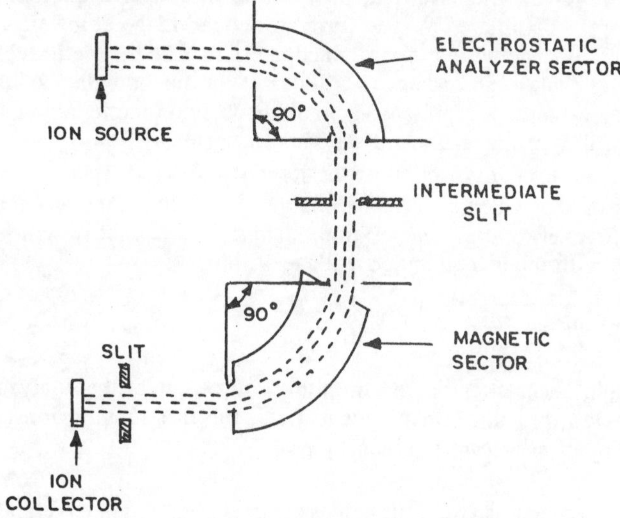

Fig. 20.3. Neir-Johnson double focussing system.

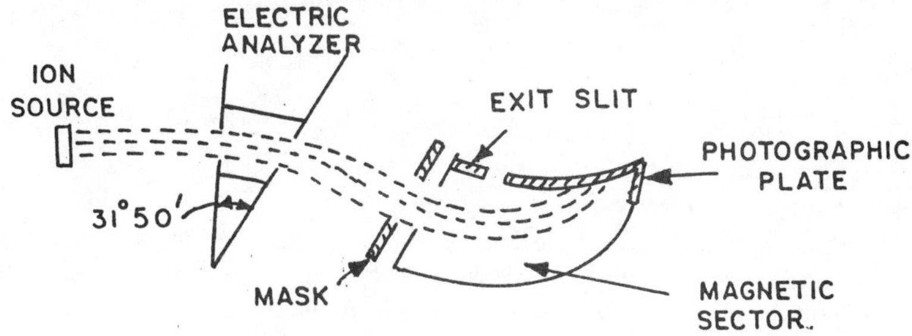

Fig. 20.4. Mattauch-Herzog double focussing system.

On the contrary high resolution mass spectrometers possess two analyzer sectors and use double focussing technique.

The double focussing is achieved by allowing ions to pass through an energy selector after acceleration but before magnetic analysis. This is done by incorporating a unit known as "electrostatic sector". It comprises of two curved plates across which a uniform potential difference is maintained. The ions which enter midway between the plates and having proper energy will assume a circular orbit. Two types of double focussing systems namely (a) Neir-Johnson system and (b) Mattauch-Herzog system are shown in Fig. 20.3 and Fig. 20.4 respectively.

In Neir-Johnson system there is a 90° — 95° radial electrical analyzer followed by a 60° or 90° magnetic analyzer. With this type of arrangement, the ions leaving the electrical sector converge at a narrow exit slit placed between the two analyzers. The magnetic field is automatically varied so that at any given field strength, only ions of same m/e ratio can travel in sharp focus to a detector and read out system.

In Mattauch-Herzog system, the electrical analyzer is placed at a geometry of 31.50°. With this arrangement, the ion beam is collimated as if to form an optical image at infinity. The ions will enter the magnetic field at normal incidence with a minimum edge effect. The magnetic sector is placed at an angle of 135°, thereby allowing each ionic species to a focus at the far boundary of the field. The net effect of this arrangement is that all masses are focused simultaneously on the focal plane which makes possible direct photographic recording of the masses of the various species.

The equations involved in the dispersion of the ionic beam into a spectrum are derived below :

Let m be the mass of the ion, and e be its charge. The initial kinetic energy for the ion will be negligible. Let the kinetic energy after acceleration become v, this energy will be equal to electrostatic energy acquired in passing through the applied voltage V.

$$\therefore \frac{1}{2} mv^2 = eV \text{ or } v^2 = \frac{2eV}{m}$$

The fast moving ionic beam after having the ionic source enters the analyzer tube. In the analyzer tube, the ions are subjected to a uniform magnetic field, the fast moving ions pick up a trajectory of circular path whose radius of curvature is given by $r = \frac{mv}{eH}$

Where r = radius, H = magnetic field, m = mass, e = charge and v is velocity.

$$\therefore \quad r^2 = \frac{m^2 v^2}{e^2 H^2} \quad \text{or} \quad v^2 = \frac{r^2 e^2 H^2}{m^2}$$

$$\therefore \quad \frac{2eV}{m} = \frac{r^2 e^2 H^2}{m^2} \qquad \left(\text{because } v^2 = \frac{2ev}{m}\right)$$

$$\text{or } 2V = \frac{r^2 e H^2}{m} \quad \text{or } 2Vm = r^2 e H^2$$

$$\therefore \quad \frac{m}{e} = \frac{H^2 r^2}{2V}$$

From the above equation we draw the following observations :

(a) the radius r of the circular path (i.e. deflection) is dependent on ; V the accelerating voltage, H the strength of the magnetic field, m/e the mass-to -charge ratio of the ions and (b) for the ions accelerated by a fixed voltage V, the deflection caused by a magnetic field H is proportional to the m/e ratio of ions. Therefore at fixed values of V and H all the ions of the same mass (say m_1) will follow same circular path and record the same mass value (m_1) on the spectrum and another set of ions with identical mass (say m_2) will be recorded at a different mass value m_2. In a way, we can say that the analyzer tube functions like a monochromator and causes the dispersion of ions.

The ions that are produced should not collide with each other or with molecules because that would produce inter-ionic, inter-molecular or ion-molecule reactions. Further if the vacuum is not efficient, there is erosion of electron producing filament and broadening of the ion-beam. A vacuum of 10^{-6} to 10^{-7} torr is needed for the ion source to prevent undue scattering by collision of ions with residual gas molecules.

The ions are accelerated by application of electrostatic field and then are deflected by application of a magnetic field through an angle of 60°, 90°, 120° or 180°

A schematic diagram of a 180° magnetic deflection mass spectrometer is shown in the Fig. 20.5.

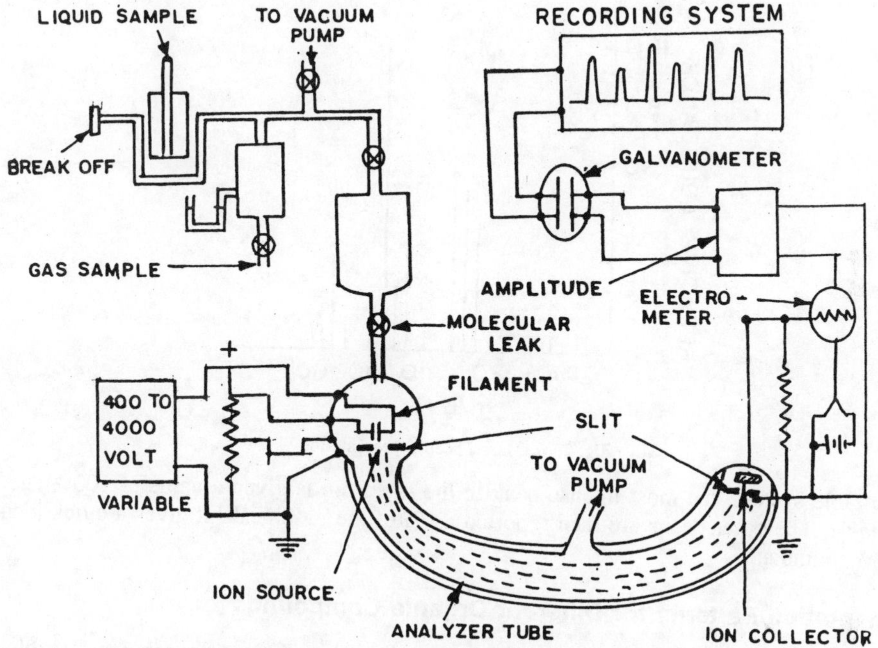

Fig. 20.5. Schematic diagram of a 180° magnetic deflection mass spectrometer.

(iii) Detection and Recording : The two commonly used techniques of detection and recording of ions in mass spectrometry are by (a) photographic method and (b) by use of electron multipliers. A photographic detector has the advantage that it can record all the ions simultaneusly and can give a better resolution than electrical detector but it does not give good relative abundance of isotopes.

The use of electron multipliers is similar to photomultiplier tube used in a conventional U.V- visible spectrophotometer except that it uses a beryllium -copper collector plate as a primary cathode. Such a type of cathode responds to ions rather than to photons.

The pen and ink type of recorders are slow for mass spectrometers work. The common arrangement involves the use of 3 to 5 galvanometer mirrors which deflect the beam of U.V. radiation into a UV sensitive recording paper as ions are collected on the electron multiplier.

However, microprocessor based mass spectrometers with computer and printer-plotter attachements have been available in the market for the last several years.

20.4 Spectral Presentation

In a mass spectrometer, the molecules of a sample are ionized and then fragmented into different masses. The detector registers these ions and produces signals according to the abundance and mass/charge ratio of the ions produced. Therefore, a mass spectrum of a particular compound is a graphical record of its fragmentation pattern. There are two simple ways of presentation of a mass spectrum (Fig. 20.6), namely: (a) bar graph or a (b) % table. In the bar graph system, the relative intensity is plotted as ordinate and the m/e along abscissa and gives a pictorial impression

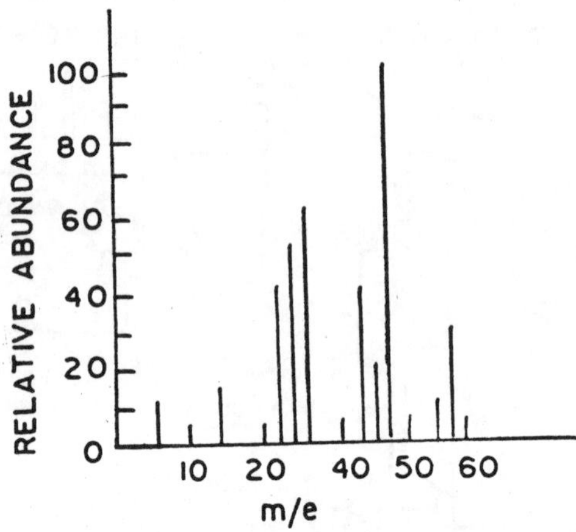

Fig. 20.6. Mass Spectral presentation

In the % table system, the most intense peak in the spectrum is given a value of 100% and is called the "*base peak*". The other peaks are then reported as % of the base peak. It gives a quick idea of mass number and % abundances.

20.5 Fragmentation Patterns for Different Organic Compounds

The main purpose of the mass spectrometer is to convert the unknown sample into measureable products that can indicate its original structure. Thus the fragmentation patterns of an unknown molecule can give some clue to its identity.

For the purpose of establishing the structure of an organic Compound, we want to obtain its molecular weight and molecular formula. For a large majority of organic compounds, the molecular wieght can be obtained directly from the spectrum. In these compounds the molecular ion produced by the initial ionization process is stable enough to reach the detector. The molecular weight of such compounds can be read directly from the spectrum by noting the highest *mass peak* (M) whose relative intensity is independent of the pressure. The intensity of this peak is related to the chemical stability of the molecule. An intense M peak may suggest the possibility of a conjugated olefinic, aromatic or polycyclic compound. On the other hand a weak M peak may indicate acetals, tert. alcohols, branched chain alcohols etc. The obundance of the molecular ion will depend on the bond strengths of the various individual bonds contained in the parent molecule. The other factors like polarizability, inductive and steric effects, resonance, hyperconjugation, energy of transition for fragmentation and lastly the stability of the fragments produced will also affect the abundances of the molecular and other fragment ions. An approximate order of decreasing stability of ions is stated as; aromatic > heteroaromatic, conjugated obfins, st. chain hydrocarbons, amiaes, ketone, aldehydes, amines, esters, ethers, nitriles, primary alcohols, tertiary alcohols and acetals.

Some common examples of fragmentation patterns for various classes of organic compounds are discussed below :

Hydrocarbons

(a) Alkanes : The straight chain alkanes show low intensity molecular ion peaks and their intensity decreases with increasing chain length, the very intense being in the C_1—C_5 range. They rarely eliminate CH_3 groups and therefore peak corresponding to M-15 are absent or of low intensity. The removal of groups like C_2H_5, C_3H_7 etc from the molecular ion give peaks at mass C_nH_{2n+1} (i.e. m/e = 29, 43, 57, 71, 85). These peaks are intense in the C_2 to C_5 range. The peaks at 43 or 57 are base peaks due to propyl ion ($C_3H_7^+$) and butyl ion ($C_4H_9^+$). on the other hand intensites of 14 mass unit i.e. CH_2 dereases with increasing weight of the fragment. The mechanisms for fragmentation of a few hydrocarbons is shown below :

(i) Straight chain :

$$CH_3—CH_2—CH_2—CH_2—CH_2—CH_3 \xrightarrow[\text{ionization}]{-e} CH_3 \overset{+\cdot}{—} CH_2—CH_2—CH_2—CH_2—CH_3$$

Parent ion

↓ hemi-heterolysis

$$CH_2 + CH_2-CH_2-CH_3 \xleftarrow{\text{Heterolysis }+} CH_2-CH_2-CH_2-CH_3 + CH_3CH_2$$

(ii) Branched chain :

$$CH_3—CH_2—\underset{CH_3}{\overset{CH_3}{\underset{|}{\overset{|}{C}}}}—CH_3 \xrightarrow[\text{ionization}]{-e} CH_3 \overset{+\cdot}{—} CH_2—\underset{CH_3}{\overset{CH_3}{\underset{|}{\overset{|}{C}}}}—CH_3 \qquad \underset{CH_3}{\overset{CH_3}{\underset{|}{\overset{|}{C}}}}\overset{+}{—}CH_3 + CH_3\dot{C}H_2$$

(iii) Cycloalkanes :

Cyclohexane $\xrightarrow[\text{ionization}]{-e}$ (ring radical cation, +•, with α, β, γ positions) $\xrightarrow[\text{(ii) Heteolysis of } \beta r\text{-bond}]{\text{(i) hemi hetroysis}}$ $\overset{+}{C}H_2CH_2CH_2\dot{C}H_2$ + C_2H_4

(b) Alkenes : The spectra of alkenes is usually difficult to interpret but they readily lose a π electron to produce a molecular ion. The intensity of M peak decreases with increasing molecular weight. The most intense peak is due to a stable charged species produced by allylic cleavage as :

$$H_2C—CH—CH_2—R \longrightarrow H_2C^+—CH= CH_2 + R^o$$

$$m/e = 41$$

The outcome of the allylic cleavage is formation of fragmentsat 41, 55,69,83 with generalformula $C_n H_{2n-1}$ (i.e. allylic carbonium ions.

(C) Aromatic hydrocabons : They usually show stronger molecular ion peaks than n-paraffins. The alkylbenzenes cleave at the bond β-to the ring and show a base peak at m/e at 91 due to the formation of tropyllium ion.

(i) $C_6H_5-CH_2R \xrightarrow[\text{ionization}]{-e} [C_6H_5-CH_2R]^{+} \xrightarrow{-\dot{R}} C_6H_5-CH_2$

Rearrangement → tropylium ion ($C_7H_7^+$), m/e = 91

(ii) $C_6H_5-CH(CH_3)-R \xrightarrow[\text{ionization}]{-e} [C_6H_5-CH(CH_3)-R]^{+} \xrightarrow{-\dot{R}}$

$C_6H_5-\overset{+}{C}H-CH_3 \xrightarrow{\text{Rearrangement}}$ methyltropylium ion (CH_3)

$C_6H_5-CH_2-CH_2-CH_2-R \xrightarrow[\text{ionization}]{-e} [C_6H_5]^{+}-CH_2-CH_2-CH(H)-R$

$\longrightarrow$ $C_7H_8^+$ (m/e = 92) + $CH_2=CH-R$

The tropyllium ion may undergo further fragmentation and show peaks at 65 or 39.

m/e = 39 ← m/e = 91 → m/e = 65

Alcohols

The molecular ion peak M, is very small or absent, usually abundant in secondary than in primary and tertiary alcohols. The molecular ion is formed initially by removal of the non-bonding electron from oxygen and then fragmentation into stable products. e.g. ethyl alcohol shows M-1 peak at m/e = 45 by a the α-elimination, of H but M–15 peak at m/e = 31 is more intense as the removal of a larger group is favoured.

$$CH_3-CH_2-OH \xrightarrow[\text{ionization}]{-e} CH_3-\overset{\overset{H}{|}}{\underset{\underset{H}{|}}{C}}-O-H$$

$$CH_3 + H_2C=O^{+}-H \quad (m/e = 31) \qquad\qquad CH_3-C^{-}=O-H + H \quad (m/e = 45)$$

The primary alcohols show very low intensity M – 2 and M– 3 peaks in addition to M –1 peaks as indicated below.

$$R-\overset{\overset{H}{|}}{\underset{\underset{H}{|}}{C}}-O-H \xrightarrow[\text{ionization}]{-e} R-\overset{\overset{H}{|}}{\underset{\underset{H}{|}}{C}}-\overset{\bullet+}{O}-H \xrightarrow{-H} R-\underset{\underset{H}{|}}{C}=\overset{+}{O}-H \xrightarrow{-\dot{H}} \quad (M-1)$$

$$R-\underset{\underset{H}{|}}{C}=\overset{\bullet+}{O} \xrightarrow{-H} R-C\equiv O$$
$$(M-2) \qquad\qquad (M-3)$$

All primary alcohols except methanol and high molecular weight secondaryand tertiary alcohols lose water (H_2O) and exhibit peaks at M – 18.

$$R-CH(H\cdots\overset{\bullet+}{O}H)-(CH_2)_n-CH_2 \longrightarrow \left[R-CH-(CH_2)_n \text{ (bridged by } \overset{H_2}{C}\text{)}\right]^{+\bullet} + H_2O$$
$$M-18$$

$$\overset{+\bullet}{HO} \leftarrow H,\ H_2C,\ CHR,\ \text{C(H)(H)}-\text{C(H)(H)} \longrightarrow \underset{M-28}{H_2C=CH_2} + \underset{M-46}{CHR=CH_2} + H_2O$$

Phenols and Aromatic Alcohols

The molecular ion peak M, in phenols and aromatic alcohols is of strong intensity though in phenols, it forms the base peak. The phenols also show low intensity M –1 peak dueto lose of Hydrogen which is strong in cresol and benzyl alcohol.

OH, CH_3, p-Cresed; −e; OH, CH_3; −H; OH; CH_2OH; CHOH, H; −e; CH_2OH, Benzyl Alcohol

The main route of fragmentation in phenols and benzyl alcohol involves the loss of CO and CHO giving rise to peaks at M – 28 and M – 29 respectively.

(i)

OH; −e; OH; O, H, H; m/e = 99 (M) 100%; H, H; + CO; m/e = 66 (M−28); + H; m/e = 65 (M−29)

(ii)

CH_2OH; −e; CH_2OH; m/e = 108; − H; OH, H; (M−1); C≡O$^+$, H, H; −CO; H, H; m/e = 79 (M−29); m/e = 77 (M−31); OH; m/e = 107 (M− 1); OH, H, H; −CO; H, H; m/e = 79 (M−31)

It is usually found that cresols, catechols, resorcinol, hydroquinones and methyl substituted benzyl alcohol undergo a loss of water and show M – 18 peaks.

$$\text{(o-methylbenzyl alcohol: } C_6H_4(CH_2OH)(CH_3)) \xrightarrow{-e} \left[C_6H_4(CH_2OH)(CH_3)\right]^{+\cdot} \text{ (M)} \longrightarrow \left[C_6H_4(=CH_2)_2\right] \text{ (M-18) } 100\%$$

Aldehydes and Ketones

The procedure in the carbonyl Compounds involves a loss of one of the lone pair of electrons of the oxygen. This is followed by the fragmentation of the molecular ion so produced either through a α – Cleavage or if a concerted migration of γ--hydrogen to oxygen is possible through a β-cleavage. In the α-cleavage, the bond between the C = O group and γ– carbon to oxygen is possible through a β-cleavage. In the α-cleavage, the bond between the C = O group and α-carbon is broken by a homolytic cleavage so that the + ive charge is retained by the oxygen containing fragment to generate an oxonium ion.

$$\begin{matrix} R \\ R_1 \end{matrix}\!\!>C=O \xrightarrow{-e} \begin{matrix} R \\ R_1 \end{matrix}\!\!>C=\overset{+\cdot}{O} \xrightarrow[\text{homolytic}]{\alpha\text{ – cleavage}} R_1-C\equiv O + \dot{R}$$

In the condition when γ-hydrogen migration is possible, β-cleavage results in the formation of an olefin and a charged enol — this is known as Maclafferty rearrangement.

$$R_2(H)\overset{\gamma}{C}H-\overset{\beta}{C}H(R_1)-\overset{\alpha}{C}H_2-C(=O)-R \xrightarrow{-e} [\text{six-membered H}\cdots O \text{ arrangement}] \xrightarrow[\text{Rearrangement}]{\beta\text{-Cleavage}} R_2-CH=CH-R_1 + CH_2=C(\overset{+}{O}H)-R$$

(a) Aldehydes : They show M peaks which are prominent in aromatic compounds because of the presence of resonance stabilization. The intensity of the M–peaks in aliphatic aldehydes decreases with compounds containing more than 4 carbon atoms. The M–1 peak intensities in aldehydes are as much as M peaks and is due to the loss of H radical through a homolytic α -cleavage.

$$R-\underset{\displaystyle H}{\underset{|}{C}}=O \xrightarrow{-e} R-\underset{\displaystyle H}{\underset{|}{C}}=\overset{+}{O} \longrightarrow \underset{(M-1)}{R-C\equiv O} + H$$

There is a presence of strong peak at m/e = 29 (base peak) which is due to α – cleavage and the formation of a formyl ion of H– $C^+ \equiv O$.

$$R-\underset{\displaystyle H}{\underset{|}{C}}=\overset{+\bullet}{O} \longrightarrow \underset{m/e\,=\,29}{H-C\equiv O^+} + \dot{R}$$

In higher aldehydes starting from butyraldehyde, a base peak at m/e = 44 is formed which is due to β-cleavage.

$$H_3C-CH_2-CH_2-\overset{O}{\overset{||}{C}}-H \xrightarrow{-e} \left[H_2C(\gamma)\cdots H\cdots\overset{+}{O}=CH,\ H_2C(\beta)-CH_2(\alpha)\right] \longrightarrow \underset{m/e\,=\,44}{CH_2=C(H)-\overset{+\bullet}{O}H} + CH_2=CH_2$$

(b) Ketones : The parent ion peak M, is of medium intensity, it is usually greater for low molecular weight than for higher molecular weight ketones. They produce stable R – C ≡ O^+ ions through α – cleabvage as indicated below.

$$\begin{matrix}R\\ \quad\diagdown\\ \quad C=O\\ \quad\diagup\\ R_1\end{matrix} \xrightarrow{-e} \begin{matrix}R\\ \quad\diagdown\\ \quad C=\overset{}{\underset{+\bullet}{O}}\\ \quad\diagup\\ R_1\end{matrix} \xrightarrow{\text{Homolysis}} R_1-C\equiv\overset{+}{O}+\dot{R} \text{ if } R > R_1$$

$$\xrightarrow{\text{Homolysis}} R-C\equiv\overset{+}{O}+\dot{R_1} \text{ if } R_1 > R$$

$$\xrightarrow{\text{Heterolysis}} R-C\equiv\dot{O}+R_1^+$$

The homolytic cleavage produces masses with m/e = 43, 57, 71 while in heterolysis masses with m/e = 15, 29, 43, 57 are formed. In aliphatic methyl ketones, a fragment $CH_3\ C \equiv O^+$ with m/e = 43 will thus be obtained through α – cleavage. An aromatic ketone like acetophenone undergoes a fragmentation pattern as shown.

$$C_6H_5-\overset{O}{\overset{||}{C}}-CH_3 \xrightarrow{-e} C_6H_5-\overset{\overset{+}{O}}{C}-CH_3 \xrightarrow{-\dot{C}H_3}$$

$$\underset{m/e\,=\,105}{C_6H_5-C\equiv\overset{+}{O}} \longrightarrow \underset{m/e\,=\,77}{C_6H_5^{+}} + CO$$

The ketones containing a chain of 3 or more carbons also undero Mac Lafferty rearrangement via a b-cleavage as was the case in aldehydes, e.g. propyl methyl ketone.

(i)

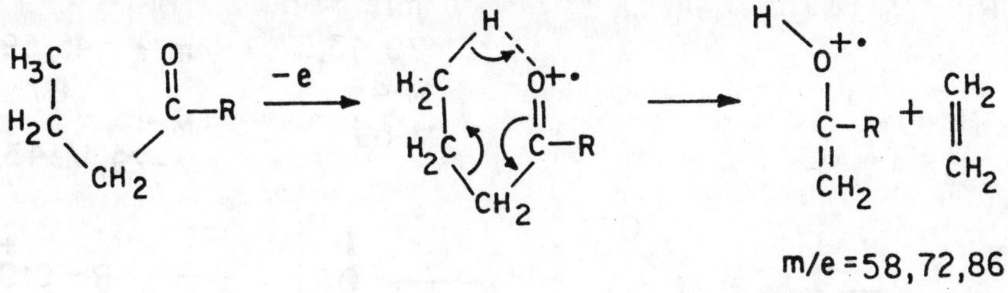

$m/e = 58, 72, 86$

(ii)

$m/e = 58$

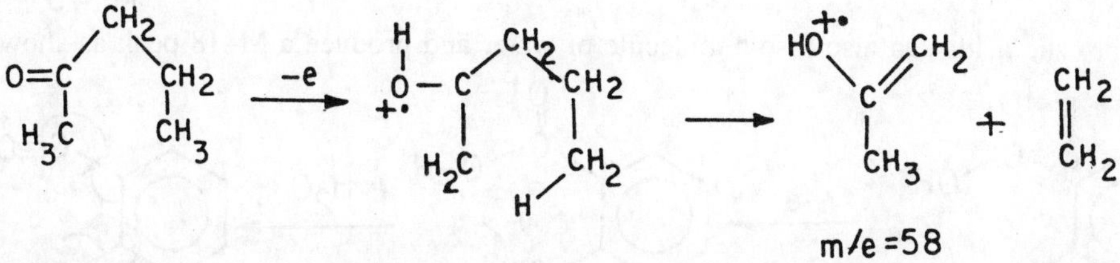

Carboxylic Acids

The aliphatic monocarboxylic acids and their esters exhibit weak molecular ion peak M, with its intensity decreasing along with molecular weight. They also show Mac Lafferty rearrangement involving a bond β-to carbonyl group with a rearrangement of γ– hydrogen. Conseuqently aliphatic acids show a base peak.

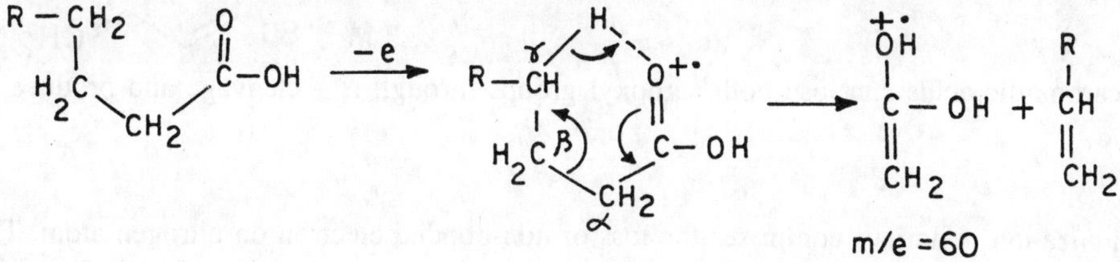

$m/e = 60$

Methyl Esters $\xrightarrow{-e}$ $CH_2{=}C(OH)OCH_3^{+\bullet}$

$m/e = 74$

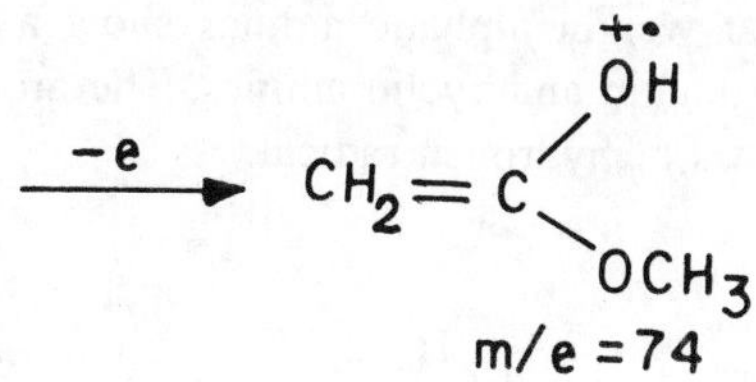

at m/e = 60, whereas all methyl esters of straight chain carboxylic acids exhibit a base peak at m/e = 74. The cleavage of α– bond to carbonyl can four different types of ions.

$$R-C(=O)-OR_1 \xrightarrow{-e} R-C(=O^{+\bullet})-OR_1 \longrightarrow \overset{+}{R} + C\equiv O(-OR_1)$$

$\overset{+}{R}$: m/e = 15, 29, 43, 57, M-45, M-59

$C\equiv O(OR_1)$: m/e = 45, 59, 73, 87, M-15, M-29, M-43

$$R-C(=O)-OR_1 \xrightarrow{-e} R-C(=O^{+\bullet})-OR_1 \longrightarrow \overset{+}{O}R_1 + R-\overset{+}{C}\equiv O$$

$\overset{+}{O}R_1$: m/e = 17, 31, 45, 59, M-43 M-47

$R-\overset{+}{C}\equiv O$: m/e=43, 57, 71, M-17, M-31, M-45

The carboxylic acids can also lose a molecule of water and produce a M–18 peak as shown below.

$$\text{o-toluic acid} \xrightarrow{-e} [\text{molecular ion}]^{+\bullet} \xrightarrow{-H_2O} \text{ion with } \overset{+}{C}\equiv O \text{ and } \dot{C}H_2 \leftrightarrow C_6H_4(=C=\overset{+\bullet}{O})(=CH_2)$$

M = 136

m/e = 118 (M–18)

The dicarboxylic acids can lose both carboxyl groups through α – cleavage and produce a peak at M–90.

Amines

The initial ionization in amines comprises the loss of non-bonded electron on nitrogen atom. The – NH_2 group releases electrons more easily than the – OH group, consequently amines show a lower ionization potential. The high molecular weight alphatic amines show a weak to absent molecular ion peak M, whereas it is strong in the aromatic and cyclic amines. The aromatic and low molecular weight amines display a M–1 peak due to loss of hydrogen radical.

(i)

$$CH_3-NH_2 \xrightarrow{-e} H-\underset{H}{\overset{H}{C}}-\overset{+\bullet}{N}H_2 \longrightarrow H_2C-\overset{+}{N}H_2 + \dot{H}$$

(m-1)

(ii) $C_6H_5{-}NH_2 \xrightarrow{-e} [C_6H_5{-}NH_2]^{+\bullet} \longrightarrow C_6H_5{-}\overset{+}{N}H + H$

Amines can also rupture a bond β-to nitrogen and generate various types of ions as shown below.

(i) $R{-}CH_2{-}NH_2 \xrightarrow{-e} R{-}CH_2{-}\overset{+}{N}H_2 \longrightarrow \rangle C{=}\overset{+}{N}H_2 + R$

m/e = 30, 44, 58, 72, 86

(ii) $C_6H_5NH_2 \xrightarrow{-e} [C_6H_5\overset{+}{N}H_2] \xrightarrow{-HCN} [C_5H_6]^+ \longrightarrow C_5H_5^+ + H$

m/e = 66   m/e = 65

(iii) N-methylpyrrolidine $\xrightarrow{-e}$ [ion] $\longrightarrow$ $H_2\dot{C}{-}N(CH_3){=}CH_2$ + $CH_2{=}CH_2$

$H_2C{=}N{=}CH$

m/e = 42

Nitro Compounds

They do not show molecular ion peak M, but strong peaks are exhibited at m/e = 46 and 30 due to the formation of N^+O_2 and NO^+ ions. However, aromatic nitro compounds show a strong M peak at odd mass number. In addition peaks at m/e = 30 due to NO^+ and M – 46 and M-58 are also observed.

$C_6H_5NO_2 \xrightarrow{-e} [C_6H_5NO_2]^{+\bullet} \xrightarrow{-NO_2} C_6H_5^+ \longrightarrow \overset{+}{C_4H_3}$

m/e = 123 (M)   m/e = 77 (M − 46)   m/e = 51

$M \xrightarrow{-NO} C_6H_5O^{+\bullet} \longrightarrow C_5H_5^+ + CO$

m e = 93 (M − 30)   m e = 65 (M − 58)

Halogens

The molecular ion peak M, is strong in aromatics but usually detectable in aliphatic halogen compounds. However, the intensity of M peaks for alkyl or aryl group decreased in the order I > Br > Cl > F.

A strong effect due to isotopic abundance of halogen is observed in the halogen compounds, e.g. Iodine and fluorine are monoisotopic. On the contrary chlorine and bromine occur as isotopic mixture e.g. Cl as 3 parts of ^{35}Cl and ^{37}Cl while Br as equal parts of ^{79}Br and ^{81}Br. Further, the mass spectra of ions containing one Cl atom or one Br atom show doublets at masses m and m + Z. The m +2 peak in chlorides is about 1/3 of intensity of the peak at m, whereas the m and m + 2 peaks in bromides and bromies containing n-alkyl chain of 6-Carbon atoms or more formcyclic chloronium ion or bromonium ion whereas the fluorides, iodides and branched chain halides do not form such ions.

$$R-CH_2-CH_2-CH_2-CH_2-Br \xrightarrow{-e} R-CH_2-CH_2-CH_2-CH_2-Br^{+\bullet} \longrightarrow \text{cyclic } Br^{+} + R$$

$M/e = 135$

The halides in general also exhibit peaks at M – X, M – HX, M –H_2 X and M – R as shown below.

(i) $R-X \xrightarrow{-e} \underset{(M)}{R-\overset{+}{X}} \longrightarrow \underset{(M-X)}{\overset{+}{R} + \dot{X}}$ Strong When X=Br, I

(ii) $R-CH_2-CH_2-X \xrightarrow{-e} \underset{(M)}{R-CH_2-CH_2-X^{+\bullet}} \longrightarrow R-\dot{C}H-\overset{+}{C}H_2 + HX$

(M–HX) Strong When X= F, Cl

(iii) $CH_3-CH_2-X \xrightarrow{-e} \underset{(M)}{CH_3-CH_2-X^{+\bullet}} \longrightarrow CH-\overset{+}{X} + \dot{C}H_3$

(M–R) Heaviest group on α –Carbon is lost

(iv) $R-H_2C-H_2C-CH_2-CH_2-X \xrightarrow{-e} R-H_2C-H_2C-CH_2-CH_2-X^{+\bullet} \longrightarrow \text{cyclic } (H_2C-X^{+}-CH_2-CH_2-CH_2) + R$

Ethers

They produce ions at m/e = 45, 59 and 87 like alcohols but do not show a loss of H_2O from M ion.

(i)

$$(H_3C)_2CH-O-CH(CH_3)_2 \;(M = 102) \xrightarrow{-e} (H_3C)_2CH-\overset{+\bullet}{O}-CH(CH_3)_2 \xrightarrow{-CH_3} CH_3-CH=\overset{+}{O}-CH(CH_3)H \;(m/e = 87)$$

$$CH_3-CH=\overset{+}{O}H + CH_3-CH=CH_2 \;(m/e = 45)$$

(ii)

$$(H_3C)_2CH-O-CH(CH_3)_2 \xrightarrow{-e} (H_3C)_2CH \,\vdots\, \overset{+\bullet}{O}-CH(CH_3)_2 \longrightarrow (H_3C)_2CH \;(m/e = 43) + O-CH(CH_3)_2 \;(m/e = 59)$$

In Contrast m – dimethoxybenzene gives major fragment peaks at m/e = 108 (i.e. M — CH_2O) and m/e = 109 (i.e. M — CH_2O)

$$C_6H_4(OCH_3)_2 \xrightarrow{-e} [C_6H_4(\overset{+}{O}CH_3)(O-CH_3)]\;(M = 138) \longrightarrow \overset{+}{O}CH_3\text{-cyclohexadienone} \;(m/e = 123) + CH_3$$

$$M = 138 \xrightarrow{-CH_2O} C_6H_5{=}O-CH_3 \;(m/e = 108)$$

20.6 Metastable Ions

Sometimes a mass spectrum shows few diffused, broad, low intensity peaks at non-integral masses, these are due to *metastable ions.* Suppose an ion m_o produced in the ion source is very stable, it will remain undecomposed during its passage through the accelerator and deflector to the ion collector. If m_o is very unstable, it will decompose immediately (at 10^{-13} seconds) into smaller fragments which are deflected and recorded. On the other hand the ions of intermediate stability undergo fragmentation (at 10^6/second) during or immediately after acceleration but before magnetic deflection. These ions depict weak and diffuse peaks at non-integral mass numbers. Because of the energy difference when they enter the analyzer and leave the accelerator, the metastable ion m_o is accelerated to a velocity determined by its heavier mass, but the ion deflected by the magnetic deflector is a lighter ion m^+, which is produced as per the equation $m^o = m^+ + (m_0 — m)$. It is due to this difference between the acceleration mass and its deflection mass that the product mass m^+ is not recorded at its true mass but is found at the apparent mass m^* represented as : $m^* = m^2/m_0$. The loss of kinetic energy during decomposition and variation in the life time of these ions causes the m^+ peak to be diffuse and broad.

The study of metastable ions helps in studying the mechanism involved in fragmentation and structure elucidation e.g. disopropylamine displays metastable peak at m/e = 22.8 in addition to strong peaks at m/e = 44 and 86 and a weak peak at 101.

$$(CH_3)_2CH—\ddot{N}H—CH(CH_3)_2 \xrightarrow{-e} (CH_3)_2C—H—\overset{+\bullet}{N}H—CH(CH_3)_2 \; (M) \longrightarrow$$

$$\dot{C}H_3 + CH_3—\overset{+}{=}NH—CH(CH_3)(CH_2\text{–}H) \quad m_0,\ m/e = 86 \longrightarrow \underset{m^+,\ m/e\ =\ 44}{CH_3-CH=\overset{+}{N}H_2} + \underset{\text{Propene}}{CH(CH_3)=CH_2} \quad \text{mass} = m_0 — m$$

The formation of metastable peak at apparent mass $m^* = 22.8[m^2/m = (44)^2/86 = 22.5]$ is taken as the proof for the above given fragmentation pattern of diisopropylamine which involves an α — cleavage of M to give m_0 at m/e = 86 followed by fragmentation to an ion m^+ (m/e = 44) and a neutral fragment propane of mass 42 (m_0 — m i.e. 86 — 44) by transferring a b — hydrogen to nitrogen in a homolytic process.

20.7 Determination Of Molecular Formula

Normally, the mass of the heaviest ion (i.e. molecular ion peak) in a particular fragmentation process gives us the molecular weight. But, all the elements except F, I and P have heavier isotope and these the contained in certain fixed proportion. The mass of the heavier isotope is usually 1 or 2 a.m.u more than that of the higher isotope, consequently the heavy isotopes appear on the spectrum at m/e one or more higher than the normal. Therefore the spectra of many compounds show M + 1, M + 2, and M + 3 peaks. although the intensity of these is low compared to M, but is fixed. The number of possible molecular formulas can be achieved by the study of abundances of natural isotopes for different elements. As the % of M, M + 1, M + 2 peaks are fixed for a given composition, the observed values are compared with the theoretical values. The table for calculation of values for M, M + 1, M + 2 for compounds containing atoms C, H, O, N up to the molecular weight of 500 have been calculated and are available in text books.

The % of M + 1, M + 2 in relation to M can be calculated for a compound with the molecular Formula as $C_w\ H_x\ N_y\ O_z$ by the method shown below.

The % of M + 1 peak = (1.08 × W) + (0.016 × X) + (0.38 × Y) + (0.039 × Z)

$$\% \text{ of } M + 2 \text{ peak} = \frac{(1.1 \times W)^2}{200} + 0.20 \times Z$$

Say, we have the compound with molecular formula $C_9\ H_{10}\ O_3$

$\therefore$ % M + 1 = (1.08 × 9) + (0.016 × 10) + (0.039 × 3) = 9.97%

$$\text{and } \% \ M + 2 = \frac{(1.1 \times 9)^2}{200} + (0.20 \times 3) = 1.08\ \%$$

$$\text{No. of carbon atoms} = \frac{\%\text{ of } M + 1 \text{ Peak}}{1.1} = \frac{9.97}{1.1} = 9.06$$

The molecular Formula thus obtained enables us to determine the double bond equivalent (D.B.E.) i. e. the number of double bonds and or rings in the compound.

If the general Formula of the Compound is $C_w\ H_x\ N_y\ O_z$, then

$$\text{D.B.E.} = \frac{1}{2}(2W - X + Y + 2)$$

For example consider benzene i.e. C_6H_6

$$\therefore \quad \text{D.B.E.} = \frac{1}{2}\ (2 \times 6 - 6 + 0 + 2) = \frac{1}{2}\ (8) = 4 \ \textit{i.e.}$$

3 double bonds or one ring.

Let us consider another example like,

allylamine i. e. $C_3\ H_7\ N$

$$\therefore \text{D.B.E} = \frac{1}{2}(2 \times 3 - 7 + 1 + 2)$$

$$\therefore \frac{1}{2}\ (6 - 7 + 1 + 2) = 1 \text{ i. e. one double Bond}$$

$$\therefore \quad C_3\ H_7\ N = CH_2 = \underset{}{\overset{H}{\overset{|}{C}}} - CH_2 - NH_2$$

We can take one more example like $C_4\ H_4\ S$.

$$\therefore \text{ D.B.E.} = \frac{1}{2}\ (2 \times 4 - 4 + 0 + 2) = \frac{1}{2}\ (4 + 2) = 3$$

$\therefore$ C_4H_4S =

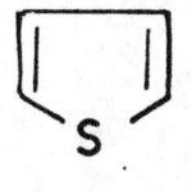

S

20.8 Rules for Determination of Mass Spectra

In addition to the procedure already described for the determination of molecular Formula and the amount of unsaturation contained in a particular compound the following rules should also be utilized in arriving at a structure of an unknown compound.

(i) The loss of 14 mass unit from molecular ions means presence of a homologue i.e. differing by CH_2 unit, but requires high energy.

(ii) In compounds having C, H, O, N the loss of 5 — 13 units is impossible — loss of many hydrogens would require high energy but loss of 3 — 5 hydrogens is possible by dehydrogenation.

(iii) Molecular weight of compounds containing only C, H (O) are *even,* so are those of molecules containing *even* number of N atoms.

(iv) Molecular weight of compounds containing C, H, N, (O) are *odd* when the number of N atoms is *odd.* For example, compounds with C, H, O lose radicals like CH_3, OCH_3 etc and *odd* mass fragments are formed. When neutral molecules are expelled i. e. H_2O, HCN, olefin, ACOH etc. *even* mass fragment is formed.

(v) Odd electron ions decompose by loss of radicals or even — electron molecules, whereas even — electron ions decompose by loss of even — electron molecules. i. e. odd electron ions contain upreared electron and include molecular ion $M^{+\cdot}$ and fragment ion $A^{+\cdot}$ formed from $M^{+\cdot}$ by loss of even — electron molecule.

20.9 Interpretation of Mass Spectra

(i) Firstly, a single electron is removed and no other bond is affected i. e. we get five ion radical with mass equal to the molecular weight. It is known at *parent ion* i.e. M peak. The strong peak in the spectrum is called *base peak* and other peaks are expressed in terms of % of the base peak.

(ii) Secondly, a single bond can split and produce principle fragments e. g.

$$\overset{+\bullet}{R - CH_4} \longrightarrow \overset{\bullet}{RH} + \overset{+}{CH_3}$$

(iii) Thirdly, a cleavage with rearrangement of hydrogen atom or a larger group can occur.

(iv) Fourthly, two electrons may get lost and give rise to an ion of apparent m/e 1/2 of true value.

(v) After establishing the parent ion peak i. e. M, the fragment peaks, we should measure m + 1 and m + 2 peaks i. e. isotopic peaks. This will give the number of C, N, O atoms. M + 1 peak is due to 1.1% of ^{13}C in normal carbon plus 0.4 % ^{15}N in normal nitrogen. M + 2 peak is due to ^{18}O isotope of oxygen and due to Si and S. Fluorine and iodine are monoisotopic, but chlorine has ^{35}C, ^{37}Cl in 3:1 ratio, while bromine has ^{79}Br, ^{81}Br in 1:1 ratio, Therefore, for chlorine, the pattern will comprise peaks spaced 2 masses apart.

Solved Examples : Methyl benzoate

$$C_6H_5 - \underset{\underset{O}{\|}}{C} - OCH_3 \longrightarrow C_6H_5 - \overset{+\bullet}{\underset{\underset{O}{\|}}{C}} - OCH_3 \xrightarrow{-\dot{O}CH_3} C_6H_5 - \overset{+}{C} \equiv O$$

m/e = 136 (M) m/e = 105

$\downarrow$ – CO

$$\overset{+}{C_4H_3} \xleftarrow{C_2H_2} \overset{+}{C_6H_5}$$

m/e = 51 m/e = 77

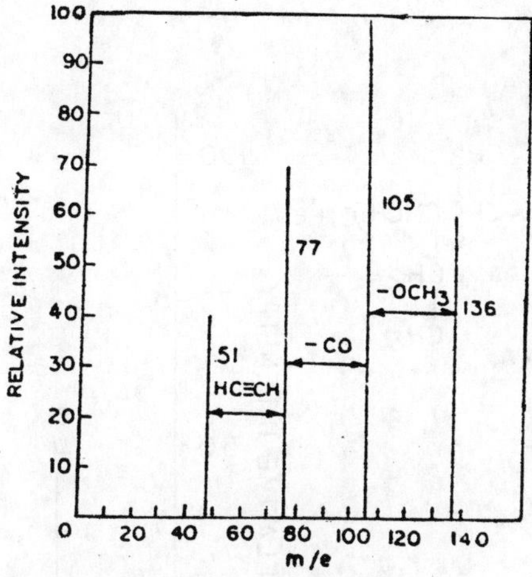

Fig. 20.7 Mass spectrum methyl benzoate

For practice purpose, examples of mass spectra (1 to 8) of organic molecules from various classes are given below.

20.10 Recent Developments

The discussion so far has been mainly concentrated on the mass spectra which are generated through electron impart technique. Such spectra sometime may show excess fragmentation and lack of molecular ion peak. Therefore other alternative techniques have been developed and have certain advantages, e. g.

(i) Field ionization and field desorption.

(ii) Chemical ionization.

The instrumentation aspects of mass spectrometry has also advanced in recent years. Thus there has been the development of Fourier — tramsform mass spectrometer,

The computer hook-up for mass spectrometry has been an interesting development as computers can identify the peaks as they are formed and also record them accordingly.

Further, the combination of gas chromatography i. e. GC/MS has proved very fruitful in quantitative analysis.

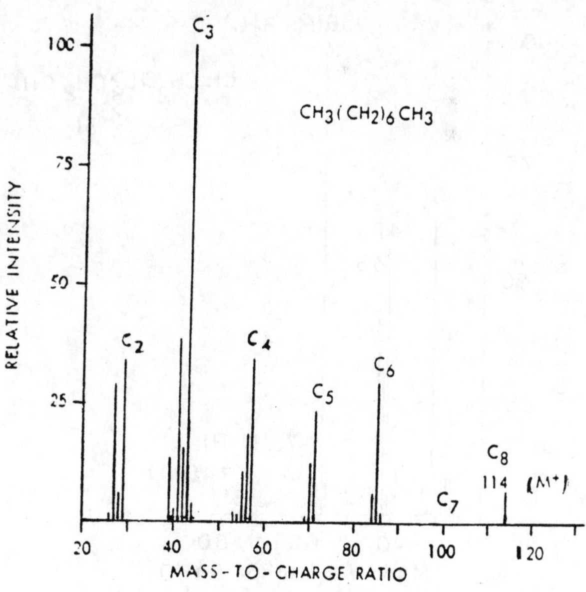

Mass Spectrum No. 1

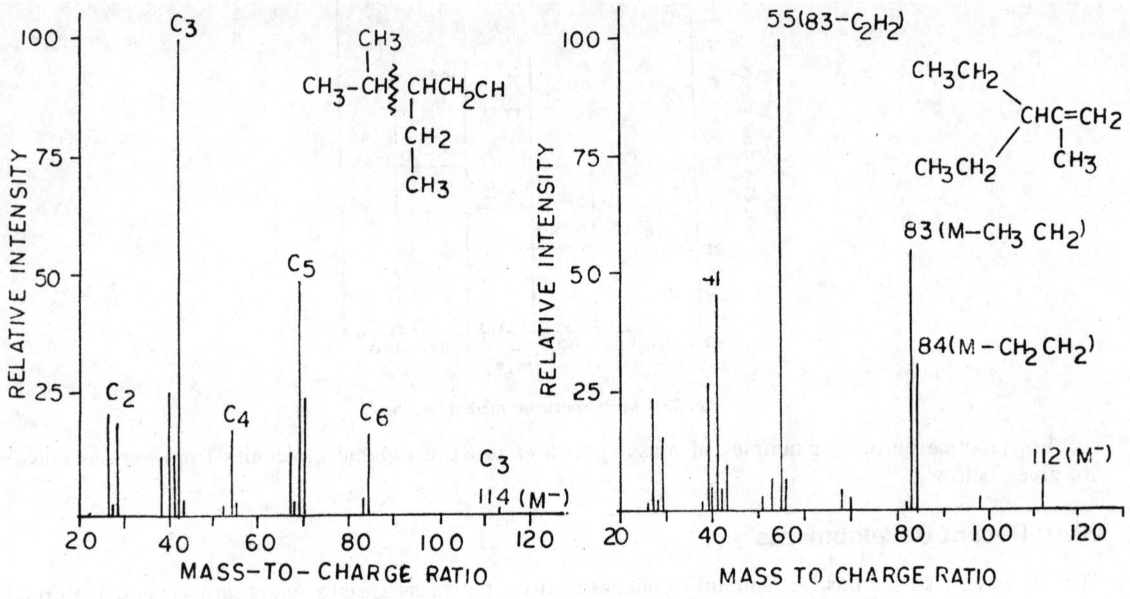

Mass Spectrum No. 2

Mass Spectrum No. 3

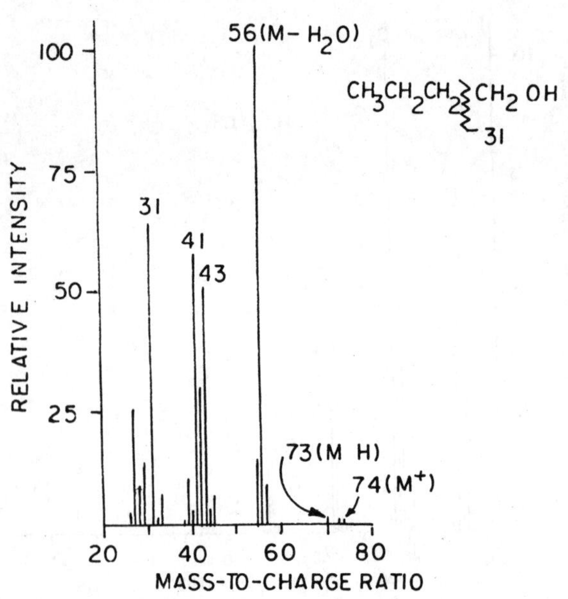

Mass Spectrum No. 4

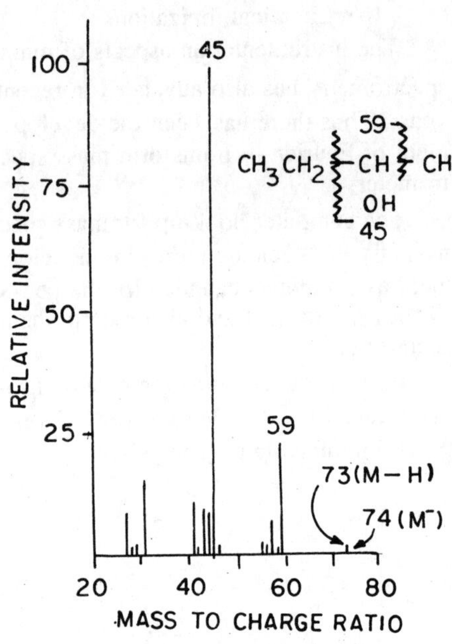

Mass Spectrum No. 5

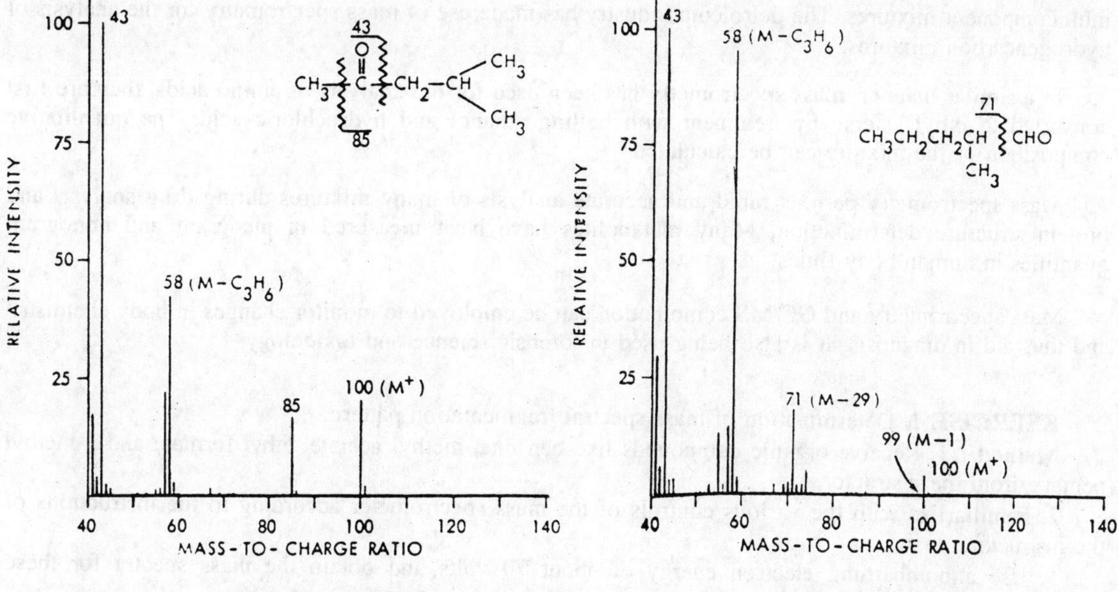

Mass Spectrum No. 6

Mass Spectrum No. 7

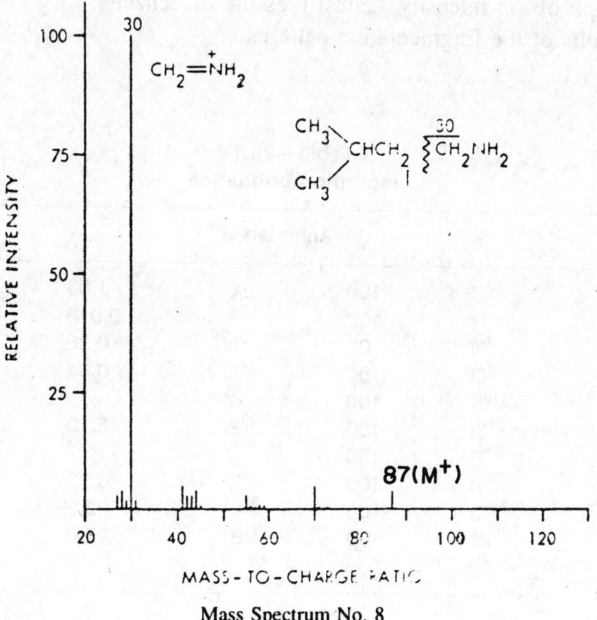

Mass Spectrum No. 8

One of the most important value of mass spectrometry has been in the quantitative analysis of multicomponent mixtures. The petroleum industry has made use of mass spectrometry for the analysis of hydrogencarbon mixtures.

In a similar manner, mass spectrometry has been used for the analysis of amino acids, they are first converted to ethyl esters by treatment with boiling ethanol and hydrochloric acid. The quantitative composition of the mixture can be calculated.

Mass spectrometry permits rapid and accurate analysis of many mixtures during drug analysis and protein structure determination. Many metabolites have been measured in picogram and nonogram quantities in human body fluids.

Mass spectrometry and GC/MS combination can be employed to monitor changes in body chemistry and thus aid in diagnosis. It is also being used in forensic science and toxicology.

EXERCISE 1. Determination of mass spectral fragmentation pattern.

Method : 1. Receive organic compounds like benzene, methyl acetate, ethyl formate and 3-methyl pentane from the instructor.

2. Familiarlize with the various controls of the mass spectrometer according to the instructions of the instructor.

3. Use a bombarding electron energy of about 70 volts and obtain the mass spectra for these compounds.

4. Compare these spectra with known spectra for these compounds in the catalogs of mass spectral data.

5. Now vary the pressure of benzene in the mass spectrometer and observe the fragmentation pattern obtained, and plot a graph of ion intensity against pressure of benzene.

6. Compare the results of the fragmentation patterns.

Table - 20.1
Isotopic Abundance

Element	Abundance					
Carbon	^{12}C	100	^{13}C	1.08		
Hydrogen	^{1}H	100	^{2}H	0.016		
Nitrogen	^{14}N	100	^{15}N	0.38		
Oxygen	^{16}O	100	^{17}O	0.04	^{18}O	0.20
Fluorine	^{19}F	100				
Silicon	^{28}Si	100	^{29}Si	5.10	^{30}Si	3.35
Phosphorus	^{31}P	100				
Sulphur	^{32}S	100	^{33}S	0.78	^{34}S	4.40
Chlorine	^{35}Cl	100	^{37}Cl	32.5		
Bromine	^{79}Br	100	^{81}Br	98.0		
Iodine	^{127}I	100				

Table - 20.2

Intensities of Isotope peaks (Relative to the molecular Ion) for combinations of Bromine and Chlorine

Halogen Present	% M+2	% M+4	% M+6	% M+8	% M+10	% M+12
Br	97.7					
Br_2	195.0	95.5				
Br_3	293.0	286.0	93.4			
Cl	32.5					
Cl_2	65.3	10.6				
Cl_3	97.8	31.9	3.47			
Cl_4	131.0	63.9	14.0	1.15		
Cl_5	163.0	106.0	34.7	5.66	0.37	
Cl_6	196.0	161.0	69.4	17.0	2.23	
BrCl	130.0	31.9				
Br_2Cl	228.0	159.0	31.2			
Cl_2Br	103.0	74.4	10.4			

Table - 20.3

Common Fragment ions

A small list of common fragment ions is indicated below.

m/e	Ions*	m/e	Ions
14	CH_2	33	SH, CH_2F
15	CH_3	34	H_2F
16	O	35	Cl
17	OH	36	HCl
18	H_2O, NH_4	39	C_3H_3
19	F, H_3O	40	$CH_2C=$ N, Ar(Air)
26	$C \equiv N$	41	C_3H_5 . $CH_2C = N + H$, C_2H_2NH
27	C_2H_3	42	C_3H_6
28	C_2H_4, CO, N_2 (air), CH = NH	43	C_3H_7,$CH_3C = O$,C_2H_5N
29	C_2H_5, CHO	44	$CH_2\overset{H}{\overset{\vert}{C}} = O + H$,$CH_3CHNH_2$,$CO_2$, $NH_2C = O$, $(CH_3)_2N$
30	CH_2NH_2, NO,	45	$\overset{CH_3}{\overset{\vert}{C}}HOH_2$ CH_2CH_2OH, CH_2OCH_3, $\overset{O}{\overset{\Vert}{C}} - OH$, $CH_3CH{-}O + H$
31	CH_2 OH, OCH_3	46	NO_2
32	O_2 (Air)	47	CH_2SH, CH_3S

(*Contd.*)

* Ions indicated as a fragment + nil (n = 1, 2, 3, . . .) are ions that arise via rearrangement involving hydrogen transfer.

m/e	Ions*
48	$CH_3S + H$
49	CH_2Cl
51	CHF_2
53	C_4H_5
54	$CH_2CH_2 \equiv N$
55	$C_4H_7, CH_2=CHC=O$
56	C_4H_8
57	C_4H_9, $C_2H_5C=O$
58	$CH_3-C(O)(CH_2)+H$, $C_2H_5CHNH_2$, $(CH_3)_2NCH_2$, $C_2H_5NHCH_2$, C_2H_2S
59	$(CH_3)_2COH$, $CH_2OC_2H_5$, $C(=O)-OCH_3$, $NH_2C(=O)(CH_2)+H$, CH_3OCHCH_3, CH_3CHCH_2OH
60	$CH_2C(O)(OH)+H$, CH_2ONO
61	$C(=O)-OCH_3+2H$, CH_2CH_2SH, CH_2SCH_3
65	(cyclopentadienyl ring) $\equiv C_5H_5$
66	(cyclopentadiene ring, +•) $\equiv C_5H_6$
67	C_5H_7
68	$CH_2CH_2CH_2C \equiv N$
69	$CH_5H_9, CF_3, CH_3CH=CHC=O$, $CH_2=C(CH_3)C=O$
70	C_5H_{10}
71	C_5H_{11}, $C_3H_7C=O$
72	$C_2H_5C(=O)(=CH_2)+H$, $C_3H_7CHNH_2$, $(CH_3)_2N=C+O$, $C_2H_5NHCHCH_3$, and isomers
73	Homologs of 59
74	$CH_2-C(=O)-OCH_3+H$
75	$C(=O)-OC_2H_5+2H$, $CH_2SC_2H_5$, $(CH_3)_2CSH$, $(CH_3O)_2CH$
77	C_6H_5
78	C_6H_5+2H, Br
80	(pyrrolyl, N–H)–CH_2, CH_3SS+H
81	(furyl)–CH_2, C_6H_9 (cyclohexenyl)
82	$CH_2CH_2CH_2CH_2C \equiv N$, CCl_2, C_6H_{10}
83	C_6H_{11}, $CHCl_2$, (thienyl)–CH_2
85	C_6H_{13}, $C_4H_9C=O$, $CClF_2$

(*Contd.*)

86 $C_3H_7C(=O)(CH_2) + H$, $C_4H_9CHNH_2$, and isomers

87 $CH_2-C(=O)-OC_2H_5 + H$

88 CH_3H_7CO (C=O), homologs of 73, $CH_2CH_2COCH_3$

89 $C(=O)-OC_3H_7 + 2H$, C_6H_5–C

90 CH_3CHONO_2, C_6H_5–CH

91 C_6H_5–CH_2, C_6H_5–CH + H, C_6H_5–C + 2H, $(CH_2)_4Cl$, C_5H_4–N

92 C_6H_5–CH_2 (ring-substituted), C_6H_5–O, C_6H_5–CH_2 + H,

93 CH_2Br, C_6H_5–OH, C_7H_9, pyrrole(NH)=C = O, C_6H_5–O, C_7H_9 (Terpenes)

94 C_6H_5–O +H, pyrrole(N)–C=O

(Contd.)

95 (furan-2-yl)–C=O

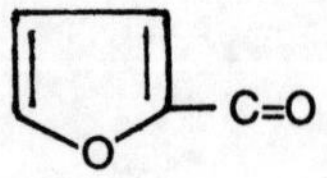

96 $CH_2CH_2CH_2CH_2CH_2\ C\equiv N$

97 C_7H_{13}, (thiophen-2-yl)–CH_2

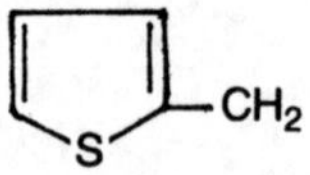

98 (furan-2-yl)–CH_2O + H

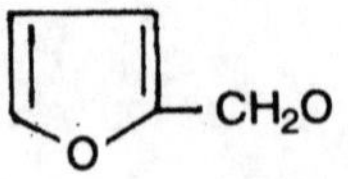

99 C_7H_{15}, $C_6H_{14}O$

100 $C_4H_9C(=O)(CH_2)$ + H, $C_5H_{11}CHNH_1$

101 $C(=O)-OC_4H_9$

102 $CH_2C(=O)-OC_3H_7$ + H

103 $C(=O)-OC_4H_9$ + 2H, $C_5H_{12}S$, $CH(OCH_2CH_3)_2$

104 $C_2H_5CHONO_2$

105 C_6H_5–C = O, C_6H_5–CH_2CH_2, C_6H_5–$CHCH_3$

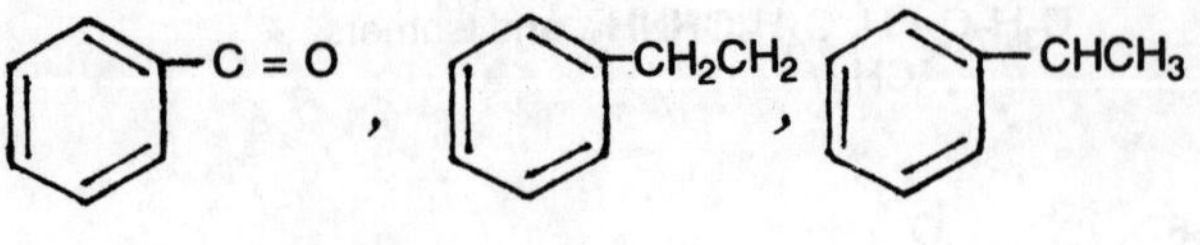

106 C_6H_5–$NHCH_2$

107 C_6H_5–CH_2O, CH_2–C_6H_4–OH, CH_2–C_6H_4–OH

108 C_6H_5–CH_2O + H, (N-methylpyrrol-2-yl)–C = O (N–CH_3)

109 (cyclohexenyl)–C = O

111 (thiophen-2-yl)–C = O

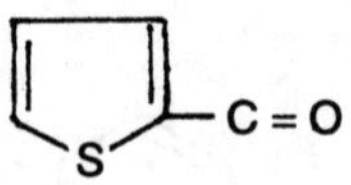

119 CF_3CF_2,

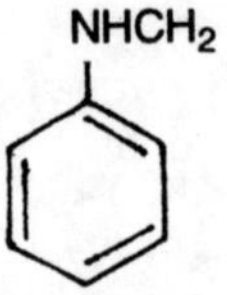

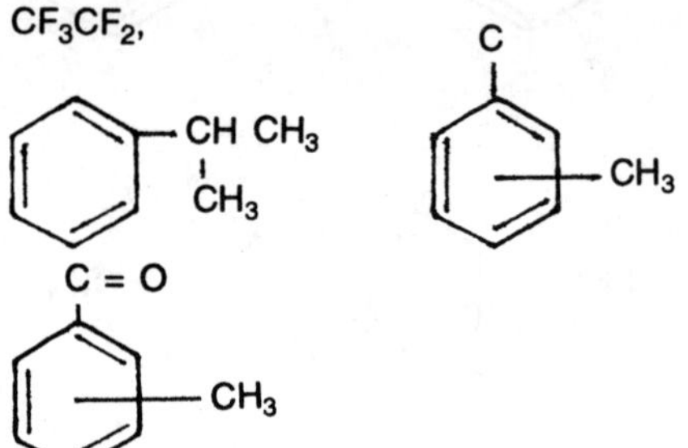

C_6H_5–CH CH_3 (CH_3), C–C_6H_4–CH_3

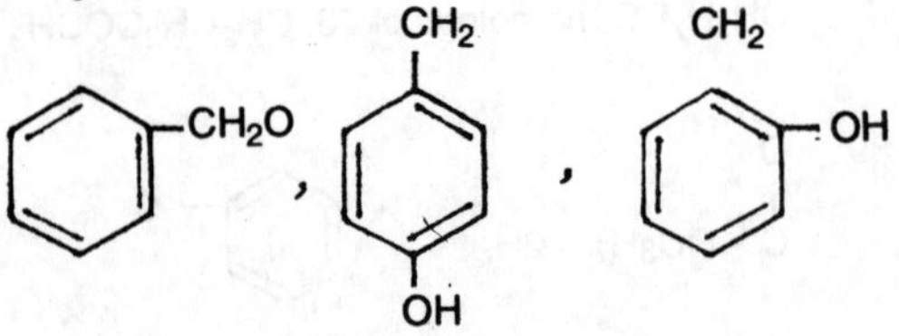

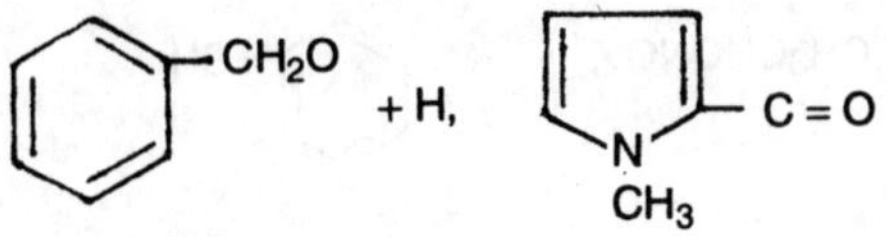

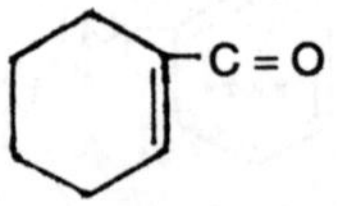

C = O–C_6H_4–CH_3

120 C = O, O (cyclohexadiene ring)

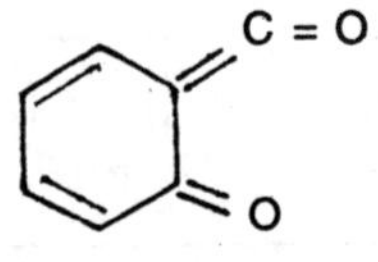

(Contd.)

121 C = O, OH,

138 CO, OH + H

123 C = O, F

139 C = O, Cl

125 S → O

149 O, C, O + H, C, O

127 I

131 C_3F_5 O=O, CH = CH

154

135 $(CH_2)_4Br$

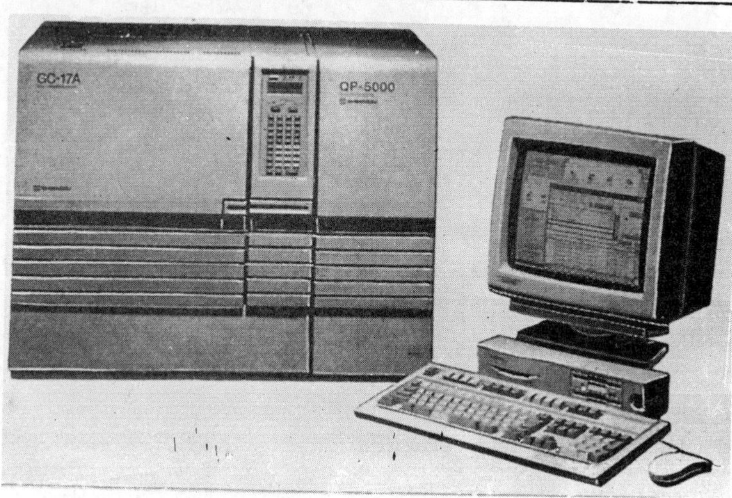

Fig. 20.8 Gas chromatograph - Mass spectrometer, Model QP-5000.
(Courtesy Shimadzu)

Table 20.4
Common Fragments Lost

This is a small list and should be used in conjunction with Table 20.3.

Molecular Ion Minus	Fragment Lost
1	H
15	CH_3-
17	HO-
18	H_2O
19	F-
20	HF
26	$CH \equiv CH$,$-C \equiv N$
27	$CH_2 = CH_2$, CO, $HC \equiv N$
28	$CH_2 = CH_2$,CO, (HCN + H)
29	CH_3CH_2–, –CHO
30	NH_2CH_2–, CH_2O,NO
31	–OCH_3,–CH_2OH, CH_3NH_2
32	CH_3OH,S
33	HS–,(–CH_3 and H_2O)
34	H_2S
35	Cl-
36	HCl, $2H_2O$
37	H_2Cl (or HCl + H)
38	C_3H_2–, C_2N, F_2
39	C_3H_3,HC_2N
40	$CH_3C \equiv CH$
41	$CH_2 = CHCH_2$–
42	$CH_2 = CHCH_3$, $CH_2 = C = O$, $CH_2 - CH_2$ (bridged by CH_2), NCO, $NCNH_2$
43	C_3H_7–, $CH_3C(=O)$–, $CH_2 = CH - O$–,[CH_3– and $CH_2 = CH_2$], HCNO
44	$CH_2 = CHOH$, CO_2, N_2O, $CONH_2$, $NHCH_2CH_3$
45	CH_3CHOH, CH_3CH_2O–, CO_2H, $CH_3CH_2NH_2$
46	[H_2O and $CH_2 = CH_2$], CH_3CH_2OH, –NO_2
47	CH_3S–
48	CH_3SH, SO, O_3
49	–CH_2Cl
51	–CHF_2
52	C_4H_4, C_2N_2
53	C_4H_5
54	$CH_2 = CH - CH = CH_2$
55	$CH_2 = CHCHCH_2$
56	$CH_2 = CHCH_2CH_3$, $CH_3CH = CHCH_3$, 2CO
57	C_4H_9
58	–NCS, (NO + CO), CH_3COCH_3
59	$CH_3OC(=O)$–, $CH_3C(=O)NH_2$,
60	C_3H_7OH
61	(three-membered ring with S–H), CH_3CH_2S–,
62	[H_2S and $CH_2 = CH_2$]
63	–CH_2CH_2Cl
64	C_5H_4, S_2, SO_2
68	$CH_2 = C(CH_3) - CH = CH_2$
69	CF_3–, C_5H_9
71	C_5H_{11}–
73	$CH_3CH_2OC(=O)$–
74	C_4H_9OH
75	C_6H_3
76	C_6H_4, CS_2
77	C_6H_5, CS_2H
78	C_6H_6, CS_2H_2, C_5H_4N
79	Br–, C_5H_5N
80	HBr
85	–$CClF_2$
100	$CF_2 = CF_2$
119	$CF_3 - CF_2$–
122	C_6H_5COOH
127	I–
128	HI

SECTION-F
SEPARATION METHODS

21

Chromatographic Methods

21.1 Introduction

Chromatography is the name given to a particular family of separation techniques. The original method was introduced in 1903 by J Swett and used in the separation of coloured substances, therefore the name. The method is used on mixtures including gases.

All chromatographic sepraration methods are similar in principle : a mobile phase passes over a stationary phase and transports the components of the mixture at diferent speeds in the direction of flow of the mobile phase. As there are repeated exchanges between the two phases, the separation of the components is a result of differential affinity of the components for the mobile phase (liquid or gas) and the stabionary phase (a solid or liquid)

If the stationary phase is a solid, the method is called adsorption chromatography.

If the stationary phase is a solid, the method is called partition chromatography. In each case, mobile phase may be either liquid or a gas. There are four types of chromatography :

(i) Liquid - solid : (a) Adsorption (b) Thin-layer (c) Ion-Exchange
(ii) Gas - Solid : (a) gas - solid
(iii) Gas - liquid: (a) Gas - liquid chromatography (GLC), (b) Capillary - column.
(iv) Liquid - Liquid. (a) Partition chromatography, (b) High pressure liquid chromatograph (HPLC)

21.2 Plate Theory

By analogy with distillation column, chromatography column may be considered to be made up of a number of theoritical plates. A *theoritical plate* is defined as a small section of the column in which equilibrium is established between the gas and the dissolved phases of a solute before the gas phase passes on to the next stage where the process is repeated. The concept of plate theory may be illustrated to a liquid - liquid extraction device and compared to a liquid - liquid chromatography — a large collection of separating funnels in which two immiscible solvents can be shaken together, allowed to separate and upper layer of solvents passed on to the next funnel. Each funnel corresponds to a theoritical plate.

If a substance A is introduced into the first stage and then shaken until equilibrium is established with two immeiscible solvents, M is the upper and mobile layer and S is the lower and the stationary layer. A will distribute itself between M and S according to partition coefficient K. M corresponds to mobile phase and S to stationary phase. M containing a portion of A is transferred to the next stage and equal quantity of M introduced into the 1st stage. The process is repeated and then transferring the layers of M from 2nd to 3rd stage and 1st to 2nd, fresh M again into 1st stage.

The process is repeated n times, during which M moves succesively from stage to stage, S remains stationary.

Distribution of A among the n stages can be obtained $(A + B)^{n+1}$ where

n = no of stages

$$a = \frac{1}{k+1}, \quad b = \frac{k}{k+1}, \quad k = \text{partition coefficient}$$

$$k = \frac{\text{Conc. of solution in 'S}}{\text{Conc. of solution in M}}$$

of V_m and V_S, Volumes of M and S are unequal k must be multiplied by V_m/V_S

21.3 Adsorption Chromatography

The most common and simple method of adsorption chromatography consists in the separation of substances in solution by filtration through a column of a finely powdered adsorbant palced in a glass tube. The two widely used techniques for the separation by column adsorption chromatography, are (i) Displacement and (ii) elution.

(i) Displacement chromatography : In displacement chromatography a solution containing the compounds to be separated is added from the top of a column of tightly packed finely powdered adsorbant (stationary phase) contained in a glass tube known of dimensions. Let us consider a solution of compounds A and B, both of which are strongly adsorbed to the column packing, but assume that B is much more strongly held than A. A solvent (mobile phase) C which is more strongly held to the absorbent than either A or B is then poured over the top of the column. The solvent C will displace both A and B from their adsorbed sites – on the column leaving them momentarily free to proceed down the column. Since B is

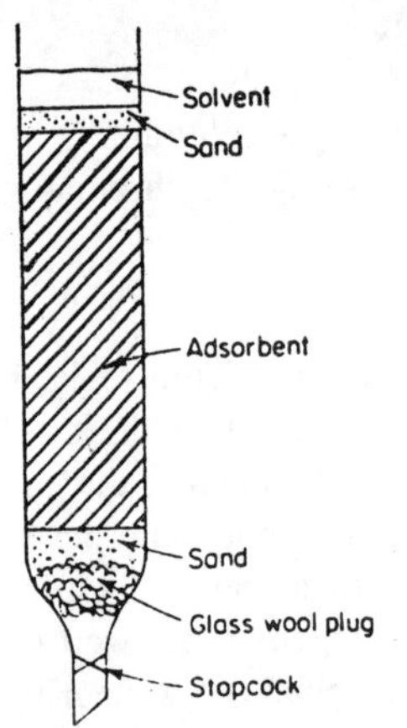

Fig. 21.1 Construction of a chromatography column

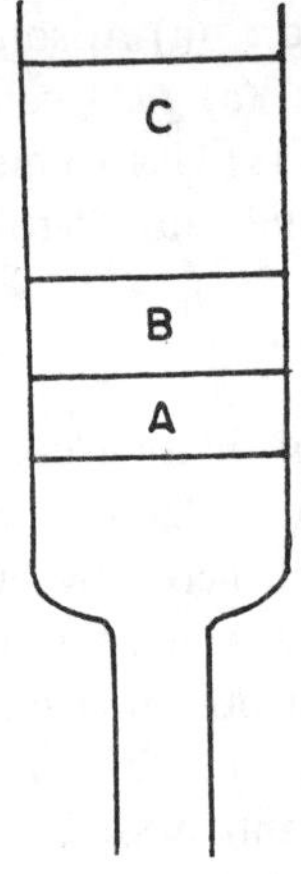

Fig. 21.2. Separation of a mixture of compounds A and B.

more strongly adsorbed than A, it will be readsorbed on the next available site of the column packing material, thus forcing A to go further down the column before being adsorbed. If more of C is added to the top of the column a continuing displacement takes place due to multiple adsorption — desorption process, the solvent C displaces B and B displaces A from the adsorbent. This procedure is good for preparative work, but because of contamination between the bands, it is not preferred for quantitative work.

(ii) Elution : Elution Chromatography uses the same type of equipment as in the displacement chromatography but with one exception. The column packing is coated with a thin film of a solvent which is strongly adsorbed to the particle surface of the packing material. This thin solvent film serves as the stationary phase. A second solvent is selected so that : (a) it does not dissolve or mix appreciably with the stationary phase and (b) does not adsorb to the surface of the packing material as is the case with stationary phase, is then passed through the column. The second solvent is called the ''mobile phase'' or the ''eluting agent''.

For example, if solution consisting of a mixture of A and B is placed at the top of the column and the mobile phase C, is added, the compounds slowly proceed down the column. As the compounds move down they distribute or partition between the stationary and the mobile phase. If more of the Compound B dissolves in the stationary phase than does compound A, after a short period of time compound B will begin to lag behind compound A because A is not being held back as much and therefore can move down the column faster. The net result is that a separation of A and B takes place. By means of this technique a complete separation of A and B is possible. Therefore elution analysis is preferred for quantitative separation.

In both the above procedures, if the substances are pigments, the separation is easily visualised and coloured bands are seen to move down the column during the development. After development, the solvents can be removed from the column, the adsorbent can be extruded from the glass tube and the coloured zones can be cut out or removed mechanically. If the substances are not coloured, the contents of the column can be arbitarily divided and the fractions can be examined by suitable analytical methods.

In elution chromatography, the development can be allowed to proceed untill the reparated compounds emerge from the column and appear in the filtrate. A series of fractions of the filtrate from the column can be collected and the separated compounds can be detected by suitable methods.

In general, the separation of compounds by either method is a function of chemical consituennts of the substances being separated, the nature of solvent system used and the nature of adsorbent. The

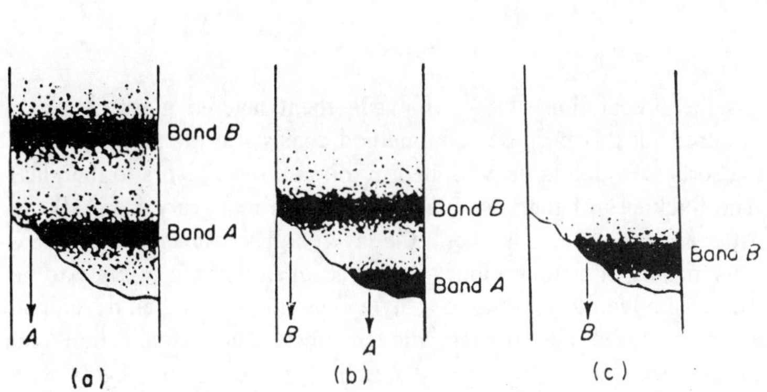

Fig. 21.3. Elution of successive bands from a chromatography column which is not square at bottom. (a) Elution of A. (b) Elution of A and B. (c) Elution of B.

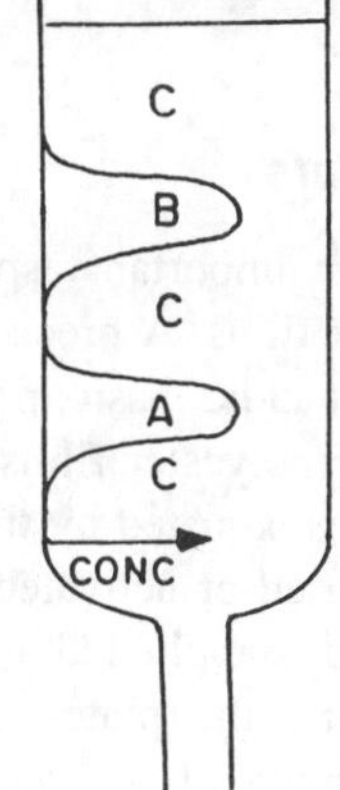

Fig. 21.4. Separation of a mixture of compounds A and B.

commonly used adsorbents are : activated alumina, magnesium silicate, florisil, calcium and magnesium oxides, calcium, potassium and sodium carbonate, calcium phosphate, fulleres earth, charcoal, talc, inulin starch and sucrose.

The solvents used are : Cyclohexane, CCl_4, Petroleum ether, benzene, various alcohols, ethers, ketones, esters, organic acids and water.

The substances that can be separated and purified are steroids, carotenoids, chlorophylls, enzymes, sugars, amino acids etc.

EXERCISE 1. Separation of Phenol and Salicylic acid by column chromatography.

Method : 1. Prepare a column of 2 cm in diameter and 30 cm long. 2. Fill the column with 83 gm of alumina (neutral, d = 3.6/cc). 3. use 9.6 ml of water and 61 ml of butanol mixture as the solvent system. 4. Determine the Rf values for the two constituents of the mixture, the partition coefficients being 0.194 and 3.42 respectively.

EXERCISE 2. Separation of Mixture of two dyes – Bromothymol blue and Metacresol purple by column chromatography.

Method : 1. Follow the steps as in the previous exercise except that t– amyl alcohol - glacial acetic acid-water mixture (4 : 1: 1) is used as the eluting solvent to separate the dyes. 2. Determine the Rf values and report the results.

21.4 Thin Layer Chromatography

Thin layer chromatography (TLC) has become a widely use method for the separation of substances in a great variety of inorganic and organic studies. The separation of solutes is carried out on a layer of adsorbent that is adhered to a flat surface of inert material like a galss plate or a polyester film. The development of the chromatographs on the glass plate or the polyester film is carried out in a manner similar to the procedure for ascending paper chromatography.

The common adsorbents used in TLC are silica gel or aluminium oxide. The method is a partition technique rather than adsorption-desorption process if the adsorbent is impregnated with a polar stationary phase.

The main advantage of TLC over that of paper chromatography is that there is less spreading of spots of separated materials and the separations take a shorter period of time. The separated substances are identified by their observed R_f values. The quantitative estimation of the separated substances can be made by comparison with reference standards and after elution of the chromatogram by suitable analytical methods.

Procedure

The most important aspect of TLC is the preparation of the Thin adsorbent layered glass plates or polyester films. A precision spreader is used for this purpose. The method consists in the preparation of a slurry (acidic, basic, neutral) of the adsorbent which is then applied in thin, uniform layers to the glass plates or polyester films or stripps. The thickness of the adsorbent layer which may vary from 100 to 2000 μ, is adjusted by the spreader. After spreading the adsorbent, the layered glass plates or film strips are air dried or activated in an oven. By means of a micropippet measured quantity of a mixture to be separated is applied along a base line near an edge of the adsorbent layer. The mixture is then developed by placing the plates or film strips in a closed chromatographic chamber. The visualization and identification of the separated constituents is then carried out by spraying the adsorbent layers with reagents for the production of colour. The colour can be further examined by fluorescence or radioactivity methods or transparency methods.

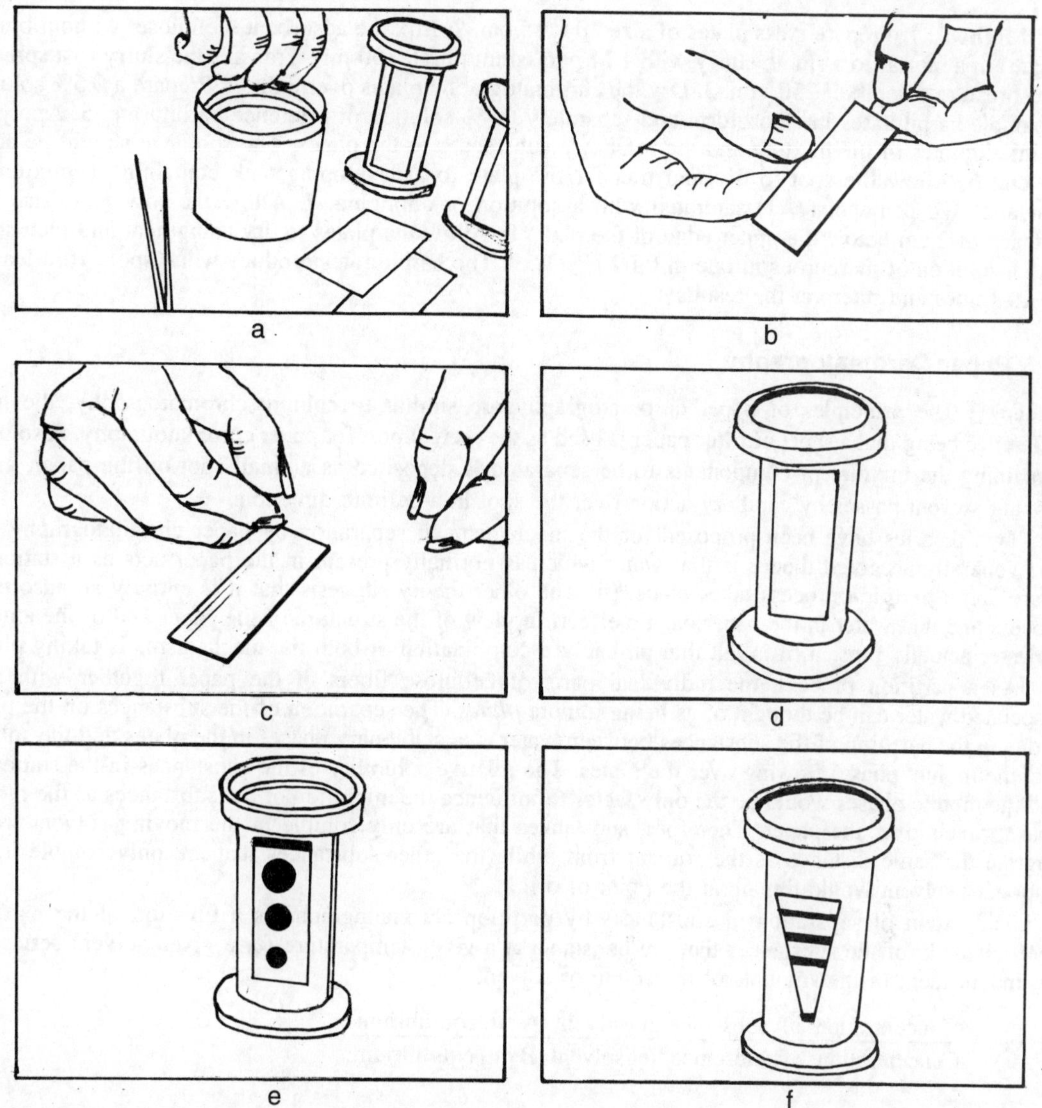

Fig. 21.5 TLC on microscope slides. (a) Two microscope slide, back-to-back, are dipped into the slurry, separated, and allowed to dry. (b) The edges are smoothed by removing a small amount of the adsorbent. (c) The sample is applied with a small capillary. Up to three samples may be applied on a single slide. (d) The chromatogram is developed in a small closed chamber for about 5 min. Jars designed for slide staining make convenient development chambers. (e) The chromatogram is visualized by placing it in a closed chamber containing a few crystals of iodine. (f) Chromatography on shaped layers results in the formation of narrow bands rather than round spots. Only one sample can be placed on a slide, but the method often results in improved separation of the components and facilitates the detection of trace components of low R_f value.

The quantification of the separated substances can be done by comparison with the standards by means of standard analytical methods.

EXERCISE 3. Separation of a mixture of Barbiturates by thin layer chromatography.

Method : 1. Prepare glass plates of size 20 × 15 cm. 2. Mix the adsorbent (cellulose, without binder, 25 gm) in a mortar to a smoth slurry with 1 M potassium nitrate (50 ml). Transfer the slurry to a spreader and spread to a depth of 250 μm. 3. Dry the chromatography plates overnight. 4. Prepare a 0.5% solution of sample barbiturates in chloroform and separately 0.4% solution of reference barbiturate. 5. Apply 5 - 10 ml aliquotes of the mixture and the reference substances to the plates. The spot size should be about 0.3 cm. 6. Allow the spot to dry and transfer the plate to a developing tank containing a mixture of n-butanol and pentanol (1 :1) saturated with a solution of ammonia. 7. Allow the solvent to rise to a distance of 2 cm below the upper edge of the plate. 8. Allow the plates to dry using heat and then spray with a solution of mercurous nitrate in 0.IN HNO_3. 9. The barbiturates produce white spots 10. Measure the R_f values and interpret the results.

21.5 Paper Chromatography

Thoery : The principles of paper chromatography are similar to column chromatography, the main difference being that a sheet of filter paper is used as the inert suport for paper chromatography. A solution containing the mixture of components to be separated is deposited as a small spot on the paper, and a moving solvent passes by capillary action over the spot in a definite direction.

Two theories have been proposed for the mechanism of separation by paper chromatography : (i) The generally accepted thoery is that water which is normally present in the paper acts as a stationary phase and a partition process takes place. (ii) The other theory suggests that it is entirely an adsorption process and that water in the paper has no effect. In view of the structure of the paper and of the amount of water actually present, it is felt that probably a combination of both the mechanisms is taking place.

As a partition process, the individual parts of cellulose fibers of the paper together with their associated water can be thought of as being minute *plates*. The separation of the substances on the paper is due to the partition of the substances between water (i.e. stabionary phase) in the plates and the solvent (i.e. the mobile phase) flowing over the plates. The relative solubility of the substances in the stationary and the mobile phases would be the only factor to influence the migration of the substances as the mobile phase travels over the paper. Therefore, substances that are only soluble in the moving solvent would migrate the same distance as the solvent front while the other substances that are only soluble in the stationary solvent would remain at the point of origin.

The extent of separation of substances by partition chromatography is a function of the partition coefficients k, of the substances that are constants at a given temperature for a given solvent series and are independent of the amounts of the solute or solvent.

$$k = \frac{\text{Concentration of substance in solvent A at equilibrium}}{\text{Concentration of substance in solvent B at equilibrium}}$$

Procedure

The paper chromatography can be performed on a large sheet of paper so that several samples of the mixture are chromatographed simultaneously or each sample may be run on strip of paper. The experiment is carried out in a closed chromatographic chamber that is saturated with the vapour of the developing solvent. The sample is delivered as a small spot by means of a micropippet along a base line near the edge of the filter paper. In ascending chromatography the edge of the filter paper where the spot is placed is immersed in the developing solvent, *which is* contained in the chamber and is drawn up the paper by capillary action. In descending chromatography, the edge of the paper where the spot is placed is suspended from a trough of developing solvent, which moves down the paper by gravity and capillarity.

The sample constituents then move along the paper at different rates due to partition and adsorption processes. When the solvent front has travelled a suitable distance the paper is removed from the chamber and dried. The chromatogram after drying is sprayed with suitable reagents that react with the sample constituents and disclose their *location* on the paper. *In case* the sample constituents fluoresce or absorb U.V light, their location can be detected with the aid of U.V. light. For the purpose of quantification the constituents *the spots produced* on the paper can be cut, solutes are eluted and then analysed by suitable means.

The chromatographic behaviour of the sample constituents is represented by the term R_f value which is based on a given set of conditions like (i) temperature (ii) solvent system (iii) manner of development (iv) the type and grain of paper. The R_f value is a characteristic of a particular substance and is defined as :

$$R_f = \frac{\text{dustabce from baseline substance travelled}}{\text{distance from baseline solvent travelled}}$$

EXERCISE 4. Separation of mixture of Amino acids by Ascending paper chromatography.

Method : 1. Receive the various amino acids from the instructor and prepare the following solutions:

(i) Solution X : a 0.1 g/100 ml mixture of cysteine, dl-∝-alanine and isoleucine.

(ii) Solution Y : a 0.1 g/100 ml mixture of glycine and cystine.

(iii) Solution Z : an unknown mixture of various amino acids from the above list.

(iv) Ninhydrin solution : A fresh 0.2% ninhydrin solution in water saturated with n-butanol

(v) Mobile Phase : 95% methanol in water by volume

2. Prepare 8″ strips of chromatographic paper (whatman No. (1) and label them at the top the same as the solutions being analysed, both known and unknown. 3. Spot small amounts of solutions of amino acids (1–2 microlitres) by means of micropippets on the filter paper about 0.5 inches from the bottom. 4. label the spots and allow them dry on a hot plate or with the air of a hair dryer. 5. Hang the strip in the chromatigraphic chamber in such a manner that the paper neither touches the walls nor dips into the solution of mobile phase kept in the bottom of the chamber. 6. Allow the system to come to equilibrium for five minutes and then allow the filter paper to just dip into the solution. 7. Allow the solvent to run to a height of about 6 inches. 8. Remove the chromatogram from the chamber, mark the position of the sulvent front with a pencil and allow it to dry. 9. Spray the chromatogram with ninhydrin solution by a sprayer in a fume-cup board. 10. Allow the paper to dry on a hot plate when purple spots will develop indicating position of the amino acids thus separated. 11. Measure the distances of movement of the developed amino acids and the solvent front and compute the R_f values. 12. Analyse the known solutions X and Y and the unknown solution Z air the above manner and interpret your results.

EXERCISE 5. Separation of mixture of Steroids by descending paper chromatography.

Method : 1. Receive the small amounts of the three steroids (Estradiol, estriol and estrone) and prepare three separate solutions having a concentration of 1 mg/ml.

2. Thereafter prepare the following solutions :

(a) Stationary Phase : 30% triethylene glycol in methanol (V/V).

(b) Mobile Phase : ortho-dichlorobenzene.

(c) 1% ferric chloride by dissolving 1 g of $FeCl_3$ $6H_2O$ in 100 ml water

(d) 1% potassium ferricyanide by dissolving 1 g of K_3 Fe $(CN)_6$ in 100 ml water.

3. Prepare 10 inch strips of whatman NO. 1 chromatography paper. With a pencil, draw a line about 2 inches from the top of the paper. Label the strip so that each system can be distinguished. 4. Dip the filter paper into a solution of triethylene glycol in methanol. Allow the paper to dry. The methanol will evaporate leaving the paper impregnated with glycol.

4. By means of a micropipette, streak the sample across the paper at the pencil mark D. The streak should be as narrow as possible. Dry the streak on a hot plate or with a dryer.

Place three layers of sample on the streak, drying thoroughly after each layer. Prepare a separate strip for each known and unknown sample.

5. Place about 10 ml of O-dichlorobenzene in the solvent tank. Insert the paper in the tank. Allow the chromatogram to develop until the solvent front is 1/8 inch from the bottom of paper.

6. Remove the paper from the Jar, mark the position of the solvent front and dry the paper.

7. Spray the paper with the colour reagent mixture of (10 ml of ferric chloride solution with 11 ml of ferricyanide). The reagent will turn the paper green but estrogens will form blue bands.

8. Measure the R_f values immediately and interpret your results.

21.6 Ion-Exchange Chromatogaphy

Theory : The main principle involved in ion-exchange chromatography is the differential affinity of charged molecules in solution for inert, insoluble charged materials. Ion-exchange chromatography is carried out by elution of the sample constituents on a column of ion-exchange material.

The earliest ion-exchange materials used are the insoluble natural sililates e.g. chabazite (Na_2 Al SiO_{12}. $6H_2O$) and Kalonite (a silicate clay material). Both of these highly porous silicates are charged materials because they contain sodium and hydroxyl ions held in their chain like molecular structure. They will exchange their ions for ions that are small enough to penetrate the pores of their structural lattice, e.g. calcium ions will exchange for Na^+ ions in chabazite; and Cl^- ions will exchange for ^-OH ions in kalonite respectively. Accordingly chabazite is known as "cation-exchange" material and kalonite is referred as "anion-exchange material". In both the cases, the extent of exchange is dependent upon (a) the concentration of the small ion (i.e. counter ion) for exchange and (b) the relative affinities of the substrates for the counter ions and the ions held in their structural lattice.

Preparation of Resins : In the laboratory, in general, ion-exchanges used are synthetic ion-exchange resins. These synthetic resins are prepared by emulsion or pearl copolymerization of varying amounts of styrene and divinyl benzine. The resultant polymer is an elastic, three dimensional hydrocarbon and is obtained as spherical beads of uniform diameter. By varying the content of divinyl benzene the degree of cross-linking in the polymer can be controlled in a reproducible manner. Thereafter, the acidic and basic ionizable groups are introduced into the polymer matrix. The reaction for the preparation of this polymer is shown below :

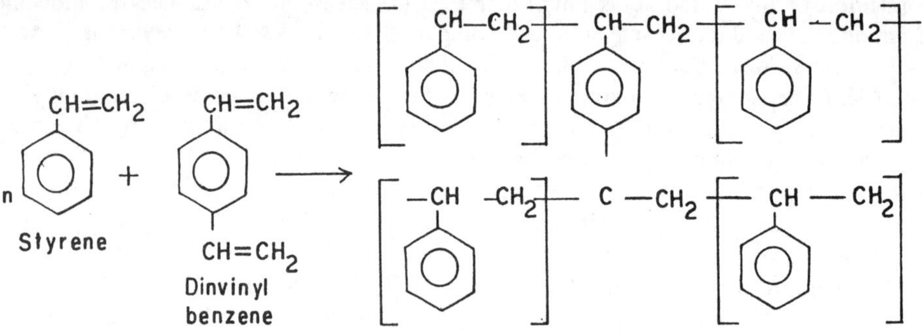

Sulphonation of the polymer produces a strongly acidic or cation exchange resin. Further addition of water to the resin causes a swelling of the resin because of the affinity of the highly polar sulphonic acid groups (SO_3H) for water and ionization takes place.

$$Res - SO_3H + H_2O \longrightarrow Res - SO_3^- + H_3O^+$$

The H_3O^+ is held strongly to the anion which is fixed in the polymer matrix and does not migrate in the electrically neutral resin unless it is repalced by another cation. Weakly acidic resins which contain-COOH groups can also be prepared and will exchange in a similar manner.

On the contrary, the anion exchange resins contain basic functional groups in the polymer matrix. An example of a strongly basic resin is Res — NR_3 X^- where X^- is usually – OH or Cl ion which will exchange for other anions. Weakly basic resins like Res— N^+H_3 X^- can also be prepared. The methods of exchange are similar to those described for cation exchange resins.

The affinity or selectivity for an exchangable ion in solution is the most important aspect of ion - exchangers. This selectivity is expressed quantitatively in terms of weight distribution coefficient D, of a particular exchangable ion which is different for various ions on the same ion- exchange resin.

$$D = \frac{\text{mM of ion per gm of dry resin}}{\text{mM of ion in solution per ml of solution}}$$

The other factors which affect the affinity of a given ion-exchanger for its exchangable ion are (i) valence states of ions and (ii) radius of the hydrated ions of the same valence state. In general, the greater the charge on the ion, the more tightly bound it will be to the resin (e.g. $Al^{3+} > Ca^{2+} > Na^+$). At each ionic valency, the smaller the radius of the hydrated ion, the more strongly it will be held by the resin (e.g. $K^+ > Na^+ > Li^+$).

The polymer matrix will also affect the affinity of an ion-exchange resin for an ionized solute. Since the accessability of the ionized solutes for exchange in the resin is related to the size of the pores in the polymer matrix, the degree of cross - linking of the resin is important. For example, cholestyr-amine resins like Dowex contains 4—10% of divinyl benzene and is referred to as 4—10% cross–linked. Thus, the lower the degree of cross–liking, the larger the size of pores in polymer matrix and greater the accessibility of ionized solutes.

The molecules of different molecular weight can be separated on ion-exchange resins depending upon the pore-size of the resin polymer matrix. For example cross-linked dextran polymers called sephadexes are classified as to the molecular weights of molecules which will be held by them. They are widely used for the separation and fractionation of peptides and proteins.

Procedure

Ion-exchange chromatography is carried out by elution of a mixture of ioinic substances on an appropriate ion-exchange resin contained in a glass column. The eluent for development of the mixture is generally either a buffer solution or a mixture. Because the ion-exchange resins vary considerably in their degree of swelling on weting, ion-exchange columns are packed after soaking the resins in water and making a slurry.

When the resin beads have settled in the column, the column is washed with buffer solution or water and can be regenerated if the resin is not in its original ionic form. Cation exchange resins are regenerated with dil HCl and anion exchange resins are regenerated with Na OH or KOH. After the regeneration the excess acid or base is washed with water from column. The level of the liquid in ion-exchange columns must not fall below the top of the resin column at any time. When the column is ready for use, an aqueous or buffer equilibrated solution of the solutes to be separated is added from the top of the column in a quanity less than the total capacity of the resin. The solutes will exchange for the ions on the resin column which is then developed by adding buffer solution or water through column. The separation of the components of the mixture takes place bacause of the differential affinity of the resin for the various ionic components of the mixture. Each component moves down the column at a different rate and emerges from the column in a pure form.

21.7 Gas Liquid Chromatography

21.7.1 Technique

Gas chromatography uses as the mobile phase an inert gas called the *carrier gas.* The stationary phase also referred to as the *liquid substrate* consists of a high bioling liquid which is used to coat granular particles (60-80 mesh) made of silicous earth or firebrick. The coated particles are placed in a tube having diameter of 0.6 cm and length of 2 meter (0.6 cm × 2 m), (1/4 in × 6 ft.) and which is made of copper, glass or stainless steel. The tube containing the coated particles is called a *column* and is mounted in the constant - temperature heating chember of a G.C. apparatus. The temperature of the column is elevated to a constant value; with the carrier gas passing through the column at a constant rate. A small quantity of liquid sample is injected through a silicon rubber septum into a heated injection port, using a needle and syringe. The components of the sample volatilize here and are carried to the column by the carrier gas. The components of the smaple are then partitioned between the liquid substrate and the gas phase and are transported through and down the column at different rates depending on the physico-chemical properties of the sample, liquid substrate, solid support and operating conditions of the GC apparatus.

When a component of the sample finally reaches the end of the column, it passes through a detector (for example thermel conductivity ceil) through an electric bridge circuit to a strip chart recorder. Here a peak is recorded on the chart paper. The position of the peak on the chromatogram is characteristic of the component.

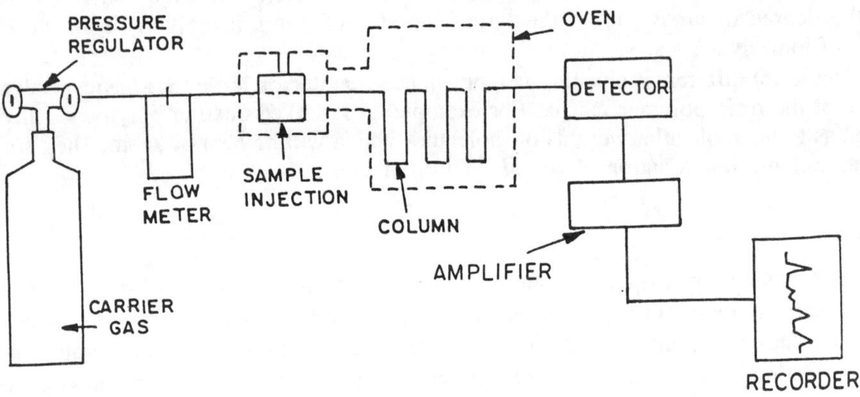

Fig. 21.6 Schematic Diagram of a G.L.C.

All the gas chromatographs are used as per above technique, the essential parts are shown in the schematic diagram (Fig. 21.6). In general, they consist of:

(i) Pressure regulator and flow meter for carrier gas,

(ii) A sample injection system

(iii) Separation column,
(iv) The thermal compartment or oven,
(v) Detection system and
(vi) Strip-chart recorder or any other type of device for indicating the out put of the detector say an integrator or a computer.

The purpose and functions of the essential parts of the G.C. apparatus are discussed below:

21.7.2 Pressure Regulator and Flow Meter

The operating efficiency of a G.C. is dependent on the maintenance of a highly constant carrier gas flow rate. Carrier gas from the cylinder tank passes through a flow meter, a few feet of metal capillary restrictors and a gauge. The flow meter with a range of 0 - 200 ml/min, indicates flow rate in the reference side of the detector (thermal conductivity cell). Flow rate is adjustable and is controlled by the pressure regulator.

Contaminants in the carrier gas may affect column performance and detector response when ionization detectors are used. A trap containing molecular sieve (5A) is sufficient for removal of impurities and H_2O vapour.

21.7.3 Sample Injection System

The sample is introduced in a reproducible manner, sample must not decompose nor create pressure surges and vaporize instantly. Liquid samples are injected by hypodermic syringes through a self - sealing silicon rubber septum (compressed by means of a threaded nut) into a heated metal block (flash evaporator). The metal block which encloses the capillary is heated by a controlled resistance heater. Here the sample is vapourized as a plug and carried into the column by the carrier gas. The needle tip should be made to get well down into the heated block ahead of column. The sample size used is small from 1 to 10 μl.

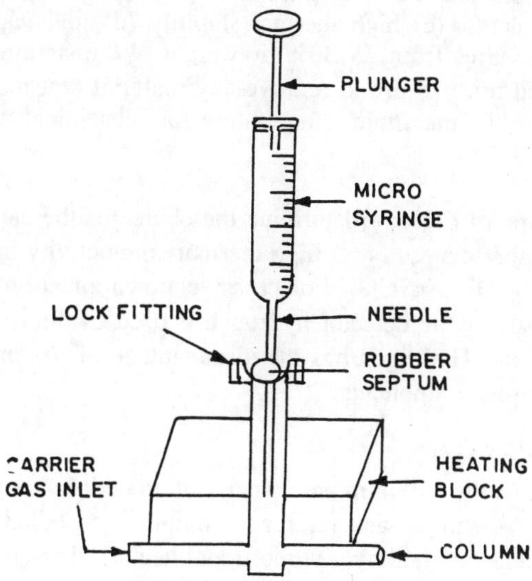

Fig. 21.7 Injection system for GLC.

The solid samples are dissolved in volatile liquid or temporarily liquified while gas samples are injected by a gas sampling valve or gas tight syringe.

21.7.4 Column

The main part or most important part is the column - packed or capillary in which separation is effected. The packed column is commonly 4 mm (i.d) tubing of stainless steel, copper cupronickel or glass either bent in a u-shape or coiled. Lengths run from 120 cm to 150 m.

Solid support available are diatomaceous earth (Fire brick) chromasorb P & W, silica gel, molecular sieve, alumina and activated charcoal. The range of particle size suitable being 60/80, 80/100 or 100/120 mesh material.

The liquid phases suitable for separations by GLC are listed below:

paraffin oil	Suitable for paraffins, olefins halides	Temp limit being 150°C
Silicone oils	Suitable for paraffins, olefins, ester, ether	
Polyglycols (Carbowaxes)	Suitable for Amines, nitriles, ketone, ester alcohol, ether, aromatic compounds	Tamp limit 100-200°C
Apiezon-L grease	Suitable for polar type of molecules	Temp limit 300°C

The requirements of a liquid phase are (a) good solvent properties for components, (b) differential partitioning of sample components, (c) high thermal stability (d) low vapour pressure at the column temperature. The liquid phase varies from 2 - 30% by weight of the stationary phase.

The column is conditioned prior to use to remove any material that may come off when packing is first heated for several hours at the maximum temperature for subsequent use.

21.7.5 Carrier Gas

The availability, purity and type of detector determine the choice of the carrier gas. Helium is preferred for thermal conductivity detector because of its high thermal conductivity but is expensive. Other carrier gases that can be used are N_2, H_2, Ar, CO_2. For cross section ionization detector Ar can be used. If flame-ionization detector is used as the detector hydrogen is used as the fuel along with air while Ar or N_2 can be used as the carrier gas. Hydrogen has the disadvantage of *fire* and explosion hazard and also can react with unsaturated simple components.

21.7.6 Thermal Compartment or Oven

An airbath chamber surrounds the column and air is circulated by a blower through the thermal compartments. A matched set of sample and reference column is installed in the thermal compartment continuously varying the wattage supplied by a proportional heater. There is separate heater for vaporizer and detector block. One can have linear or non-linear temperature control programme for sample and reference columns. The temperature control system must be sensitive to changes of 0.01°C and should control to 0.1°C.

The temperature one wishes to employ for the separation of components of a sample is dictated by (i) the degree of separation needed and (ii) a reasonable length of time for analysis. The lower the temperature the greater the separation of various components but the retention of the components on the column increases with lowering of temperature. A temperature near the boiling points of the components of the sample may be satisfactory but the optimum temperature must be determined by trail by the analyst.

21.7.7 Detectors

The type of column used is the determing factor in the selection of detectors. For packed columns one can use (i) hot wire (thermister) (ii) thermal conductivity cell (iii) gas density cell (iv) cross section detector.

For capillary columns one can use (i) ionization gauge, (ii) Flame (iii) beta ray (iv) electron capture or (v) radio frequency. However, the latter types can also be used for packed columns if suitablly attenuated. The output must be linear with concentration i.e. linear dynamics range expresses this range and coupled with sensitivity the limits.

The purpose of the detector is to monitor the column effluent, measuring the variations in its composition. They do not identify the components of the mixture.

Most of the detectors are of differential type i.e. they give zero signal when pure carrier gas is passing through them, but when a component of a smaple is detected the signal is proportional to the concentration or mass of that component.

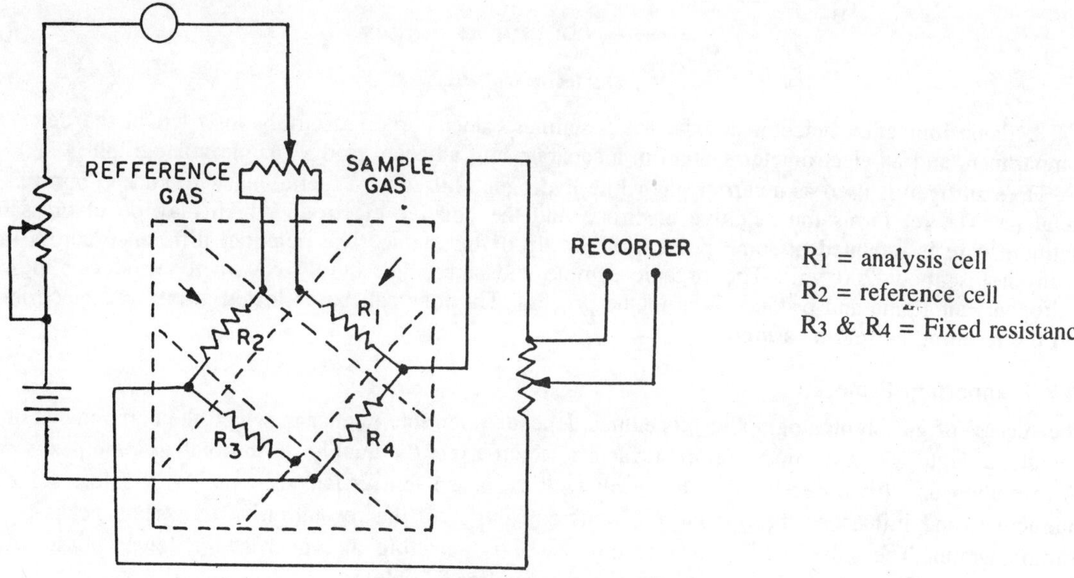

Fig. 21.8 Thermal Conductivity Cell.

In this write up, only thermal conductivity cell and flame ionization type of detectors will be discussed.

A thermal conductivity detector consists of heat sensing elements each situated in a separate cavity or a brass or stainless steel block which serves as a sink. The heat sensing elements are either thermisters or resistance wires. Filaments are fabricated from some metal or alloy with a high temperature coefficient of resistance, e.g. Pt or Kovaror tungston. The filaments within the cell form a wheatstone bridge that detects the difference in thermal conductivity between the stream of carrier gas that contains the sample components and the reference stream of pure carrier gas before the injection point. This difference in thermal conductivity generates a signal that is amplified to drive a recorder pen to a proportional height on a strip chart recorder.

21.7.8 Ionization Detectors

The chief principle of operation of ionization detector is based on the conduction of electricity by gases. At normal temperature and pressure a gas behaves like a perfect insulator; but if electrically charged atoms molecules or free electrons are present, their free motion in the direction of an electrical field renders the gas conducting.

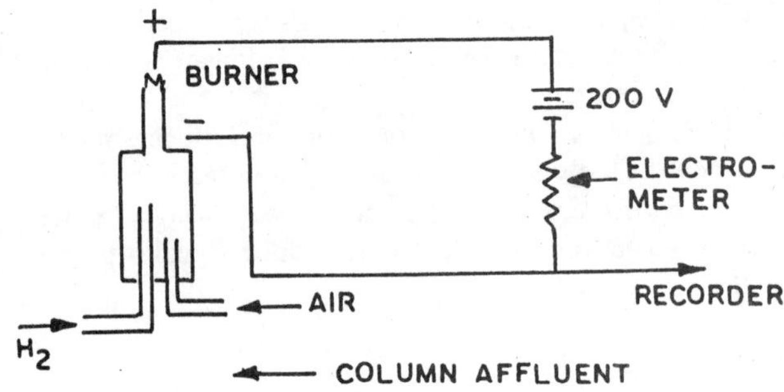

Fig. 21.9 Ionization Detector.

A flame ionization detector consists of a stainless steel burner assembly installed in the detector compartment and an electrometer system in a separate unit adjacent to the gas chromatograph.

Here nitrogen is used as a carrier gas while hydrogen is used as a fuel along with air and burnt at a metal jet. The jet forms the negative electrode and the positive electrode which may be of brass or platinum wire is mounted at some point near the tip of the flame. The potential difference across the electrodes is about 200 volt. The organic sample substances are pyrolyzed when introduced into a hydrogen - air flame and produce ions in the process. The ions can be collected at charged electrodes and the resulting current measured.

21.7.9 Important Factors

The success of gas chromatographic procedures depends upon the manner in which the components of a mixture seperate. The two most important factors which affect the quality of chromatographic peaks are (i) resolution and (ii) broadening of the peak width. The solvent efficiency deals with solute solvent interactions and influences the relative positions and therefore the resolution of the solute peaks on a chromatograph. The solvent efficiency is optimized by selecting an upper and a lower phase with distribution coefficients which promote increased separation of solutes.

On the contrary, column efficiency deals with peak broadening and depends upon the solvent, solute, temperature, flow rate and sample size. The broader the peak, the less efficient the column operation. The peaks sould be narrow at the base and well defined.

In gas chromatography, column efficiency is evaluated in terms of "height equivalent to a theoritical plate" i.e. HETP. This concept has been borrowed from distillation process where it was used as a means of evaluating distillation column performance. In gas chromatography the number of theoritical plates are determined by injecting a suitable solute on the column, measuring the distance X and peak width Y on the chromatogram and calculating N by substituting these values into equastion 1.

$$N = 16\left(\frac{X}{Y}\right)^2 \qquad (1)$$

Where X = distance from point of injection to peak maximum (Fig. 21.10)

Y = width of base of peak drawn as a triangle

HETP is related to N as indicated in equation 2.

$$\text{HETP} = \frac{\text{column length}}{N} \qquad (2)$$

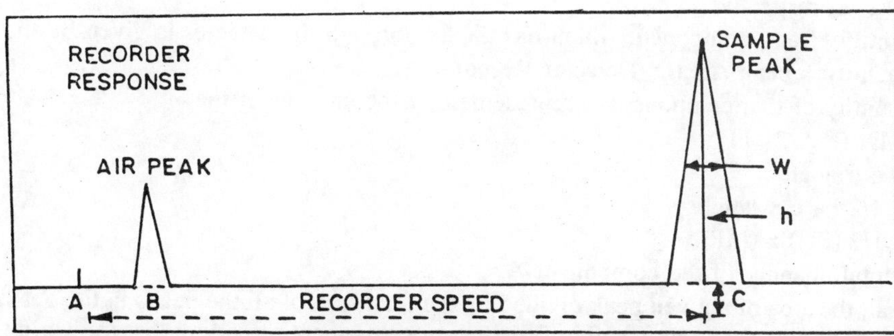

Fig. 21.10 Gas chromatogram.

The smaller the HETP value, the more efficient the column.

A = Point of injection, B = air peak, C = peak max.

h = peak height, W = peak width at half height

AC = retention.

Further, it has been found that HETP varies with flow rate and the factors which affect peak broadening and column efficiency during chromatography are : (i) multipath effect (A) molecular diffusion (B) and resistance to mass transfer (C) These are combined into an equation called Van Deemter equation (3) shown below:

$$\text{HETP} = A + \frac{B}{\mu} + C\mu \qquad \text{........(3)}$$

Where μ = linear gas velocity and is measured as:

$$\mu = \frac{\text{length of column}}{\text{retention time of air , Cm/s}}$$

21.7.10 Quantitative Analysis

The most commonly used terms in GLC are *retention time* and *Retention Volume.*

Retention time (t_r) is defined as the time required by an average molecule of component to pass from the point of injection through the column to the detector. It is found from the chromatogram by measuring the distance from the point of injection i.e. A (Fig. 21.10) to the peak maximum C and multiplying this value by the reciprocal (mint/ml) of the recorder speed.

Thus $t_r = \dfrac{\text{Dist. from A to C}}{\text{Recorder speed}}$ ....(4)

Retention volume V_R is defined as the volume of carrier gas necessary to carry an average molecule of the componant from the point of injection of the detector. It is found by multiplying the retention time by gas flow rate of the carrier gas.

Thus, $V_R = t_r \times$ (flow rate of carrier gas) .... (5)

However, because of various operating variables one may use relative retention x which is given by the equation.

$$\frac{x_2 - x_a}{x_1 - x_a} \quad \text{......... (6)}$$

where x_2 = retention from point of injection for test sample, x_1 for the standard and x_a for inert compound like air respectively.

The quantity of any component which has passed through the detector is given by the equation.

Total quantity = peak Area X Detector Response

Total quantity of that component is represented by the area under the peak LMN (Fig. 21.11)

LMN is a triangle

Area = 1/2 base x height

= 1/2 (LN) x (MP) -----(7)

= total quantity of the component A

In general, the area of a given peak divided by the total area of all the peaks in the gas chromatogram will approximately give the % by weight of that given component providing that the various components are similar in structure and their thermal conductivities are nearly the same.

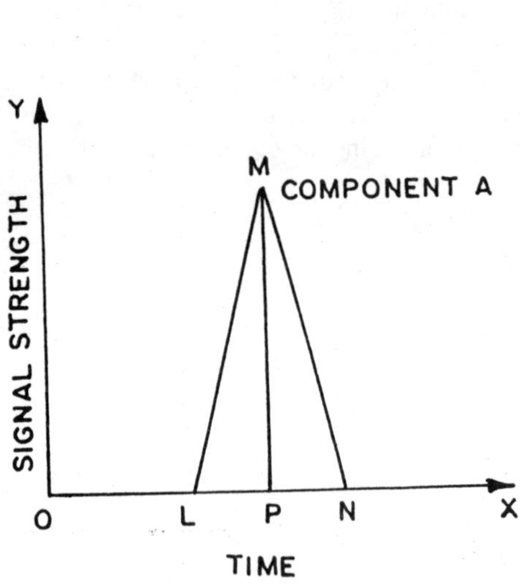

Fig. 21.11 Total quantity of component A

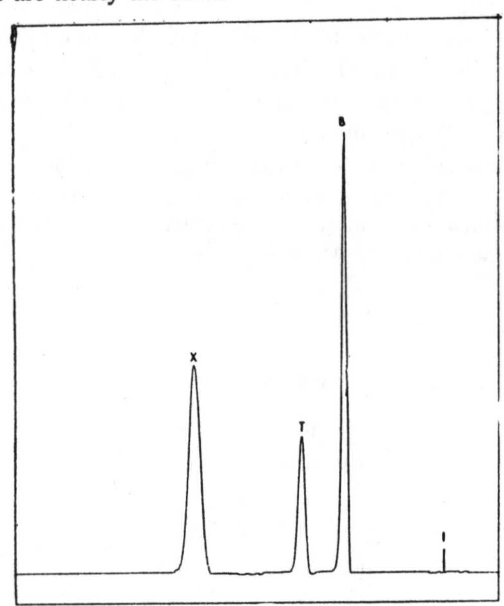

Fig. 21.12. Gas-liquid chromatogram of benzene (B), toluene (T), and xylene (X) on a 5 ‹ ft, 20% Carbowax 20 M column at 140°. The small peak labeled I indicates the point of injection of the sample

EXERCISE 6. Estimate the composition of a synthetic mixture prepared from benzene, toluene and xylene.

(i) Determine the retention time and retention voleme for each constituent.

(ii) Calculate the % weight, % volume and % mole for each constituent of a synthetic mixture..

(iii) Report all the parameters used for setting the G.C. apparatus.

EXERCISE 7. Determine the percentage of component A in the given synthetic mixture. (Follow the instructions given by the instructor).

(i) Report all the parameters, used, to set the G.C. apparatus for the experiment.

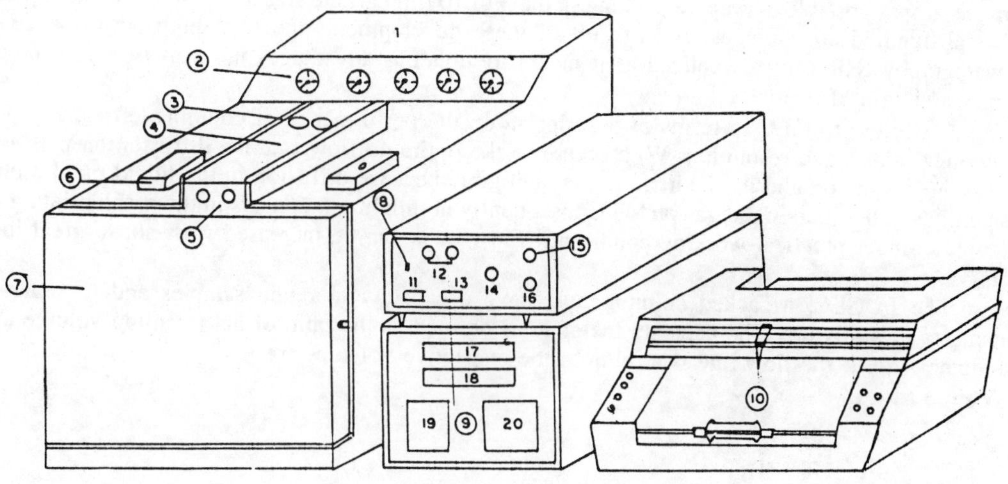

Fig. 21.13 AIMIL-Nucon Gas Chromatograph
(Courtesy of AIML, India)

Legends

S.No.	Description	S. No.	Description
1.	Flow Control Housing	11.	Mains
2.	Pressure Gauges	12.	Balance
3.	Top Removable Lid	13.	Polarity
4.	Ionization Detectorn	14.	Current
5.	T.C.D./Catalyst Chamber	15.	Mark Event
6.	Injector	16.	Attenuator
7.	Oven Door	17.	Digitoscope
8.	F.I.D./T.C.D. Controls	18.	Led's
9.	Temperature Controllers	19.	Function Keys
10.	Recorder	20.	Numerical Keys

21.8 High Performance Liquid Chromatography

21.8.1 General

It should be understood that the early method of liquid chromatography developed by Tswett was performed in glass columns having diameters of 1 to 5 cm and lengths from 50 to 500 cm. The diameter of the particles of the solid stationary phase was in the range of 150 to 20 μm, but the flow rates were low, about few tenths of a mililitre per minute. Efforts to increase the flow rates with the aird of vacuum or punping did not prove effective because increase in flow rates also lead to increase in plate height beyond the minimum in the plate height versus flow rate curves and thus efficiencies were low.

Later, it was realized that the increase in the column efficiency could be obtained if the particle size of the packings was lowered. Technology for packings with particle size as small as 10 μm was developed. Soon after it was possible to prepare packing in the 3 to 10 μm particle size and pumps to obtain pressures of several hundred atmosphares. As a result of these developments the term high performance liquid chromatography (HPLC) was realized as it meant tremondous advantages in terms of speed, precision, accuracy and ease of operation.

HPLC is close to GLC in terms of description on the performance of columns, efficiency in terms of theoritical plates and resolution. With regard to the optimum flow rate the diffusion term B/μ in the Van Deemter equation and its modification is negligible because diffusion in the liquid mobile phase is considerbly smaller than in the gas phase. Consequently no minimum appears in the graph relating HEPT to flow rate under practical working conditions. Flow rates can be increased with not to great increase in HETP.

Just like in GLC, a packed column must have a capacity to retain samples and to separate the components of a mixture. The capacity factor K′ is defined as the ratio of net retention volume (V_N) to void vlume (V_o). If the flow rate is a ml/mint the respective volumes are

$$V_N = a(t_r - t_o)$$

$$V_o = at_o$$

$$\text{and } K' = \frac{V_N}{V_O} = \frac{T_r - T_O}{t_O}$$

The type of chromatogram shown below is used for calculation (Fig. 21.14)

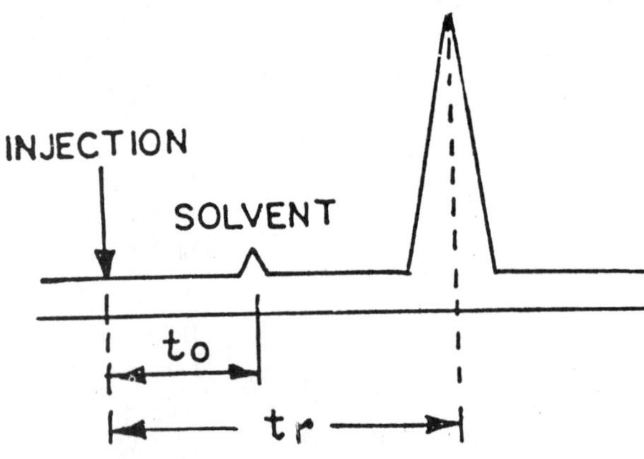

Fig. 21.14. A typical gas chromatogram.

Further, we know $$K' = K\frac{V_N}{V_O}$$

Where, K = distribution coefficient

V_N = Volume of stationary phase

V_o = volume of mobile phase (Void Volume)

When $K' = O$, Components elute in Volume V_o and no separation is possible.

The separation of two components depends upon their relative capacity factors and a separation factor α that is defined as

$$\alpha = \frac{V_2 - V_O}{V_1 - V_O} = \frac{V_{N_2}}{V_{N_1}} = \frac{K_2'}{K_1'}$$

sz

The resolution (R_S) of two closely spaced peak is given by the formula below :

$$R_S = \frac{1}{4}\left(\frac{\alpha - 1}{\alpha}\right)\left(\frac{K_2'}{K_1' + 1}\right)\sqrt{N}$$

Where N = no of theoritical plates.

The resolution can be improved by altering solvent composition. If this fails, a particular adsorbant paking, partition or ion-exchange columns may be tried.

To-day HPLC has become one of the most popular methods of analytical separation techniques. Thus it has ability to give accurate quantitative separation for amino acids, proteins, nucleic acids, hydrocarbons, antibiotics, pesticides, various types of inorganic sulbstances as well as non-volatile and thermally labile materials.

21.8.2 Components of the Instrument

A modern HPLC apparatus is equipped with the following components :

1. Mobile Phase Reservoirs and solvent Treatment Systems : The reservoirs may be made of glass or stainless steel containing up to 500 ml of solvent. They are also provided with means for removing

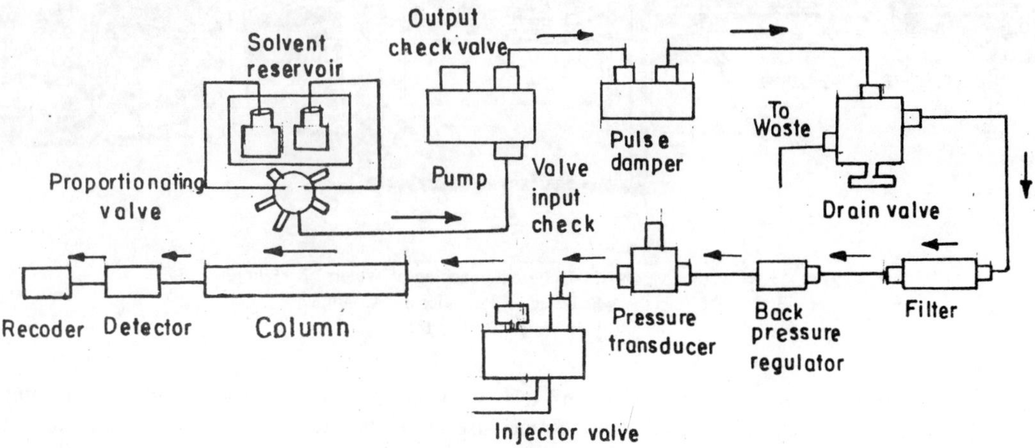

Fig. 21.15 Components of HPLC

dissolved gases like oxygen and nitrogen which may form bubbles in the column and the detector systems. The degasing can be done by means of a vacuum pump or the solvents may be filtered by a Vacuum pump which will remove both impurities as well as gases.

A separation that involves a single solvent of constant composition is called *"Isocratic System"*. Separation can also be performed by *"Gradient elution"* in which two or more solvent systems that differ in polarity are used. The ratio of the two solvents can be varied in a programmed way. The gradient elution programme can produce similar effects as that by temperature programming in gas chromatography.

2. Pumping systems : The main requirements of pumping systems are : (a) generation of pressures up to 60000 psi; (b) pulse-free out-put; (c) flow rates ranging from 0.1 to 10 mL/mic; (d) flow control and flow reprodibility of 0.5% or better. (e) corrosion - resistant components (seals of teflon or stainless steel). Three types of pumps having their own advantages and disadvantages are available — these are (a) reciprocating types (b) displacement type (c) pneumatic or constant pressure type.

Reciprocating Pumps : The most commonly used are reciprocating pumps. They consist of a small chamber in which the solvent is pumped by the back and forth motion of a motor - driven piston; the solvent being in direct contact with the piston. The reciprocating pumps produce a pulsed flow which has to be damped as it is manifested as a base - line noise on the chromatogram. The reciprocating pumps have the advantage of having small internal Volume (35—400 μl), high output pressures (up to 10,000 psi), Their constant flow rates independent of column back - pressure and solvent viscosity and finally their ready adaptability to gradient elution.

3. Flow control : The pumping system are provided with computer controlled devices which can determine the pressure and accordingly increase or decrease the speed of the pump motor.

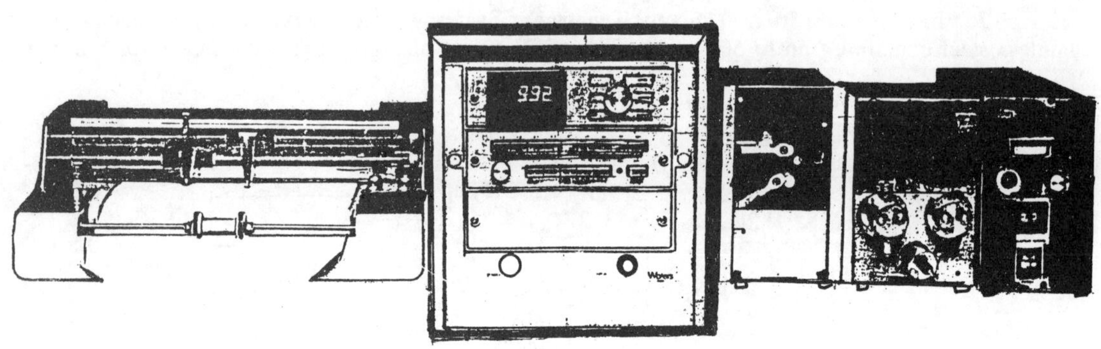

Fig. 21.16 Waters M240 HPLC System consiting of Waters 501 Pump, U6K Injector, 440 Detector, Recorder and Column (Courtesy of Waters (India) Ltd.)

4. Sample Injection System : It is necessary to have a set up so that reproducibility of the sample into the Column packing can be ensured. The volumes used must be very small e.g. few tenths of a μL, 500 μL. One should be able to introduced the samples without depressurizing the system. The most commonly used sampling methods are sampling valves or loops. The sample size varies from 5 to 500 μL. Sampling loops of this type permit the introduction of samples at pressures up to 7000 psi.

5. Columns : The columns are constructed from smooth - bore stainless steel tubing. Heavy - walled glass can also be used but are restricted to lower pressures of about 600 psi. The columns range in length from 10–30 cm. However, column length can be increased by coupling two or more columns together when needed. The inside diameter of the columns is from 4 to 10 mn. The most common particle size of the packing is 5 to 10 μm. The general dimensions of a column are 25 cm length, 4.6 mm inside diameter and packed with 5 μm particle. Such a column will have from 40,000 to 60,000 theoritical plates per meter. Micro columns with inside diameter of 1 to 4.6 mm and packed with 3 to 5 μm particles are available. Such columns contain as many as 100,000 plates/meter and have the advantage of speed and minimal solvent consumption.

A short guard column is attached to the analytical column for removing particulate matter and contaminants from the solvents. The guard column also serves to saturate the mobile phase with the stationary phase so that losses of this solvent from the column are minimized. The guard column should have to same packing material as the analytical column, the packing particle size may be larger to minimize the pressure drop.

The control of column temperature is not necessary and are operated at ambient temperature. However, instruments are available which are equipped with systems where temperature can be controlled above ambient to 100 to 150°C.

6. Column Packings : Two common types of packing materials are available for liquid chromatography :

(a) Pellicubar and (b) Porous.

The pellicular packing consists of spherical, non-porous, glass or polymer beads with diameters of 30 to 40 μm. A thin, porous layer of silica, alumina or an ion-exchange resin is deposited on the surface of these beads. In some cases, an additional coating is applied, which consists of a liquid stationary phase that is held in place by adsorption. The beads can be treated chemically to give an organic surface layer.

The other type i.e. porous are composed of silica, alumina, or ion-exchange resin having diameters from 3 to 10 μm.

7. Detectors : In case of liquid chromatography there are no detectors which as versatile and of Universal applicability such as thermal conductivity or flame ionization detectors as used in GLC. Three types of detectors are used in liquid chromatography. These being : (a) those which respond to a mobile - phase bulk property modulated by the presence of solutes; (b) detectors that respond to some property of solutes that is not possessed by the mobile phase ; (c) detectors that show a response to solutes after removal of the mobile phase. Of the various types of dectors used in liquid chromatography 71% are based on U.V. absorption, 15% by fluorescence, 5.4% by refractive index and 4.3% by electrochemical methods.

Ultraviolet Detectors : Various types of U.V. detectors are available in the market. Choice depends on the type of work and sophitication of the instrument. One of the common type of U.V. detector being filter photometers with a mercury lamp as the source. Filters to cut lines at 254, 250, 313, 334 and 365 nm can be employed. Deuterium or tungsten filament sources with interference filters are also available for species as they are eluted from a column. Scanning type of sphectrophoto-meters which encompass both U.V. and visible region are available. In this manner spectral data for each chromatographic peak can be collected as well stored. Even arrangement for quantitative determination as well as three dimensional plots can also be obtained.

Infrared Detectors : Two types of infrared spectrophotometers are available. The range of wavelength being from 2.5 μm or 4000 to 690 cm^{-1}. Fourier transform type I.R. is also being offered for use in H.P.L.C.

A simple I.R. instrument can be operated at one or more single wavelength setings or the spectra for peaks can be scanned by stopping the flow at the time of elution. The limitation for use of I.R. detectors is the low transparency of some of the solvents particularly water and alcohols.

Fluorescence Detectors : Filter fluorimeters and spectrofluorimeters can be used for HPLC. The simple type employ a mercury excitation source and one or more filters to isolate a band of emited radiation. Of course the sophisticated type use xenon lamp as the source and a grating monochromator to characterise the fluoriscent radiation. The main advantage of this method is their high sensitivity and of course can be applied to samples that fluoresce. As such fluorescent compounds are encountered in the analysis of pharma-ceuticals, natural products, climical samples, petroleum products. The scope of the method can also be enlarged by converting samples to fluorescent derivatives e.g. phenols, amino acids and amines can give fluorescent derivatives.

Refractive Index Detectors : Differential type of refractive index detector in which the solvent passes through one-half of the cell on its may to the column, the eluate then flows through the other chamber. The two compartments are separated by a glass plate mounted at an angle such that bending of the incident beam occurs if the two solutions differ in refractive index. The resulting displacement of the beam with respect to the photosensitive surface of the detector causes variation in the output of the signal which is then amplified, recorded and thus provides the chromatographic peak. The refractive index type of detectors have the advantage of responding to nearly all solutes and thus serve as general type of detectors. They are reliable and are also unaffected by the flow rate.

In addition to the above described optical detectors a variety of electro-chemical detectors as well as mass spectrometric detectors have been developed. They have their own advantages depending the needs of the types of analysis that one may be involved in.

21.8.3 Mobile Phase

Many different types of mobile phase are available for HPLC. The proper choice among these solvents will depend upon a series of trial-and-error experiments in which chromoatograms are obtained with various solvents and solvent combintions untill satisfactory results are obtained. However, the mobile phase for HPLC should have following qualities :

(a) It should have high purity
(b) It should easily available at a reasonable cost.
(c) A boiling point that is 20-50°C above the column temperatures.
(d) It should possess low viscosity.
(e) It should have low reactivity i.e. should not react with solutes or polymerize in the presence of column packing.
(f) It should not be miscible with stationary phase.
(g) It should have compativbility with the detector.
(i) It should not be flammable or have toxicity.

The capacity factor k′ for the sample components should be in a suitable range. For a two or three component system sample, the solvent should have a capacity factor k′ should have a range of 2 to 5 while for a multicomponent system this range should be from 0.5 to 20. Several solvents or solvent combinations should be tried that will have suitable capacity factors.

Types of Mobile Phase : In case of gas and exclusion chromatography the mobile phase are of non-interactive type and therefore the retention times are independent of he composition of the mobile phase. On the contrary the mobile phase for partition, adsorption and ion-exchange chromatography are interactive type in the sense that they interact electrostatically with the sample components. Therefore, the retention times will be influenced by the type of solvent used. This implies that the solvents require a proper balance of intermolecular forces among the three active participants in the separation process, namely the solute, the mobile phase and the stationary phase. These interactive forces can also be interpreted in terms of the polarity of each of the reactants. The polarities of the various organic compounds have the following order : alcohol > amines > amides > aldehydes > Ketones > esters > ethers, water being more polar than these functional groups.

In general good chromatographic separations can be obtained by matching the polarity of the analytes to that of the stationary phase and then a mobile phase of different polarity is chosen.

Normal and Reversed-Phase HPLC : In general two types of HPLC techniques are distinguished. These are based on the relative polarities of the mobile and stationary phases. The procedure which incorporated highly polar stationary phases like alumina or silica surfaces or polar liquids such as triethyleneglycol supported by silica particles; while a non-plar solvent like hexane or isopropyl ether served as the mobile phase. This type of liquid chromatography was called *normal-phase chromatography*. Here the least polar component is eluted first. But when the stationary phase is non-polar such as a hydrocarbon, and the mobile phase is polar like water, methanol, acetonitrile the procedure is called *reversed-phase liquid chromatography*.

21.8.4 Comparison of HPLC and GLC

1. Both are efficient, highly selective and widely applicable.
2. Small amounts of samples are needed for analysis.
3. In both usually samples are not destroyed.
4. Both can be adopted to quantitative methods.
5. HPLC has the advantage that it can be applied to non-volatile and thermally unstable samples.
6. HPLC can also be applied to inorganic ions.
7. GLC is simple and inexpensive
8. GLC is rapid.
9. In GLC the resolution is very high with capillary columns.
10. GLC can be interfaced or attached to a MS.

EXERCISE 8. Determination of Aspirin and caffeine from tablet preparations by HPLC.

Method : 1. Read the HPLC equipment as per instructions from the instructor or as per operating manual. 2. Weigh and powder 20 tablets. 3. Accurately weigh a quantity of powder equivalent to one tablet : 3. Extract the drug several times thoroughly with acetonitrile. 4. Filter through a sintered-glass funnel. 5. Dilute the filtrate to 200 ml with distilled water and mix well. 6. Set the parameters on the HPLC apparatus. 7. Prepare the standard solutions of pure aspirin (18%) and caffcine (0.015%) using acetonitrile as solvent (10-15% V/V in water) 8. Inject 15 μl samples of pure samples of aspirin and caffcine into the column. 9. Elute with 10% acetonitrile. 10. Measure or record the peak heights and retention times for the standard pure samples. 11. Now, inject the assay samples for analysis. 12. Record the peak heights and calculate the quantity of aspirin and caffcine in a tablet of average weight. 13. In case, an integrator is used instead of a mechanical chart recorder, the retention times and percentages will be printed as output.

EXERCISE 9. Determination of methyl testosterone in a tablet preparation by HPLC

Method : 1. Ready the HPLC apparatus as per instructions from the instrutor or as per operating manual. 2. Fix the C_{18} Corasil II column. 3. Set the parameters on HPLC apparatus. 4. Condition the column by flushing it with HPLC grade methamol (60%, 0.5 ml/min.). 5. Weigh and powder 5 tablets. 6. Take accurately weighed quantity of powder equivalent to one tablet in a 25 ml volumetric flask. 7. Add 10 ml of distilled water and shake until the tablet is dispersed. 8. Add 15 ml methanol, shake well for several minutes and dilute with water up to the mark. 9. Filter any solid particles through a sintered-glass funnel. 10. Inject 10 μl of the clear solution into the column. 11. Allow to elute with 60%

MeOH-H_2O mixture and record the peaks. 12. Compare the peak height with that of the standard pure sample. 13. Calculate or read the amount of the drug in the tablets.

20.9. High Performance Thin Layer Chromatography

No clear definition for high performance thin layer chromatography (HPTLC) has been put forth by the proponents of high performance thin layer chromatography. However, the following differences and advantages may be noted for high performance thin layer chromatography.

(a) In high performance thin layer chromatographic plates, the adsorbent particles have lower and narrow particle size distribution as well as reduced thickness than the one used in thin layer chromatographic plates.

(b) The starting spot diameter in high performance thin layer plates are not more than 1 mm and small amounts between 0.005 μg and 0.5 μg (5-500 ng) are used.

(c) High performance thin layer chromatography involves special development chambers e.g. "V" chamber for circular and anticircular chromatography.

(d) The development distance in HPTLC are between 2 to 6 cm.

(e) The resolution on HPTLC plates can be increased from 10 to 30%, but with longer development distances efficiency decreases because of lower phase velocities.

(f) High performance thin layer chromatography has advantage over conventional TLC because HPTLC assayl are fully automated and can be more accurate.

(g) The high performance thin layer chromatography calibration curves are usually linear in contrast to conventional TLC.

(h) The substances sensitive to light or oxygen cannot be a problem to analyse by HPTLC than with TLC and Volatile substances can be also be analysed.

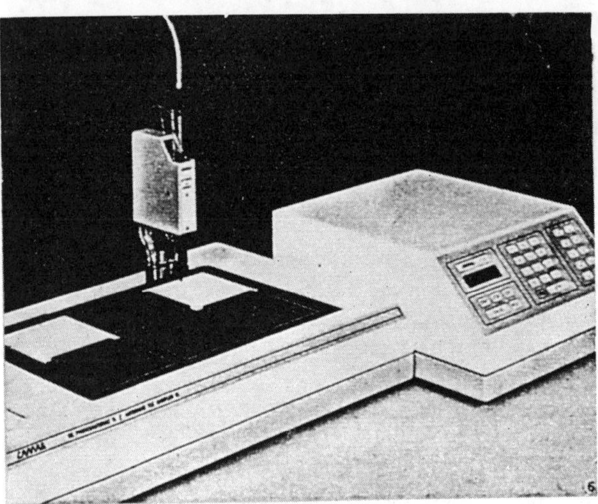

Fig. 21.17. CAMAG Automatic TLC Sampler II: for fully automatic sample application in quantitative TLC analysis.
(Courtesy of Anchrom Enterprises, india)

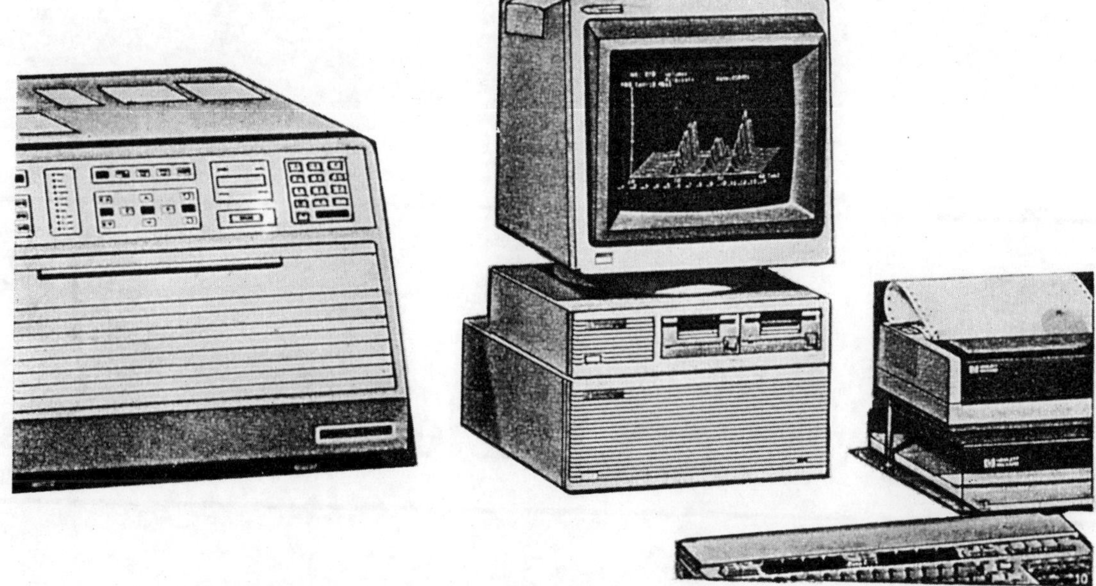

Fig. 21.18. CAMAG TLC SCANNER II with Computer Control and CAMAG Evaluation **Software**.
(Courtesy of Anchrom Enterprise, India)

The theoritical principles and the methodology involved in HPTLC are the same as in conventional TLC but the former is instrumental based (Fig. 21.17 and 21.18).

The samples are applied on the separation layers using an instrument which ensures accurate positioning and precise volume. The sample fractions can be quantified directly by scanning the chromatograms with a light beam in the visible or U.V. range of the spectrum and measures absorbance or fluorescence by diffuse reflectance. With the incorporation of TLC scanner having computer control and evaluation software HPTLC becomes fully automatic, convenient and very powerful for analysis work. Further, ready-to use TLC plates with adsorbants on glass, aluminium or plastic foil becomes an added advantage over conventional TLC. In the light of the above stated factors HPTLC can be a method of choice for many analysis tasks though the equipment is expensive.

EXERCISE 10. Quantitative determination of salicytic acid derivatives.

Method : Familiarise yourself with the functions and operations of the HPTLC instrument and its methodology from the manual or an instructor. Prepare three calibration standards of salicylamide (25 ng/μl) in ethanol-hexane (1 : 1). In a similar manner prepare 5 different solutions of samples in ethanol-hexane (1 : 1). Spot 14, 15, 16 μl of calibration standard and 15 μl of the sample solution by spray on technique with Linomat bandwise with bandlength of 6 mm and 4 mm apart on HPTLC precoated plates, Merck silica gel 60F 254 of 20 × 10 cm size. Allow the TLC plates to develop in a CAMAG twin-trough chamber containing cyclohexane-chloroform-acetic acid (60 : 5 : 5). With the aid of a CAMAG TLC Scanner II measure the absorbances of the TLC plates at 260 nm. The TLC scanner is maintained at a speed of 1 mm/sec, monochromator bandwidth of 30 mm and slit dimension of 0.3 × 3 mm. Separately determine the linearity of the three external standards of concentrations from 300 ng to 400 ng for salicylic acid and salicylamide and 600 ng to 800 ng for acetyl salicylic acid and use them for calculation of the unknowns. Determine the R_f values and the concentration of the samples. Prepare your results.

22

Electrophoresis

22.1 General

Electrophoresis was originally defined as the movement of a colloidal particle under the influence of an electric field. As the techniques and procedures were developed and became advanced, this definition is now applicable to any charged particle. The other names proposed for electrophoresis are electromigration, ionography, electrorheophoresis etc.

Depending on the sign of the net charge, charged particles and macromolecular ions will migrate either to cathode or to anode. Differences in migration velocities provide a powerful means for the separation and analysis of substances which are difficult to fractionate by other methods. The migration velocity of a particle, when the field acting on it is 1 volt cm^{-1} is called its *electrophoretic mobility*. The dimensions of mobility are in cm^2 sec^{-1} $volt^{-1}$, and its sign is the same as that of the net electrical charge on the particle. The mobility of a particle although is a characteristic property but it will also vary with the composition of the solution. Thus for example, the mobility of serum albumin will depend on the pH, the ionic strength and the nature of the supporting electrolyte. However, each of the migrated particle experiences a frictional resistance to its mvoement and will attain some maximum velocity of migration. Therefore, if a mixture of charged particles or macromolecules is exposed to a constant field strength, the maximum velocities attained will be different for particles of differing net charge. In addition to net charge and field strength, the other factors affecting will be molecular size and shape, pH and the composition of the solvent medium.

Now-a-days electrophoresis can be used for the separation of amino acids, proteins, steroids, rubber emulsions, clay suspensions and inorganic substances like copper nitrate, cadmium nitrate, silver nitrate etc.

22.2 Theory

Although the discussion of principles, apparatus, and techniques described in this chapter will be limited to paper electrophoresis but these are also applicable to other forms of electrophoresis. Currently, three main types of electrophoretic techniques in practice are :

(i) free boundary electrophoresis,
(ii) continuous or curtain electrophoresis,
(iii) zone electrophoresis.

Among these, zone electrophoresis is most commonly used for both analytical and preparative purposes. It is applicable to proteins and other charged soluble substances. The advantages being very good resolution, simplicity of technique, instrument speed and identification of separated samples.

An understanding of the principles of electrophoresis will depend on the establishement of relationship between the mobility and various parameters like electrical charge, frictional coefficient and the effect of composition of the solvent medium.

22.2.1 Origin of Charge

In colloidal particles, such as proteins the charge originates from the ionization of the functional groups of which they are composed . These functional groups can give rise to ions of both polaritics i.e. at acid pH they become positively charged whereas at basic pH they are negatively charged. The pH at which there is a zero electrophoretic mobility is called the *isoelectric point.* Whereas the pH at which the net charge due to ionization is zero is called the *isoionic point.* The two pH's may not coincide with each other. The isoelectric point may be caused due to possible adsorption of free ions like Na^+ or Cl^-. The ion adsorption can modify the net charge of protein molecules and hydrophobic surfaces like hydrocarbon droplets. The anions cause most of the adsorption whereas cations being hydrated are not usually adsorbed.

22.3 Migration of Ions in an Electric Field

When a charged particle is dissolved in a conducting liquid medium and is subjected to the influence of a uniform electrical field, it will attain a constant rate of migration. The positively charged particles will move towards the cathode whereas the negatively charged towards the anode. The rate of movement of these ions is determined by the motive force to which they are subjected. This will be given by the product of the net charge on the particle and the field strength (X) i.e. X = E/S Where E is the potential gradient applied (potential differences in volts between the test probes) spaced 'S' cm apart.

The charged particles, when placed in an electrical field are exposed to four forces, the resultant of which is a steady-state characterized by a constant electriphoretic migration velocity.

The two main forces are : (i) the electrophoretic attraction K_1 defined as K_1 = QE where Q is the charge of the electrokinetic unit and E is the potential gradient, and (ii) the Stokes friction K_2 defined as $K_2 = f_2\mu$ where f_c is the frictional coefficient of the particles. For a rigid spherical type particle

$$f_c = 6\pi\eta a$$

Where η is the viscosity of the solvent and a is the radius of the spherical particle.

The other two additional forces which arise due to the presence of small electrolyte molecules in the medium are (iii) electrophoretic retardation (K_3) and (iv) relaxation effects (k_4). The electrophoretic retardation (K_3) is produced by the electro-osmotic flow of small ions of the solvent caused by the attraction exerted by the electrical field.

During the migration towards the respective electrodes, the hydrated ions will carry with them their associated water molecules. This assemblage comprises of water molecules held directly in the solvation sheath plus additional layers of water molecules attracted and held by the inner layers. Thus, it is possible for hundreds of solvent molecules to be dragged along by each migrating ions. The opposing flows caused by the cations and anions does not compensate as the cations carry more water than anions. The net flow is almost always towards the cathode and varies linearly with the voltage gradient. The value of this electrophoretic retardation (K_3) is treated as a mobility correction to be added for anions and subtrated for cations.

The electrophoretic retardation force is calculated by Huckel's equation expressed as

$$K_3 = (\varepsilon\zeta - Q)E$$

Where ε is dielectrice constant and ζ is the zeta potential i.e. the potential at the surface of shear.

The relaxaiton effects (K_4) is brought about by the distortion of the ionic atmosphere caused due to differences in the movement of the counter ions and the colloidal particles as a consequence of which each particle is no longer in the centre of its atmosphere.

In a steady state condition which is achieved after the application of the electrical field, the sum of these four forces equals to zero and the electrophoretic velocity μ becomes:

$$\mu = \frac{QE + K_3 + K_4}{f_c}$$

If we ignore K_4 in the above equation the electrophoretic mobility can be expressed in terms of velocity and field strength as :

$$\mu = \frac{\mu}{E} = \frac{QE + K_3}{6\pi\eta a}$$

Thus the electrophoretic mobility of an ion is defined as the linear distance (d) travelled by the migrant ion in time t in a field of unit potential and is generally calculated by the following equation :

$$\mu = \frac{d}{t} / \frac{E}{S} = \frac{dS}{ET} \text{ cm}^2 \text{ Volt}^{-1} \text{ Sec}^{-1}$$

22.3.1 Resolution

It can be defined in terms of sharpness of the zones occupied by different migrant species in the supporting media after electrophoresis is completed. In order to separate two conponents effectively, it is necessary to allow migration to continue until one component has travelled at least one thickness of the volume that the sample initially occupied i.e. the starting zone. Therefore we can write :

$$\mu = \frac{dS}{Et}$$

$$d = \mu t . \frac{E}{S}$$

As a result of diffusion, there is spreading of the zones and consequently resolution of each migrant species diminishes with time. Thus after time t the difference in the distance travelled will be equal to :

$$d_1 - d_2 = (\mu_1 - \mu_2) / (E/S)\, t$$

Diffusion being time dependent and proportional to the square root of time, its effect can be minimized by applying the highest possible potential gradient.

22.4 Buffer, pH and Ionic Strength

The electrophoretic mobility is greatly affected by the pH of the electrolyte because the net charge carried by most species is pH dependent. If the sample is a weak acid or base, the pH will control its degree of ionization. The net mobility of a partly ionized solute in solution is given by the equation :

$$\mu' = \frac{\mu K_a}{[H^+] + K_a}$$

Where K_a is ionizing constant. Thus one can measure μ for a substance under conditions where conization is complete and k′ at a known pH at which ionization is not complete and then calculate the ionization constant K_a. Consequently it will also be possible to separate two incompletely ionized acids depending upon the differences in their apparent mobilities.

22.5 Instrumentation Aspects

In the case of paper electrophoresis, there are four main techniques which involve the use of paper as a stabilizer. These are known as (i) Sand witch (ii) Ridgepole, (iii) horizontal Strip and (iv) solvent immersion techniques. Commercially, various types of electrophoretic apparatuses are available. In this chapter, the sandwitch technique, which is commonly used will be described as it is simple to work with. A schematic diagram of the sand which technique is shown in the Fig. 22.1.

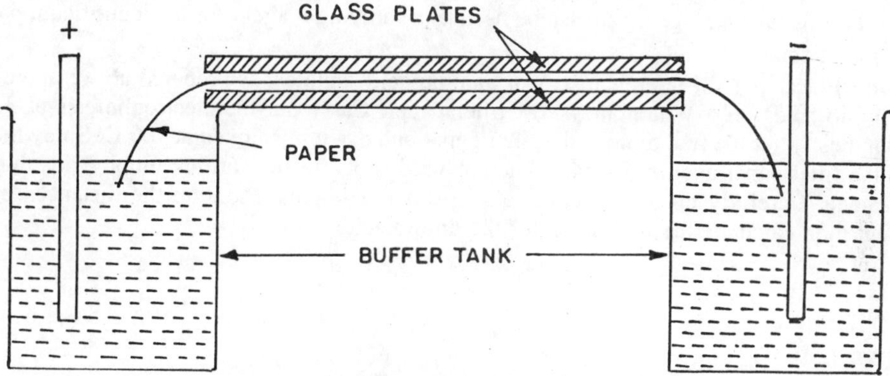

Fig. 22.1. "Sandwitch" type of electrophoresis.

The material to be separated into its constituents is spotted onto the centre or one end of a sheet of filter paper which is saturated with buffer solution. The paper is placed between glass plates or on metal plate and connected to electrode vessels. The metal plate can have arrangement for cooling by circulation of water to maintain constant temperature and prevent evaporation of buffer. The entire system can be placed in a box or chamber. Each end of the paper dips into a container holding a few hundred millilitres of buffer solution. (Wicks, made from the same paper can be used to allow the paper to get soaked with buffer solution). An electrode is placed in each container holding the buffer solution, one being connected to the positive terminal of a DC source and the other to the negative terminal. A potential of say about 5 to 10 volt/cm may be applied and if charged particles are present in the material they will move towards the terminal opposite charge.

EXERCISE 1 : Separation of Mixture of Indicators.

Method : By means of capillary tubes spot small amounts of solution of bromocresol green, bromophenol blue, methyl red and a mixture of unknown indicators on a Whatman No. 3 MM filter paper. Perform the electrophoresis at 2.0 KV for 30 minutes using a buffer prepared from 0.IM acetic acid and 0.IM sodium acetate (pH 4.5). After the run, remove the filter paper and allow it to dry in an oven. Mark the location of the each zone of the indicator thus separated on the paper. Measure the distance of travel for each indicator spot and calculate the mobility for each of them. The above experiment can also be performed in a buffer comprising 0.6 M formic acid, 0.IM aqueous ammonia and 0.IM ammonium acetate (pH 9.0)

EXERCISE 2 : Separation of a Mixture of Amino Acids .

This experiment requires the preparation of amino acid standards, buffer solution and ninhydrin reagent which are described below.

(i) Amino Acid Standards : These are prepared by making 0.05 M solutions in a 10% isopropyl alcohol solution. In case of solubility difficulties 1-2 drops of concentrated HCl can be added to the solutions.. For example samples of glycine, alanine, histidine, lysine, glutamine, serine, tryptophan can be prepared and used for separation studies.

(ii) Buffer Solution : A buffer solution with a pH of 2.0 can be obtained by mixing 31.2 ml of formic acid and 59.2 ml of glacial acetic acid and making up the final volume to 1 litre with distilled water. This buffer solution is stable and can be stored for 1 month in a refrigerator.

(iii) Ninhydrin Reagent : Dissolve 100 mg of ninhydrin in 3 ml of ethyl alcohol and make up to 50 ml by addition of ethyl ether. Mix the solution well and use it immediately. A 0.5 ml of collidine in 49.5 ml of ninhydrin reagent can also be used as a spraying reagent for the identification of different amino acid spots.

Method : Place spots of reference standard amino acid samples, as prepared above and a mixture of unknown amino acids on a Whatman 3 MM filter paper. Carry out the electrophoresis at 3.50 KV for about 45 minutes. Alter the run, remove the filter paper and dry it in an oven at 100°C. Spray the ninhydrin reagent on the filter paper and dry it again. The coloured spots for the various amino acids thus separated will be obtained. Carefully mark the zones for the separated spots. Measure the distances of travel for the spots and then calculate the mobilities for the amino acids.

SECTION-G
RADIOCHEMICAL METHODS OF ANALYSIS

23

Methods Using Radioisotopes

23.1 General

To begin with, in order to understand the applications of nuclear chemistry to analytical chemistry, it may be fruitful to review some basic concepts of nuclear structure and laws of radioactive growth and decay.

The atom is known to consist of a dense nucleus containing protons and neutrons and surrounded by electrons which follow certain paths of motion. However, according to Heisenberg it is impossible to determine at the same time the energy and position of the electron. An electron belonging to a given level of any atom may be found anywhere in the space so long as it is still found associated with that atom.

Although the picture that nucleus is made up of protons and neutrons was adopted but it was also found that the neutron was not a *stable* particle. Inside the nucleus it can remain stable for billions of years ; but when it passes out of the nucleus, it has a short life-a half-life of about 13 minutes before it decomposes into a proton and an electron.

A British physicist, Dirac made a suggestion that the entire universe is a single quantum system i.e. there are a vast set of energy levels just as there are simpler set of levels in an atom or a more complicated set in a metallic crystal. He pointed out that in addition to *particles* like electron and proton, the universe must also contain anti-particles. Thus the existence of positron having same mass as electron but a positive charge was established. In fact, the presence of antimatter which did not influence the ordinary matter was also postulated. In this manner, it has been hypothesized that there are various type of ''particles'' in the universe at the top level where they acquire energy and carry out various types of motion of the matter around us. These various kinds of *particles* are highly interrelated through force fields that determine the energy of interaction. These various kinds of force fields are designated as (i) strong nuclear force (ca. 10^{-31} cm) (ii) electromagnetic interaction varying as the inverse square of the distance, (iii) weak nuclear interaction (ca. 10^{-13} cm) and lastly (iv) the gravitation, varying as the inverse square of distance.

The '*particles*' are classified based on the type of interaction with which they are involved. Some of the common ones are listed below in Table 23.1.

Table 23.1
Chart of Nuclides

Particles & Symbols	Charge	Spin
Electron, e or β	–1	1/2
Positron, e^+ or $β^+$	+ 1	1/2
Proton, P	+ 1	1/2
Neutron, n	0	1/2
Neutrino ν	0	1/2
μ Mesons $μ^-$ & μ+	–1, + 1	1/2
π Mesons $π^-$, $π^0$, $π^+$	–1, 0, + 1	0

There are seven particles with zero rest mass, namely : antineutronoʹ, antineutrono, positron, Photon, electron (0.5 Mev) neutrino and neutrinoʹ. Particles with a rest mass of 106 Mev are two lepton i.e. the antimoun and moun. Next in the order of rest mass are mesons i.e. $π^-$ $π^o$ & $π^+$ (rest mass, 100 Mev). The particles with a rest mass of 900 Mev are neutron, proton, antineutron, antiproton. Above them are baryons which were discovered some two decades ago.

From the periodic table we have learnt that hydrogen atom contains one proton on its nucleus, helium contains two, lithium three and so on with atomic number being equal to the number of protons in the nucleus (as well as the number of electrons outside the nucleus). We also know that hydrogen may exist in one of the three forms called *isotopes* which differ in the number of neutrons in the nucleus along with protons. Hydrogen, with mass number one, contains only one proton and is referred to H^1. The hydrogen atom with mass 2 (H^2 or D) is called *deuterium.* It contains a neutron and a proton. The hydrogen-3 (H^3 or T) is called *tritium.* It contains two neutrons and a single proton. The atomic number is referred by the letter z and the mass number i.e. total number of particles in the nucleus by the letter A. Although the chemical behavior of on atom is related to the number of protons but all elements have isotops which are characterized by differing number of neutrons. Generally, it is observed that at lower atomic numbers there is a 1:1 correspondence between the numbers of neutrons and protons. As one moves to higher atomic numbers, there is a marked predominance of neutrons over protons.

23.2 Binding Energy

A cording to Einsteins equation of $E = mc^2$ there is an equivalence of energy with mass and consequently whenever energy leaves an atom it takes with it a little mass; and therefore the mass of the atom left behind is less. As we move across the periodic table from hydrogen to the haevier nuclei, these nuclei have increasingly less energy than separate protons and neutrons of which they are made, which is true until we reach nuclei with mass about that of iron. Beyond iron, a comparism of observed atomic weights with the sum of the masses of protons and neutrons indicates that the energy of the nucleus rises up again towards the sum of the energies of separate particles. This difference in energy between the observed mass of the nucleus and the sum of its separate particles is known as the *binding energy* or *mass defect* and is denoted by Z^{Δ} N^A (Neutron mass + proton mass = deutron mass + binding energy)

Thus for hydrogen : $1^{\Delta}{}_{0}{}^{A} = 7.3$ Mev

Neutron : O^{Δ} $1^1 = 8.1$ Mev

The binding energy released for an isotope in forming the nucleus (A, Z, N) is given by :

$$W = \frac{c^2}{n} [Z(1^m o^1) N(o^m 1^1) - N^A]$$

$\therefore$ W = Z ($1^{\Delta}o^{1}$) + N ($o^{\Delta}1^{1}$) - Z $^{\Delta}$ N^{A}

The binding energy per nucleon in the nucleus is known as binding fraction (f) and is given by :

$$f = \frac{1^{\Delta}o^{1} + o^{\Delta}1^{1}}{2} + \frac{N - Z}{A} \cdot \frac{o^{\Delta}1^{1} - 1^{\Delta}o^{1}}{2} - \frac{1}{A} Z^{A}N^{A}$$

A graph is plotted for the values of f against the values of A for hydrogen to uranium. This plot gives the average value of energy released per nucleon when an isotope in question is formed.

From the above graph it has been found that the greatest release of energy is in the neighbourhood of iron (Fe) i.e. these nuclei have very high stability. Thus the nuclei which are lighter, have a tendency to join together by *fusion* to form heavier nuclei near iron. On the other hand there is a tendency for heaviest nuclei like u to split by *fission* producing nuclei closer in figure to iron.

23.3 Radioactivity and Nuclear reactions

There are more than 1000 unstable or radio isotopes known to occur in nature. These have nuclei with excess energy and degrade through the process of radioactivity to a lower energy level at a characteristic rate.

The naturally occuring radioelements can be divided into three groups, namely : (i) thorium series, (ii) uranium series and (iii) the actinium series.

The excess of nuclear energy may be discharged by ejection of a highly energetic particle like α or β-*particle* and in some cases through γ - ray.

23.3.1 Beta Ray Emission

Since an alpha particle is identical to a nucleus, it has a mass of 4 and consists of 2 protons and 2 neutrons. Thus, when an α-particle is emitted the mass number of the daughter nuclide will be four units less than that of the parent. Although most of the large nuclei exhibit alpha radioactivity but radioactivity can be produced in all of the elements with suitable nuclear reactions. Suppose we decide to choose a sample of aluminium for the propose of producing a nuclear reaction, this can be done by irradiation with neutrons. The initial reaction can be written as shown $Al^{27} + n^{1} \rightarrow [Al^{28}]$ indicating that Al^{28} first forms an excited or high - energy state. The potential energy level diagram for this reaction is indicated in Fig. 23.1.

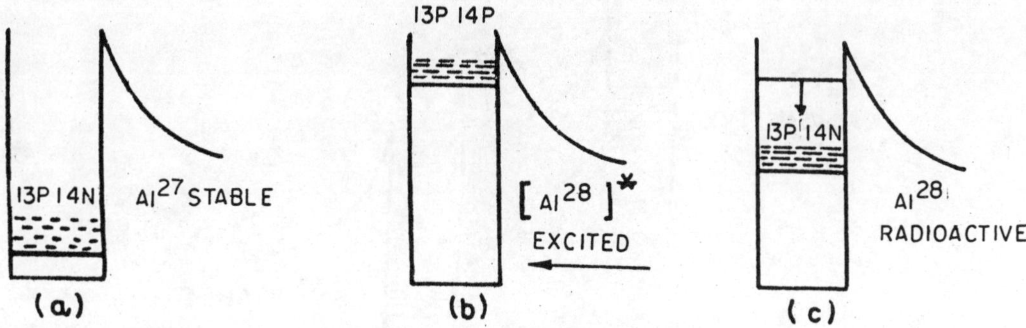

Fig. 23.1. Potential energy level diagram for neutron capture.

The Al ^{27} contains 13 proton & 14 neutrons which are placed at a low level showing stable nucleus. When neutron is introduced the condition corresponds to the excited $[Al^{28}]^*$. The question then arises as to how does the excited $[Al^{28}]^*$ give up its excess energy to come down to a lower state. This is possible to occur in several ways. The most convenient way of emitting the excess energy for $[Al^{28}]^*$ would be by photons of γ-radiation ($10^{-12} - 10^{-10}$ seconds) to become unexcited Al^{28} (Fig. 1c). The *other* various possible ways of losing excess energy for $[Al^{28}]^*$ are indicated below.

$$Al^{2+} + n^1 \longrightarrow [Al^{28}]^* \longrightarrow \begin{cases} Al^{28} + \gamma & \text{........ ..(a)} \\ Mg^{27} + p^1 & \text{........ .(b)} \\ Na^{24} + \alpha^4 & \text{..........(c)} \\ Al^{26} + Zn^1 & \text{..........(d)} \end{cases}$$

The above reactions show that transmutation can also occur giving rise to new elements. In the above reactions, (a) is an exorgonic reaction whereas (b) , (c) and (d) are endorgonic reactions. In the reaction (a) 8 Mev of energy i.e. total energy of γ-ray is given off where as in reactions (b), (c) and (d) energy equal to 2.1, 2.7 and 11 Mev respectively has to be supplied. The above changes can be also be described in a shorthand from as :

$$Al^{27}\ (n, \gamma)\ Al^{28},\ Al^{27}\ (n, p)\ Mg^{27}, \text{ etc, etc.}$$

By a similar procedure, one can show :

$$U^{235} + n^1 \rightarrow [U^{236}]^* \rightarrow Ba^{140} + Kr^{94} + Zn^1$$

A look at the periodic table shows that aluminium has only one stable nuclide i.e. Al^{27}, magnesium has three stable isotopes, $Mg^{24, 25, 26}$, sodium has on one stable isotope i.e. Na^{23} whereas silicon has three stable isotopes i.e. Si^{28}, Si^{29} and Si^{23}. On the other hand Na^{24}, Mg^{27}, Al^{26} and Al^{28} can be produced by nuclear bombardments as these nuclei are not found free in nature and they need to lose excess energy before becoming stable. The stable isotopes possess a preferred neutron-proton ratio and this ratio increases as one goes to higher atomic numbers. The above types of ratio-active atoms can become stable by the emission of a neutron to give a adjacent lighter nucleus of the same element. But, this does not occur, instead a proton and an electron are given off. The proton remains in the nucleus while electron immediately leaves the atom. This kind of transformation is called a *negative beta decay*. The above stated process can be explained by the following reaction :

$$P^{31}\ (n, \gamma)\ P^{32} \text{ or } S^{32}\ (n, p)\ ^{32}$$

Further ; $$P^{32} \longrightarrow S^{32} + \beta^-$$

The above process can also be depicted by an energy diagram (Fig. 23.2).

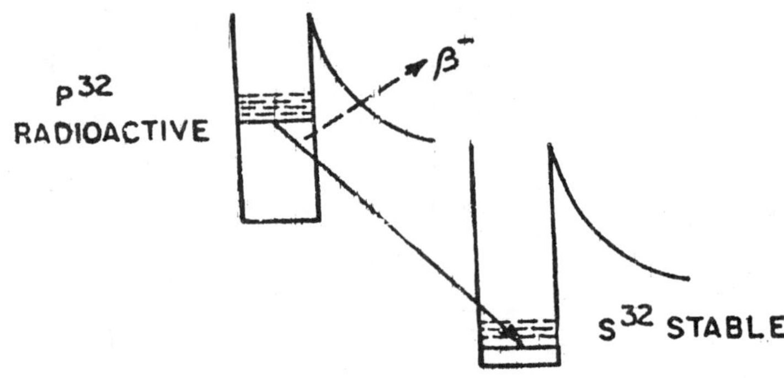

Fig. 23.2. Energy level diagram, $\bar{\beta}$—rays emission.

It is to be noted that in addition to the emission of a β^- particle, another particle is also ejected during the transformation of neutron for the purpose of energy balance. This particle is called the neutrono, ν. Thus the complete neutron transformation can be written as :

$$n^1 \longrightarrow p^1 + \beta^- + v$$

23.3.2 Gamma Ray Emission

In the above, we have explained that when a nucleus has a neutron-proton ratio higher than that possessed by its stable isotopes, β–ray emission occurs. But, in certain cases a nucleus still contains an extra energy after the neutron transformation has taken place. For example a stable Co^{59} can be changed to Co^{60} by addition of a neutron. Further, Co^{60} can cool down by β- ray emission to Ni^{60} but not to its lowest possible energy state. Thus, this energetic Ni^{60} gives off rest of this excess energy as gamma ray. This is depicted by means of the energy level diagram (Fig. 23.3).

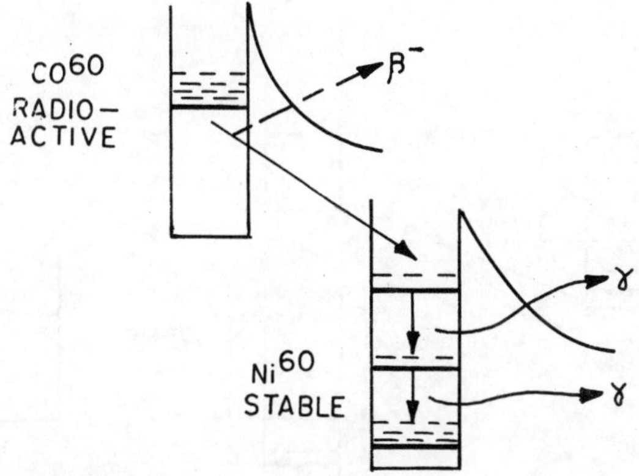

Fig. 23.3. Energy level diagram, β–ray emission with gamma ray emission.

23.3.3 Electron Capture and positron Emission

We have seen that among the nuclei which have high neutron-proton ratios, the only way to come to a stable condition is by giving off a β^-–particle. But, if the radioactive nucleus has too few neutrons in comparison with the number of protons in the stable atoms of the element, it cannot reach stability by this mechanism. For such cases, there are two ways by which a nucleus can reach stability. One of these is called *electron capture* in which case the nucleus traps an electron from one of the orbital levels and combines with to form a neutron, a neutrino is also emitted as shown in the equation ;

$$p^1 + e^- \longrightarrow n^1 + V^o$$

As such no radiation is given off in electron capture, but X - radiation is observed when an electron galls into the vacancy to replace the captured electron. This type o f transformation is depicted in the Fig. 23.4.

The other possibility occurs in cases when ground state of the daughter nucleus is at last 1.2 Mev below the radioactive level. In such cases, this excess energy can be converted into a positive electron as shown by the equation : $p^1 + 1.02 \text{ Mev} \longrightarrow n^1 + \beta^+ + V^o$. The positron does not remain in the nucleus and is ejected. This reaction can compete with electron capture process if sufficient energy is available in the nucleus. The energy level diagram for this transformation is shown in Fig. 23.5.

The above described transformations are summarised in the Table -23.2.

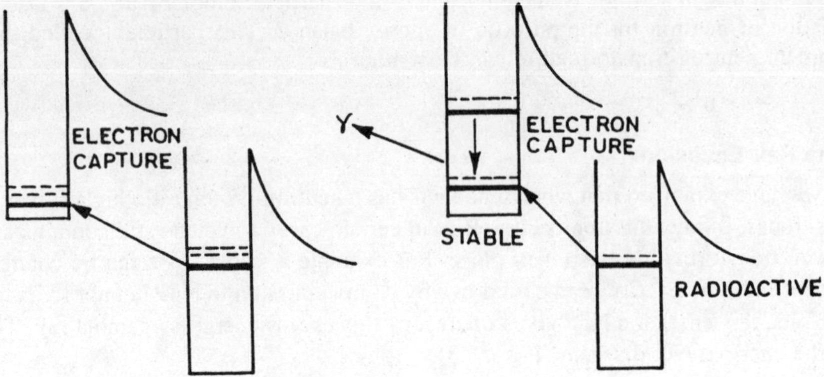

Fig. 23.4. Energy level diagram, electron capture.

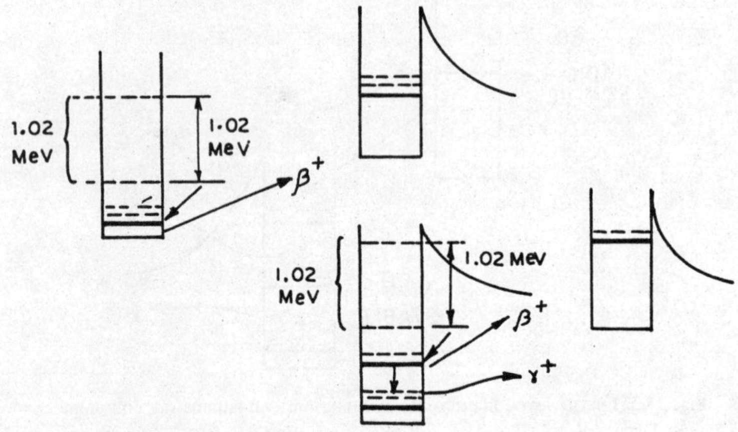

Fig. 23.5. Energy level diagram, positron emission with gamma emission.

Table 23.2

S.No.	Transformation	Nuclear Condition	Nuclear rearrangement	Emitted radiation
1.	α – decay	Excess mass	2p + 2n ejected	α (He nucleus)
2.	β^- decay	neutron : Proton ratio too high	$n \rightarrow p + e^- + \nu$	β^- (electron)
3.	β^+ decay	neutron : proton ratio too low	$p \rightarrow n + e^+ + \nu$	β^+ (positron)
4.	Electron capture	neutron : proton ratio too low	$p + e \rightarrow n + \nu$	None
5.	γ–emission	excited nuclear species	Transition to ground state	γ – ray

23.4 Background Radiation

One of the aspects concerning the measurement of radiation is the background of natural radiation which is always present. Normally, earth receives a steady stream of cosmic radiation (each with 10^{10} - 10^{13} ev) which is observed as gamma radiation on earths surface. The other contribution comes from the naturally radioactive isotopes in the earth, air, water and in the body. The largest amount of radioactivity in the air comes from radon, thoron and their daughters (about 10^{-10} microcurie per cm^3 of air). They are brought down as a natural *fall out* by rain and temperature inversions. Drinking water contains Ur, Ra and Em in concentrations of 10^{-9} - 10^{-10} microcurie per cm^3 . Milk contains 6×10^{-8} microcurie of K^{40} per cm^3. The average human body contains an equilibrium concentration of about 190,000 disintegrations per minute of K^{40}, 150,000 disintegrations per minute of C^{14} and 140 disintegrations per minute of radium which correspond to the presence in the human body of about 10^{20}, 10^{14} and 10^{11} atoms of K^{40}, C^{14} and Ra^{226} respectively.

23.5 Unit of Radiation

The unit of measurement of radioactivity deals with decay of radioactive materials. The radioactive materials decay when they change from a radioactive nucleus to another nucleus which may be either stable or radioactive. These usually involve emission of alpha particle, negative or positive beta particle, electron capture and gamma ray. The term *curie* along with its multiples and submultiples has been introduced as a unit for measure of the amount of radioactive material in a sample. It is defined as a source which decays at the rate of 3.700×10^{10} disintegrations per second (dps). A millicurie is a sample decaying at 3.700×10^{7} dps and a microcurie decays at the rate of 3.700×10^{4} dps.

23.6 Interaction of Radiation with Matter

The study of interaction of radiation with matter permits us to detect and measure the radiation.

Suppose an alpha particle strikes an atom, it may interact with the negatively charged electron of the atom. If the alpha particle does not come too close to the atom, the attraction may be such that the electron is only lifted from one energy level to the other level in the atom. The process is called *excitation.* When the source of excitation is removed, the electron will return to the lower level, giving off energy as X-ray. If the alpha particle approaches very close to the atom, it may remove the electron completely from the atom thus producing an *ion-pair.* The ion pair may exist for a short period of time before the two parts are neutralized.

When a negative β- particle passes near an atom, it also will interact with the electrons of the atom. As in this case the force is repulsive, the electrons in the atom are repelled from the negative β- particle. This interaction may be small enough to cause excitation in the atom or it may be large enough to remove the electron from the atom with the formation of an ion pair. Generally, it takes from 32 to 35 ev to produce an ion pair and differs among atoms.

23.7 Quantitative Aspects or Radioactive Decay

It has been suggested that as far as the disintegration process of radioactive material is concerned that it follows a regularity in the number of atoms decaying per unit of time provided there are a large number of radioactive atoms in the sample. It has been experimentally found that the decay of radionuclides follows a 1st order rate law i.e. it is proportional to the number of radioactive atoms in the sample. This can be stated as :

$$-\frac{dN}{dt} \propto N \text{ or } \frac{dN}{dt} = -\lambda N$$

$$\text{or } \frac{dN}{N} = -\lambda\, dt \quad \text{or } \int \frac{dN}{N} = -\lambda \int dt$$

$$\ln N_t = \ln N_O - \lambda t \quad \text{or } N = N_O e^{-\lambda t}$$

$$\frac{N}{N_O} = \frac{1}{2} = e^{-\lambda t_{1/2}}$$

$$\ln \frac{1}{2} = -\lambda t_{1/2}$$

$$\ln 2 = \lambda t_{1/2} \quad \therefore \quad t_{1/2} = \frac{\ln 2}{\lambda} = \frac{0.693}{\lambda}$$

Where N_o is number of radioactive atoms at zero time, N is the number of radioactive atoms at any other time t, λ is the disintegration constant and e is the base of natural logarithms. For convenience, the time required for one half of atoms to decay is used. It is called *half life* and the symbol $t_{1/2}$ is used for it i.e. time required for the ratio N/N_o to become 1/2. A graph of this disintegration is shown in Fig. 23.6.

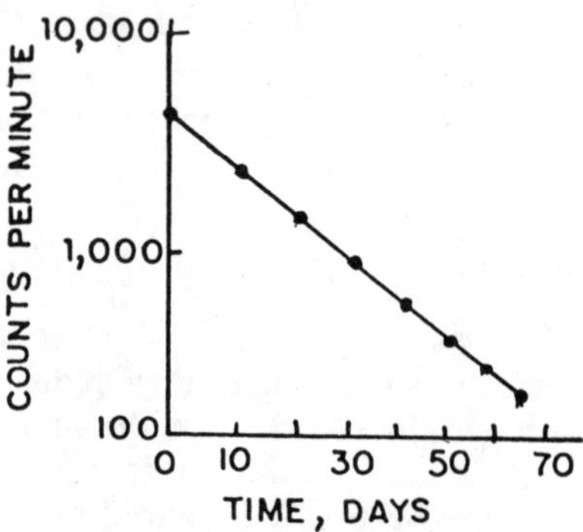

Fig. 23.6. Plot of radioactive decay.

23.8 Application of Nuclear Chemistry

The unstable isotopes play a role as *tracers* when added to a system in the chemical form. The labelled or tagged material moves with a given phase or substance and serves to establish its location and concentration.

Thus, they can be used to study the (i) mechanism of reactions (ii) metabolism of drugs (iii) toxicity of substances, (iv) biosynthesis of natural products.

The radioisotopes have also various medical and agricultural applications and use for general scientific research.

23.9 Measurement and Instrumentation Aspects

The quantitative determination of nuclear radiation is based on the measurement of (i) ionization or (ii) excitation that may be produced during the interaction of the radiation with the bound electrons of a medium.

Since the radioactive disintegration takes place in a random manner and vary in rate and energy with the nature of the substance the detector or the measuring instrument must possess the two characteristics namely; (a) rapid response and (b) sensitivity to small amounts.

The various types of detectors available for measurement of nuclear radiation can differ by following factors :

(i) Window or wall thickness (in mg cm^{-2}) and size.
(ii) Resolution time
(iii) Amplification
(iv) Background counting rate
(v) Efficiency.
(vi) Sensitivity to operating variables like applied voltage, pressure of filling gas, operating life etc.

An instrument commonly used for the detection and measurement of nuclear radiation must comprise the following two parts namely; (i) a detector for converting the energy of radiation into an electrical pulse and an electronic circuit to amplify and record the pulse to able to read it.

The various types of detectors available for the measurement of nuclear radiation can be classified as : (i) Gas ionization dectectors (ii) Scintillation detectors (iii) Solid state detectors.

These are discussed in detail below

23.9.1 Gas Ionization Detectors

The common types of gas ionization detectors available in market are ; (a). Geiger - Muller chamber (b) the proportional counter and (c) ionization chamber. The response of these detectors is based on the process of ionization of a gas by nuclear radiation. The filling gas is ionized along the path of ray or nuclear particle. The total number of ion pairs produced range from 100 to 100,000. An electric potential is applied across the electrodes in the detector which produces the electrons and the positive ions. These ions are separated and collected on electrodes before their recombination can occur and in this way a small electrical pulse is obtained. The current obtained is very small, in the range of 10^{-16} to 10^{-13} amp and it appears in the form of pulses, one pulse from each radioactive particle. A plot of the electric field versus pulse size is shown in the Fig. 23.7. A saturation current is obtained which is related to the number of ion pairs produced per unit time N by the equation i = Ne.

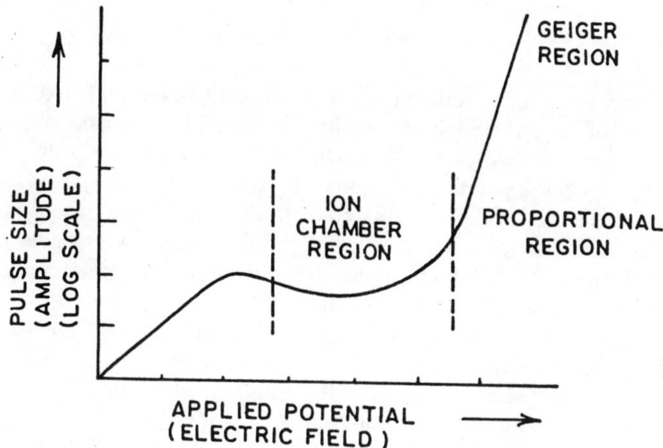

Fig. 23.7. A graph showing size of electrical pulse as function of potential applied between electrodes.

The method is actually based on the electric field gradients employed. To start with without any potential difference there would be no ion pairs or any pulse obtained. When potential between electrodes is increased, ionization is produced. A further increase in potential will not produce any greater pulse and this stage is called ion *chamber region.* When the potential is further increased, secondary ionization by collision with atoms of gas will occur. The pulse size will be larger but proportional to the primary electrons. This is known as the *proportional region.* If the potential difference is made more higher, multiple secondary ionization will occur due to production of secondary electrons. This stage is called *Geiger region.*

A cross section of the fundamental circuit of a gas ionization detector is shown in Fig . 23.8. It consists of a cylindrical cathode and an axial wire anode. The outer cylinder is 1– 2.5 cm in diameter and axial anode wire is 0.1 to 1.0 mm in diameter. All radioactive particles that penetrate the active volume i. e. space between the electrodes are counted. The field strength is inversely proportional to the radius of an electrode of circular cross section. It is high near the axial anode. The voltage gradient near the wire anode is around 1 kv cm^{-1}, therefore the electrons are greatly accelerated before collection on the anode. However, the positive ions experience a much smaller acceleration while moving towards the outer cylinder. They produce a minimum emission of photoelectrons from the cathode, when they strike the cathode.

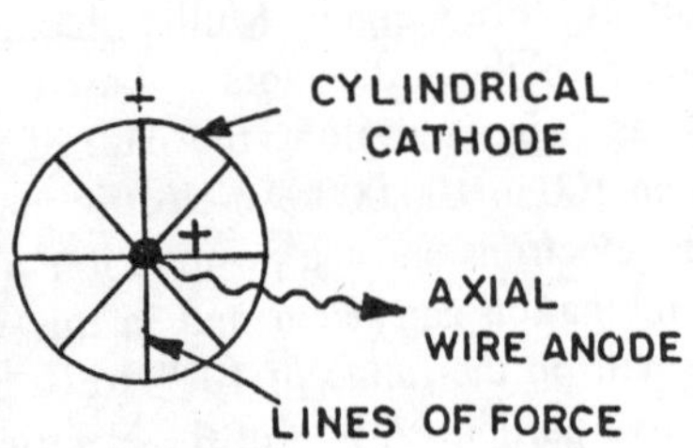

Fig. 23.8a. Cross section of a gas ionization dectector.

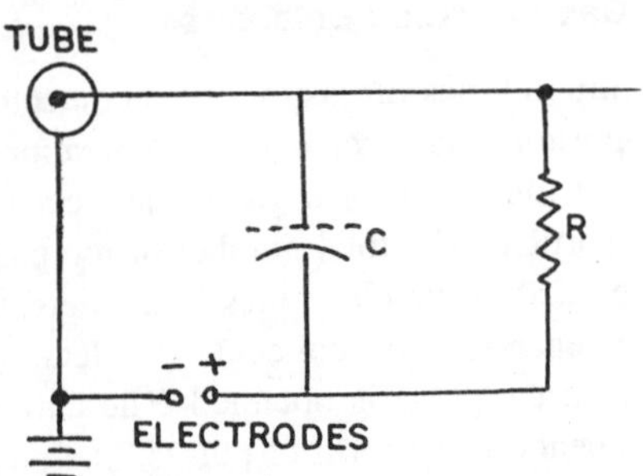

Fig. 23.8b. Fundamental circuit of a gas ionization detector

GEIGER COUNTER

It is also called a Geiger-Muller tube. A diagram showing various elements of Geiger counter is shown in Fig. 23.9.

It consists of two electrodes which are enclosed in a gas-tight envelope filled to a pressure of 80 mm of argon gas and 20 mm of Cl_2, methane or alcohol. The anode consists of a central tugston wire surrounded by cylinder cathode made of copper. A window made of mica, about 2.5 cm in diameter and 2—3 mg cm^{-2} in thickness forms the point for the entry of radioactive particles. When an ionizing particle enters the active volume of Geiger counter, collision with the filling gas produces an ion pair. This is followed by migration of these particles towards the appropriate electrodes under the voltage gradient. Because the mobility of electrons is very high, under the influence of the potential gradient, they acquire sufficient velocity to produce a new ion pair of ions on collision with another atom of argon. under these conditions which are repeated several times each original ionizing particle entering the volume of the counter produces an avalanche of electrons travelling towards central anode. When electrons strike the anode, photons are emitted, and spread the ionization throughout the tube. These produce a continuous discharge which fills the whole of the active volume of the counter in less than a microsecond.

Each discharge builds up to a constant pulse of 1—10 volts. As the pulse size is very large, a simple

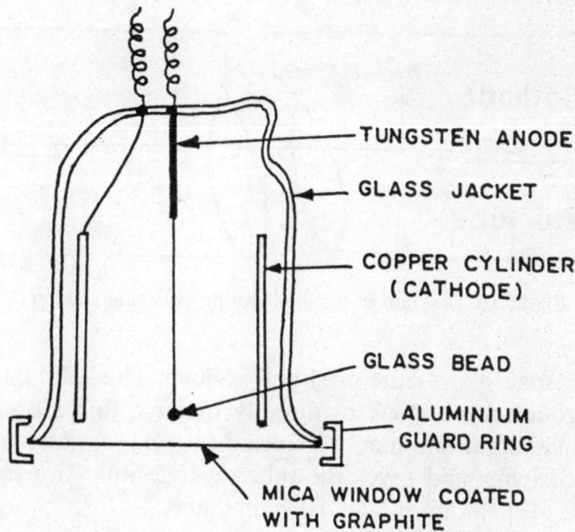

Fig. 23.9. components of a Geiger-muller tube.

circuit is required and the signal can be transmitted directly to a scalar or a rate meter without any amplification.

During the period when the electron avalaunche is collected on the anode, the positive ions being heavier take more time to reach the cathode. This travel time is about 200 μ seconds and thus the positive ions provide a virtual sheath around the anode thereby lowering the potential gradient to a point where the counter remains insensitive to the entry of further ionizing particles. This gives rise to a *dead time* for the counter (200-270 μ seconds).

Since the halogen or organic molecules have a lower ionization potential than orgon, after a few collisions the ions travelling towards the cathode comprises only these ions. These positive ions do not give rise to photons on neutralization at the cathode unlike the argon ions. Consequently photons which could initiate a fresh discharge are prevented from forming and the counter becomes *self quenching*. The filling gas is ultimately exhausted (i. e. quenching agent) on being neutralized at the cathode and therefore the counter life is limited to 10^8 counts. (15000 counts/mint) The advantage with halogen ions is that they do not dissociate, have indefinite life and also the operating voltage is less. The G. M. tube has an-excellent sensitivity for β—particles but for γ—particles it is less sensitive.

23.10 Proportional Counter

The proportional counters have been slowly replacing the Geiger counter as they are more versatile and precise for measurement of radiation. This is because as they are designed for constancy of gas amplification and this amplification is dependent on the energy of the entering radiation. There are three types of designs utilized for proportional counters i. e. (i) closed tube type similar to Geiger counter (ii) a windowless or (iii) thin window flow meter.

The windowless or thin window flow meter is constructed with a 2 π geometry i. e. 50% of radiation emanating from a thin sample enters the active volume. The cathode is hollow hemispherical in shape and an anode in the form of a small loop of wire, which is inserted into the cathode cavity through an insulator. The sample is placed at the centre of the base of the hemisphere. A second hemispherical detector can be positioned at below to obtain a 4π geometry and thus a more reliable counting can be achieved.

The windowless or thin window type of proportional counter contains a continuous stream of counter

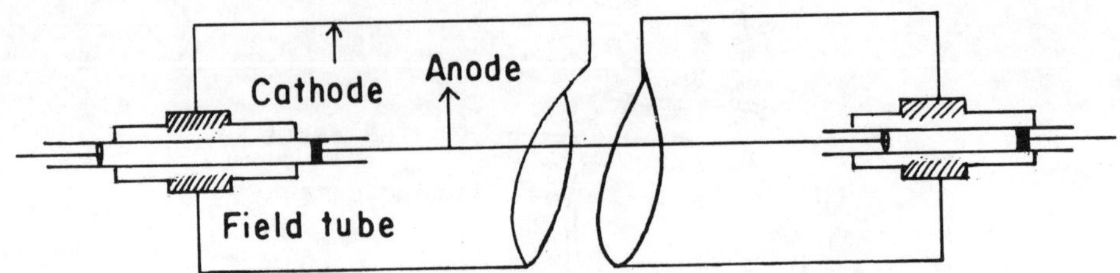

Fig.23.10. Diagram of a cylindrical proportional counter.

gas and is operated at the atmospheric pressure or slightly above. The solid or liquid samples are mounted on a slide and introduced through an air lock or directly under a thin aluminium or aluminium coated plastic film. However, the volatile sample may be carried into the counter on the gas stream. The flow of gas minimizes the effect of leaks and gives the tube an indefinite life time. The filling gas utilized may be methane or a mixture of 90% argon and 10% methane.

In the windowless or thin film proportional counter, the output pulses are small when compared to those from Geiger counter and therefore external amplification to enhance the pulses becomes necessary.

The proportional counter is useful for alpha particle counting as their ionizing power is greater than β—particles.

23.11 Scintillation Counters

Among the various types of counting equipment available for measurement of nuclear radiation, scintillation counter is the best.

The scintillation counter comprises of a scintillator and a multiplier phototube. The scintillator is a crystalline or liquid material that interacts with the entering ionizing particles to produce fluorescent radiation. As the number of photons released per particle is moderate, the output has to be amplified. Therefore, the scintillator is attached to a photocathode face of a multiplier phototube or connected to a Lucite optical coupler which produces a good optical transmission. The scintillator and phototube should be transparent in the optical range of fluorescence i. e. in the near U.V. range. For the detection of α—particles, a very thin (1 mm) layer of transparent phosphor namely, ZnS screen with Ag as an activator is used.

For the measurement of β—particles, a liquid scintillation system is used. The liquid scintillator consists of two components; (i) a solvent e. g. toluene, xylene and (ii) a dissolved phosphor called primary solute or flour (2, 5 — diphenyl oxazole) PPO, [2, 2 – p – phenylene — bis-(5—phenly oxazole)] POPOP, The sample is dissolved in the medium. Single crystals of anthracene, transstilbene and NaI are also used.

Since the measurement of radiation in this method is based on the process of fluorescence, care should be taken to minimize quenching. Quenching will lower the amount of light per pulse

Liquid scintillation system allows the detection of low energy β—particles from isotopes of 14_C and 3_H as it surrounds the sample and offers an easy geometry for their counting.

For the detection of γ—ray, NaI crystals are used as scintillators. Because of high atomic number of iodine, it is efficient in the absorption of γ—rays and thus produces a large output of pulses. But, it has the disadvantage of being (i) hygroscopic, (ii) having a high refractive index (nD 1.8) and (iii) having long resolving time (0.3 μ seconds)

A block diagram showing main components of a scintillator counter are shown in the Fig. 23.11.

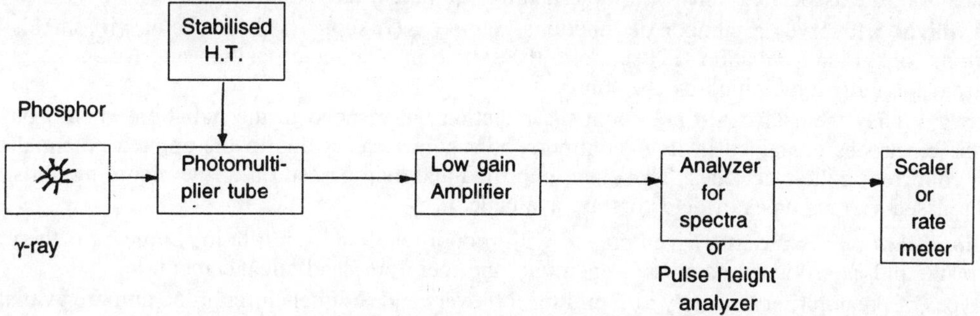

Fig. 23.11. Block diagram of a scintillation counter.

It should be remembered that for the case of a particular phosphor, the number of photons released is proportional to the energy absorbed. usually the crystal is placed in a light tight enclosure of aluminium foil which also serves as a reflector.

NaI transparent single crystals containing 1% thallium (Tl) are used. They have high density and high atomic number and are good for α— and soft β— particle determination.

Zinc sulphide (ZnS) in the form of semi-transparent deposit on a glass flat is useful for α—particle counting but is too thin for β—and γ—radiations.

However, CSI in the form of large transparent thallium can also be used as they have a longer light decay time (~ 10^{-5} seconds) but they are expensive. They are suitable for all types of radiations.

Other types of phosphor like anthracene as a solid solution in a plastic (e. g. polystyrene) or a 2% solution in polystyrene is also suitable for the counting of α, β and γ—ray detection.

The light flash is of the order of 10^{-6} seconds for an inorganic phosphor and 10^{-8} seconds for an organic phosphor.

A schematic diagram for a scintillation counter is shown in the Fig. 23.12 below.

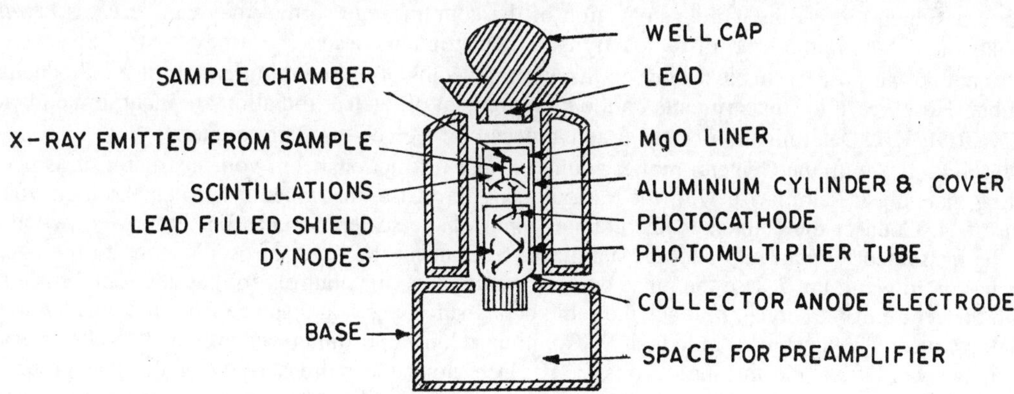

Fig. 23.12. A schematic diagram of a scintillation counnter.

After having discussed individually the various types of equipment available for the measurement of nuclear radiation, the associated units of a the counting equipment are explained below.

Lead Shield : It serves a number of functions, namely : (i) supports the detector, (ii) shields the detector from background radiation (iii) supports the source in a suitable position and (iv) protects the operator from the radiation emitted by the source.

Detector : They themselves do not count the radiation but respond to the radiation when it passes between the electrodes contained in it. A continuous discharge occurs due to the applied potential and pulses are collected at the electrodes. These are amplified and then passed on to the recording units. As already discussed various types of detectors are available.

Pre-amplifiers : They are usually employed with proportional and scintillation counters if the main amplifier or the pulses produced have low sensitivity and therefore need enhancement.

Two types of preamplifiers, namely : (a) emitter followers and (b) quenching probe unit are available.

High Tension Supply : A suitable high voltage supply (HV or EHT) different from the normal mains supply is needed for a detector to respond to the nuclear radiations and this supply must be stabili ed against the fluctuations in the mains supply.

Amplifier : Simple non-linear amplifiers of fixed gain or linear amplifiers of variable gain which have capacity to amplify pulses to the same desired extent and keep the relative pulse sizes constant are generally used for energy measurement.

Discriminator Unit : A discriminator has a function to block the passage of all pulses below the set amplitude and prevent unwanted pulses entering the circuit. Such type of pulses are usually the noise signals and the weak pulses.

Pulse Height Analyzer : It consists of two discrimator units set at different levels and arranged in such a way as to reject all pulses below the level set on lower discriminator and above that on the higher discriminator and therefore pulses with a magnitude between the two levels are allowed to pass into the circuit.

Scalers and Ratemeters : A scaler is a pulse counter and can be attached to a G. M., proportional and scintillation counter. The quantity measured is the number of pulses emitted by the detector in unit time i.e. counts per minute (cpm) or counts per second (cps).

In a ratemeter, an integrating circuit is designed to measure the average counting rate. The output from the integrating circuit is displayed on a meter or passed on to recording unit. Ratemeters are generally designed to give an audible indication of the counting rate so that they can serve as *monitors* in the laboratory giving the level of radioactivity on a continuous basis.

It is not the purpose of this text book to discuss the details of all the requirement of a radiochemical laboratory. However, a few experiments on the measurement of nuclear radiation are incorporated below:

EXERCISE 1. Determination of radio-active decay by Geiger—muller counter.

Method : 1. Set up the Geiger—muller counter as per instructions from your instructor or as per the operating manual. 2. Familiarize with the various controls of the instrument. 3. Keep the high voltage switch off. 4. Connect the counter to the counter input of the scaler. 5. Turn on the power switch and allow the instrument to warm up and get stabilized. 6. Connect the input of oscilloscope to the counter and turn it on to warm up. 7. Use the pulse generator and adjust the controls so that horizontal trace runs through the centre of the screen. 8. Place the radio active substance at a distance from the counter so that a counting rate of 2000 cpm is obtained. 9. Continue taking one minute counts at 25 volts intervals, increasing upward from the threshold voltage. 10. Determine the radio activity of the background by taking five one-minute counts at the mid point of your plateau. 11. Plot on a graph paper the variation of pulse height with voltage and variation of count rate with voltage. 12. Read the dead time for the counter from oscilloscope. 13. Now, adjust the controls such that the count rate is about 200 cpm. 14. Interpret the results and get a statistical accuracy of 1%. 15. Incorporate the background correction.

EXERCISE 2. Determination of γ—radiation by a scintillation counter.

Method: 1. Place the scintillation counter instrument into operation according to the instruction given by instructor or as per operating manual. 2. Receive the source of gamma radiation from your instructor and check that the source selected has a counting rate not more than 1000 cpm. 3. Place the source beneath the end-window Geiger counter. 4. Between the source and the counter insert a 0.5 cm aluminium absorber to eliminate any beta radiation. 5. Turn on the Geiger counter scaler and high voltage to the counter tube. 6. Determine the counting rate of the source and the rate for the background. 7. Now turn on the main power switch of the scintillation counter and keep the photomultiplier tube setting at minimum. 8. Adjust the sensitivity of the scintillation counter and check the background count rate. 10. Now place the radioactive source at the same distance from the scintillation counter as it was from the end window of the Geiger-tube in the previous measurement, and use the 0.5 cm aluminium absorber. 11. Determine the counting rate for the source and also for the background. 12. Vary the photomultiplier tube voltage at different settings and measure the counting rate as a function of applied voltage. 13. Repeat the same step without the source. 14. Interpret your results.

EXERCISE 3. Determination by a Liquid scintillation counter and Isotope dilution technique.

Method : 1. Place the liquid scintillation instrument in operation as per instructions from instructor. 2. Check that the light in both channels are operating and that the setting is on high voltage. 3. Open the deep-freeze unit and check that the sample table is in the unload position. 4. Position a carbon—14 radioactive standard into the sample table and press the load button. Set gate A to 10.0 v, gate B to 50v, and gate C to 100 v. Move the switch under gate C to the left position so that upper gate is operative. Set the switch under gate B to position— 2. The red and green lights should be on between A and B and B and C respectively. Thus the red channel is gated from 10 to 50 v and green channel is gated from 10 to 100v. 5. Turn the high voltage switch to on position, allow for warm up and then set the voltage control on the photomultiplier tube to position-4.6. Check the tube voltages on the control panel, both of them should be at 850 v and the amplifier settings for both channels should be at 1. 7. Now turn from manual to time and set 1 minute time on the clock. Record the one minute count from the red channel. Repeat it four more times. Now, take one 5-minute count and compare the data. 8. The above controls are for carbon—14 determinations and will change for other nuclides. 8. Weigh out 10.0 gm of banzoic acid and dissolve it in 500 ml of hot water. Add to this exact amount of 0.10 gm of labelled benzoic acid. This benzoic acid is labelled with carbon—14 in the carboxyl group and has a specific activity of 10,000 dps/g. 9. Cool the solution after it has been thoroughly mixed. Filter and recover the recrystallized benzoic acid. 10. Repeat the recrystallizations four times until benzoic acid becomes quite pure and is dried. 11. Now accurately weigh 50 mg from this pure, dry benzoic acid and dissolve it in 10.00 ml of scintillator solution (the scintillator solution is prepared form 100 gm naphthalene, 7 gm PPO, 50 gm POPOP in 1 litre of 1, 4-diaxane) in a volumetric flask. 12. Take five 5 gram scintillator bottles and place in them 5.0, 2.00, 1.40, 0.80 and 0.40 ml of the 10.00 ml of pure benzoic acid in scintillator prepared in the previous steps. To earth of the bottles add sufficient scintillator solution so that they are 80 % full. 13. Place each bottle in the scintillation counter and take a ten-minute count for each sample. 14. Plot the graph for counting rate vs concentration. 15. Calculate the percentage of benzoic acid present in the original sample.

SECTION-H
MISCELLANEOUS TYPES OF INSTRUMENTAL METHODS OF ANALYSIS

24

Particle Size Analysis

24.1 General

When dealing with the quality of drugs it should be kept in mind that we are not only concerned with the purity but also with such other properties which may affect its efficacy or safety. The crystal structure and particle size of a drug can influence the absorption and consequently lead differences in toxicity or clinical response. Therefore, a detailed study of the solid state properties of a drug is necessary and comprises the determination of (i) melting point (ii) particle size distribution (iii) rate of solution (iv) equilibrium solubility and (v) polymorphism etc. Among these the particle size distribution and shape of solid will determine the powder flow characteristics and the degree of fineness will affect the physical stability of suspensions. Further more in case of inhalation aerosols, particles above 5 μm are not easily transported to the required sites in the respiratory tract whereas particles below 1 μm are exhaled. The requirement of particle of particle size are essential for proper dissolution of drug substances in general, and for aerosol preparations for deposition in the respiratory tract. The present chapter will deal with methods for the determination of particle size

24.2 Theory

In the case of spherical particle the size of the particle is defined in terms of diameter. On the contrary, powders are difficult to define by means of one parameter alone because of variation in shape from flakes to elongated particles. Generally speaking, size of a particle will depend upon the method of measurement and the conventions adopted in defining particle size. The important principles used in the classification of particles and the corresponding methods of measurement are described the Table 24.1.

Table 24.1. Classification of particles

	Method	Principles of Similarity
1.	Microscopic examination	Geometry
2.	Sieving	" "
3.	Sedimentation	Hydrodynamic
4.	Elutriation	" "
5.	Coulter Counter	Volume
6.	Gas Permeability	Surface properties
7.	Adsorption	" "

So far as spherical particles are concerned the results obtained by the above methods will be same because of their symmetry. On the contrary since the irregular particles cannot be defined in geometrical terms, their volume and surface area cannot be accurately determined. Therefore an irregular particle will be assigned different sizes by the above methods and the discrepancy between the results will increase as the particle departs from the sphericity. But at the same time the size of an irregular particles as measured by the diameter of a sphere that exhibits the same properties as the particles, e.g. sieving refers to particles of imaginary spheres which will pass through sieve apertures while sedimentation refers the particles to spheres of the same density and having same terminal velocity in a particular fluid.

It is also possible to combine the sizes from different methods to give non-dimensional parameters known as "shape factors" which serve to characterise the shape of the particles. The shape factor is mainly the ratio of the mean size of powders obtained from two different methods.

The mean size is calculated on the basis of numbers of particles, weight of particles or surface area of particles.

An average diameter is the arithmetic mean diameter $\bar{d}_n$ defined for two diameters d_1 and d_2 as

$$\bar{d}_n = (d_1 + d_2)/2$$

The numerical mean diameter is defined by

$$\bar{d}_n = \frac{\Sigma n . d}{\Sigma n} \qquad (1)$$

where n is the number of particles with equivalent diameter d.

In some cases surface mean diameter can be employed as

$$\bar{d}_s = \frac{\Sigma n d^3}{\Sigma n d^2} \qquad (2)$$

because the surface area is proportional to nd^2.

The specific surface (i.e. surface area per unit weight) can be calculated from it by the following equation

$$S = \frac{6}{\bar{d}_s \sigma_s} \qquad (3)$$

Where σ_s is the density of the solid, S is the specific surface ($m^2\ Kg^{-1}$) and $\bar{d}_n$ is measured in m. This equation is strictly applicable for spherical or cubical particles.

If the weight of each fraction is noted, then the weight mean diameter is obtained from the equation:

$$\bar{d}_w = \frac{\Sigma nd^4}{\Sigma nd^3} \qquad (4)$$

If the particle density does not vary with particle size then this quantity is identical to the volume mean diameter.

On the other hand the diameter of particle of mean weight is called "mean weight diameter" and is given by the equation :

$$\sqrt[3]{\left(\frac{\Sigma\, nd^2}{\Sigma\, n}\right)}$$

24.3 Apparatus and Methodology

In this chapter one conductivity method using coulter counter which is based on the measurement of volume of particles will be discussed.

A simple diagrammatic model of a coulter counter is shown in the Fig. 24.1.

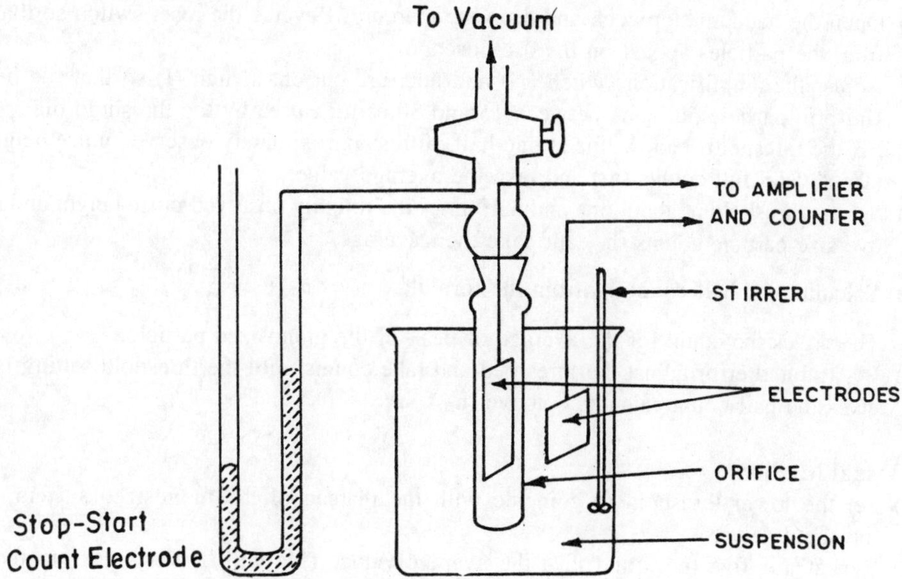

Fig. 24.1. A schematic diagramme of a coulter counter.

The method is based on the change in resistance of a solution of electrolyte produced by the presence of a particle. This is then used to calculate the volume of the particle. A suspension of the substance is placed in the beaker which has electrodes immersed in it. A second electrode is placed in the orifice tube which has a small aperture and is connected to a small vacuum pump via a stop-cock. The suspension flows through the small aperture with particle concentration such that particles travel one at a time. The passage of each particle displaces electrolyte within the aperture momentarily changing the resistance between the electrodes and producing a voltage pulse of magnitude proportional to particle volume.

The vacuum is applied in a controlled manner by opening the stop-cock, the mercury column in the manometer is drawn up the "start-stop count electrodes". When the stop-cock is closed, the mercury column rebalance and allows the suspension through the aperture so that a count can be taken on a known volume of suspension. By actuating the start-stop count electrodes a series of pulses are produced which are amplified and then fed to a threshold circuit which discriminates against particles below and permits to count those which exceed the threshold value. In this manner successive counts at different threshold levels can be obtained. This data can then be used for determining the cumulative frequency over size curve. The diameter of the particle is expressed as the cube root of the particle volume. Before, a new experiment is started it is required to calibrate the instrument by means of a reference powder of known particle size. This is because the instrument constant. will be different for each orifice tube/electrode combination on a particular model of coulter counter. Now-a-days computer based coulter counters are commercially available in various models.

EXERCISE 1. Calibration of the Instrument with a standard sample.

Method : 1. Set up the controls of the instrument as per instructions from the instructor or as per operating manual. 2. For determination of calibration factor k we can follow (a) half-count procedure :

(i) Introduce a few mgms of the mono-sized particles like ragweed pollen or paper mulberry pollen into a 250 ml beaker containing 200 ml of PFE (filtered 1% NaCl solution). Agitate with stirrer to even dispersion so that the size of the particles is between 5% and 20% of aperture diameter.

(ii) Open the vacuum stop cock and drop the mercury. Reverse the reset switch so that the pulses from the particles appear on the oscilloscope

(iii) Adjust the amplification switch (A) and aperture current switch (I) so that the height of the Uniform particle pulses is between 15 and 30 as measured by the threshold dial.

(iv) Fix the threshold shadow line at one-half of this approximately observed pulse height level and take several full counts (n_f) and take the average value.

(v) Set the threshold at about one and half times the roughly observed pulse height and take several oversize-particle counts (n_o) and take their average.

(vi) Calculate the half-count n_m from the formula : $n_m = n_o + \frac{(n_f - n_o)}{2}$

This gives the count for the average of peak of the monosized particle.

(vii) By trial and error adjust the threshold and take counts until the threshold setting is found that gives the half count calculated above (n_m).

(b) Visual Method :

(i) Set the lower threshold to coincide with the plateau of the monosized system. Record the threshold value.

(ii) Repeat this five times and take the average value. This will be very close to the half-count value and can be obtained faster.

(iii) Fill the observations in the tabular form shown below :

Lower Thresh-old Control (t_L)	Aperture current Switch (I)	Amplification control (A)	n_f	n_o	n_m

EXERCISE 2. Determination of the background count (n_o) at the preselected settings of the instrument.

Method : 1. Set up the coulter counter as per instructions from the operating manual or the instructor. Wash 150 ml and 250 ml beakers with distilled water and then rinse with particle free electrolyte (PFE, 1% NaCl). Wash the auxiliary hose inside and outside with distilled water and rinse with PFE. Take about 120 ml of PFE in 150 ml beaker and keep the auxiliary hose submerged in it.

2. Wash the aperture tube, stirrer and electrode with distilled water, rinse with PFE. Take about 200 ml of PFE in 250 ml beaker. Place the beaker on spring plateform so that aperture tube, electrode and stirrer are dipped in solution. None of these should touch the wall of the beaker.

3. Put the vacuum cork to the conical flask.. Connect to mains, and put on the vacuum pump. Open auxiliary and vacuum stop cocks together. Adjust the vacuum regulator carefully so that electrolyte from reservoir is drawn slowly. When electrolyte crosses the vacuum stop cock close both the stop cocks.

4. If the air bubbles are noticed inside he aperture, break the vacuum by removing the cork on the conical flask and open both the stop cocks. Allow the electrolyte to drain. Reconnect the vacuum at the flask and drain the electrolyte into the aperture tube. Close both stop cocks again when level crosses the vacuum stop cock. Repeat the operation till the tube is free from air bubbles.

5. Put the unit on, set the dial as below :

Lower threshold (t_L) at 40; upper threshold (t_U) fully counter clockwise; Amplifier at 64 ; aperture current (I) at 8 and manometer at 500 microlitres. Add a few mgm of sample to PFE in the sample beaker, and place the beaker on the spring platform.

6. Move the reset switch to right and then left so that all the glow-tubes read zero. Now open the vacuum stop-cock slowly. Adjust the vacuum regulator so that mercury cones slowly 1/4" – 1/2" below the start point.

7. When the level of mercury is 1/4" – 1/2" below the start point probe, close the vacuum stop-cock and bring the reset switch to R.H.S. Note the count on digital counter. This is the raw count (n').

8. Take several counts repeating the above step . Average count ($\bar{n}'$ represents the number of particles greater than the size represented by the dial settings (t_L, I, A) in 500 microlitre electrolyte.

9. Repeat the steps 6 to 8 for dial settings (t_L , I, A)

$$V = K.I.A.\ t_L \text{ and } d = 1.241\ \sqrt[3]{v}$$

Calculations :

Standard sample : 19.5 μ Ragweed

t_L = 26.4

I = 1

A = 2

Calibration factor (k) can be calculated as :

$$V = \frac{\pi}{6} d^3 = \frac{\pi}{6} (19.5)^3 \text{ Cu . } \mu = 3.882 \text{Cu } \mu$$

$$V = K \,.\, t_L \,.\, I \,.\, A.$$

$$\frac{\pi}{6}(19.5)^3 = k \,.\, 26.4 \times 1 \times 2$$

or

$$k = \frac{\pi \times (19.5)^3}{6 \times 26.4 \times 1 \times 2} = 73.4$$

Calculation of particle size (d_L) can be done as follows :

say, $t_L = 20, I = 2, A = 64$

$$V_L = k \times t_L \times I \times A = 73.5 \times 20 \times 2 \times 64 = 188,160$$

$$d_L = \sqrt[3]{6V_L} = 1.241 \cdot \sqrt{V_L}$$

$$= 1.241 \sqrt[3]{73.5 \times 20 \times 2 \times 64} = 71.1\ \mu$$

EXERCISE 3. Determination of Particle size of Powdered silica in Aqueous solutions of sodium chloride.

Method : The performance of the above determination involves two steps, (a) familiarisation and calibration and (b) the actual experimental steps. These are described separately below.

(a) Familiarisation run and Calibration of the Apparatus : Three basic calibrations are necessary for a particular aperture/electrolyte combination. These are : (i) Primary coincidence Factor 'P', (ii) aperture current expansion factors 'F' and (iii) calibration Factor "K".

(i) Primary coincidence Factor 'P' : The primary coincidence is defined as the loss of count at a particular threshold setting because of two or more particles entering the aperture simultaneously and being counted as one particle. The count loss n'' is proportional to the square of the observed count according to the equation :

$$n'' = p\left(\frac{\bar{n}}{1000}\right)^2 \qquad (6)$$

Where $\bar{n}$ = average count at each threshold setting.

p = a constant factor dependent on aperture diameter, d, in μm, and manometer volume V, in ml. is given by the equation :

$$p = 2.5\left(\frac{d}{1000}\right)^3\left(\frac{0.5}{V}\right) \qquad (7)$$

The primary coincidence must be kept down to 10% of the instrument count

A relationship between n'' and the instrument count is shown in the Fig 24.2.

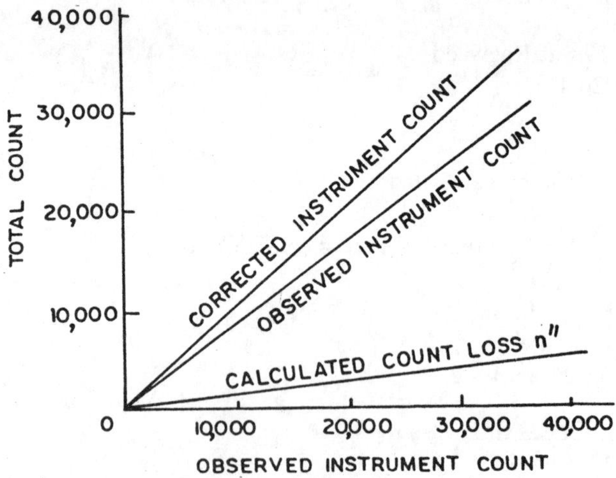

Fig. 24.2 Graph between n'', and instrument count.

(ii) Aperture current Expansion Factors 'F' : To start with, a threshold value is set as the basic scale for particle size counting but when the aperture current is set, it expands the threshold scale by a factor of 2 for each adjacent setting. The aperture current setting measures the amount of resistance introduced into the circuit and then changes the sensitivity of the threshold setting by altering the pulse height produced by each particle.

Tables of aperture current expansion factors are provided with the instrument and one must have the knowledge of resistance between the electrodes and then one can read the values of factors from the tables.

(iii) Calibration Factor 'K' : The *Calibration Factor 'F'* gives the relationship between the equivalent volume diameter and the threshold setting t'. It is represented by the equation :

$$d = k\ \sqrt[3]{(F \cdot t')} \tag{8}$$

Where F is the aperture current expansion factor.

The settings for threshold and aperture current are utilised to show the relationship between d and $\sqrt[3]{F.t'}$.

A common procedures for determining the Calibration Factor is to select monosized particles of known size; e.g. the pollen grains of hazel, which are mostly spherical and mono-sized (20 μm). The particles are dispersed in the electrolyte solution to produce a maximum count with a primary coincidence of 1-2% only. One aperture current setting is chosen and counts are taken at small increments of threshold over the whole range of threshold settings, where the count drop is more care is taken to obtain the maximum count. The threshold settings at 50% counts are read, multiplied by the appropriate aperture current expansion factors F and the value of K is obtained from the equation (8).

On completion of the calibration of the instrument the following experimental steps are adopted for the measurement of the particle size for the given sample.

(i) Prepare 500 ml of 0.9% NaCl solution and clarify the solution by filtration through a NO. 3 sintered filter under gravity or through a membrane filter using reduced pressure. (This step is necessary to reduce the background count to a small proportion. Filtration through No. 3 glass filter is sufficient when using an orifice of 100 μm).

(ii) Fill the orifice tube and the bath (beaker) with filtered vehicle. Start the stirrer and adjust the electrodes.

(iii) Open the vacuum stop-cock slowly and adjust the vacuum in such a way that the mercury in the monometer is drawn the clear of the start - stop electrodes. When the stop-cock is closed the sample is sucked through the orifice and the count is automatically made as the mercury passes the electrodes.

(iv) Prepare a concentrated dispersed suspension of the powder in the vehicle and add a small amount to the beaker. Set the gain index at 3 or 4, Aperture current setting at 10 and Threshold at 10. Read the count and repeat the count using a Threshold of 20. Set the Aperture current at 1 and Threshold at 250 and note the count. If the first two counts are large and one in agreement and the third count is negligibily small, then the orifice/electrolyte is suitable for this particular sample powder because all the particles have been taken into account.

(v) Now, rinse the beaker of suspension and rinse the aperture tube with fresh vehicle. Determine the background count of the vehicle in a clean beaker by setting the Aperture current and Threshold to obtain the maximum count as described in the step 4. Change the Aperture current and Threshold and determine counts for larger size particles. Repeat each count.

(vi) Calculate the values of equivalent diameters to correspond to the settings chosen using equation eq. (8).

(vii) Calculate the coincidence corrections to obtain the maximum count. This count should not exceed for the combination of orifice and manometer volume used.

(viii) Add more of concentrated suspension of powder to the vehicle until maximum count is slightly less than the permissible maximum count.

(ix) Count at same Aperture current and threshold settings as used for the background counting. Repeat each count twice.

(x) Check the orifice and make sure it does not become obstructed.

(xi) Calculate the results by deducting the background count and addition of count loss values and obtain a cummulative percentage oversize plot by number and by weight.

The procedure described above is appropriate for water-insoluble powders that disperse quickly in aqueous solution of sodium chloride. A small quantity of surface active agent is usually added to ensure adequate dispersion. Orifice tubes with diameters between 2 to 40% of their own diameter.

Since different models of coulter counter are commercially available their instruction and operating manual must be followed.

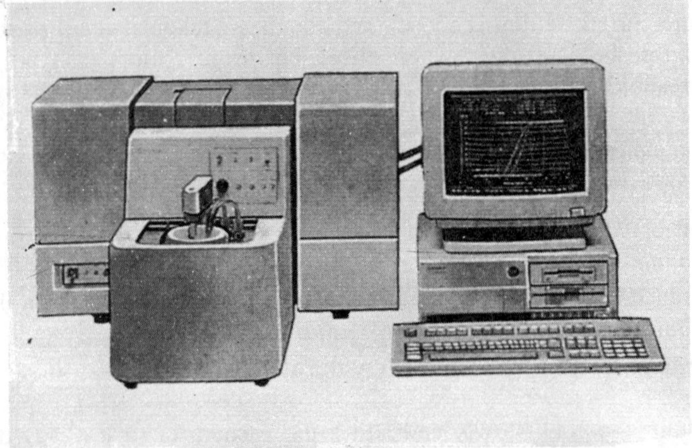

Sald 2001 Laser Diffraction Particle Size Analyzer
(Courtesy Shimadzu)

25

Differential Thermal Analysis And Differential Scanning Calorimetry

25.1 General

As pointed out in the previous chapter, the crystal form of a drug substance may influence the rate and extent of absorption and this may he reflected in terms of differences in clinical response or toxicity. The rate of solution of a solid is directly proportional to the exposed surface area and may be determined by the crystal form. A crystalline drug compound may exist in different but chemically identical forms which are called polymorphs. When the different forms of crystals arise due to inclusion of small amounts of solvent of crystallisation they are called pseudopolymorphs. The method of recrystallisation, isolation, drying and finally grinding of the drug compound may alter the form in which it exists in the dosage form. The crystalline forms of drugs, oils, fats, waxes and polymers show the property of polymorphism. The differences in the properties in the crystal forms can be studied by the procedures called ''differential thermal analysis'' (DTA) and ''differential scanning calorimetry'' (DSC).

In general, thermal analysis involves the study of temperature and rate at which materials undergo physical and chemical transitions as they are heated and cooled and changes in the weight and energy. Heat is used as the reagent and a substance taken through a wide range of temperatures.

25.2 Components of A Differential Thermal Analyzer and Methodology

A diagrammatic sketch of a common type of differential thermal analyzer is shown in Fig. 25.1.

The equipment consists of a furnace which contains a sample block having identical and symmetrically placed chambers. Each chamber contains a thermocouple positioned in the chamber and a reference material generally alumina (α — Al_2O_3) is placed in the other. The furnace and the sample

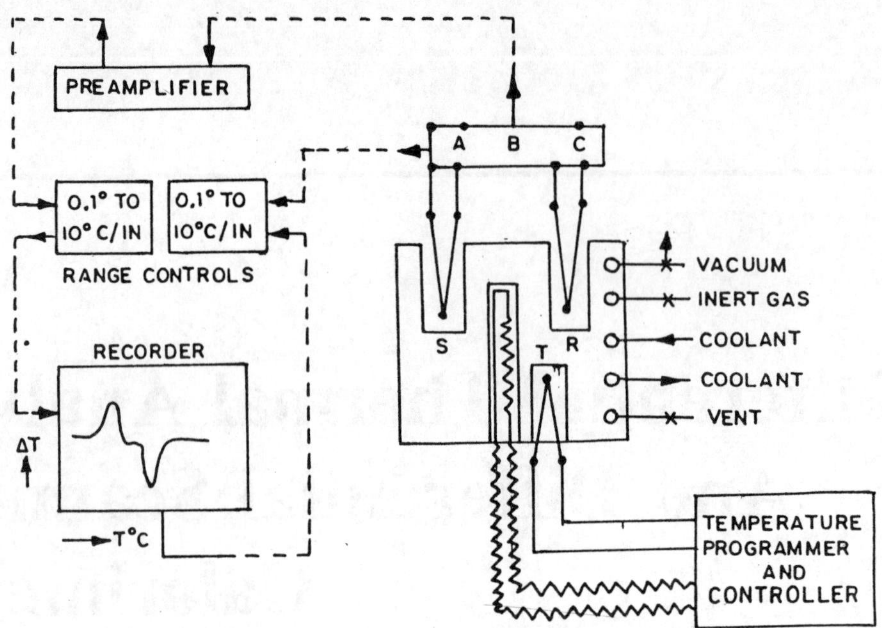

Fig. 25.1. Schematic diagram of differential Thermal Analyzer.

block are then heated at a linear rate say, 5° to 12° per minute by increasing the voltage through the heated element of a motor driven variable transformer or by a thermocouple — actuated feed back type of controller. The difference in temperature between sample and reference (i.e $T_S—T_R=\Delta T$) thermocouples which are connected in series — opposition is measured in a continuous manner. The signals obtained in micro-volt level are amplified by a d c amplifier. The difference signal is recorded on the y — axis of the millivolt recorder. The temperature of the furnace is measured by a separate thermocouple connected to the X — axis of the recorder. A typical DTA curve is shown in the Fig. 25.2. The points C and F are the temperature maxima and represent the melting points of the substance. The record is made of the temperature difference (Δ T) between the sample and a reference material against time or temperature as the two specimens are subjected to identical temperature regimes being heated or cooled at a controlled rate.

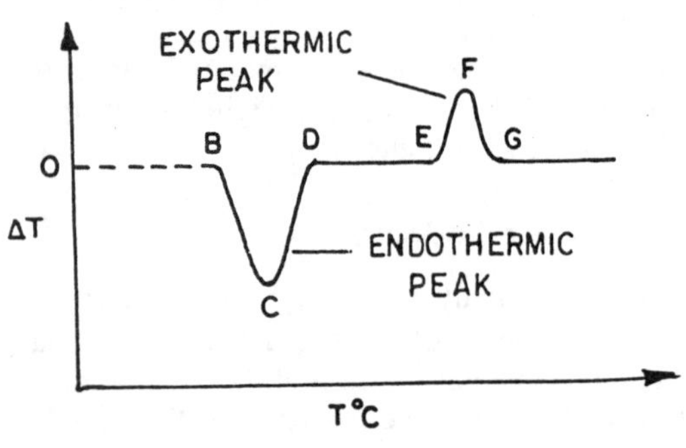

Fig. 25.2 A typical DTA curve.

The samples which can be investigated by DTA and DSC comprise powders, fibers, single crystals, polymer films, hydrated solids etc. Most of the commercial instruments have facilities for performing experiments under reduced pressure or in inert atmospheres.

25.3 Quantitative Aspects of DTA

The equation which can be utilized for determining the area under Δ T — time curve is following :

$$\frac{m\Delta H}{g\lambda_S} = \int_{t_1}^{t_2} \Delta T \, . \, dt \qquad \text{......(1)}$$

Where m is the mass in g; ΔH is the enthalpy change per g of substance; g is a constant dealing with the effect of geometry of the sample arrangement and construction on heat transfer; λ_s is the coefficient of thermal conductivity of the sample.

If A is the peak area, $\Delta H = A/K$ where $K = g\lambda_s /m$ and is temperature dependent. K should be determined over a range of temperature by using indium, tin and lead.

The factors which can affect the results in DTA are following; (i) sample weight, (ii) particle size, (iii) heating rate, (iv) atmospheric conditions surrounding the sample (v) conditions of sample packing into dishes. In general, the instrumental differences and operating condition are such that the consistancy of temperature measurement is around, ± 5 to 6° but can be improved up to ± 2.5°. So in order to achieve accuracy in recording temperature, calibration materials have to be used over a range of temperatures.

25.4 Differential Scanning Calorimetry

25.4.1 General

In this case the sample and the reference materials are heated separately. The sample and the reference temperatures are monitered separately and continuously maintained at the same level. When the sample absorbs and evolves energy, more or less power is required by the sample to allow it to be maintained at the same temperature as the reference. This differential power is recorded as a function of temperature and the peak area represents the energy of the transition. A characteristic DSC curve or a thermogram is plotted between heat flow (Cal. or J Se^{-1}) and temperature (K°) and is shown in Fig. 25.3.

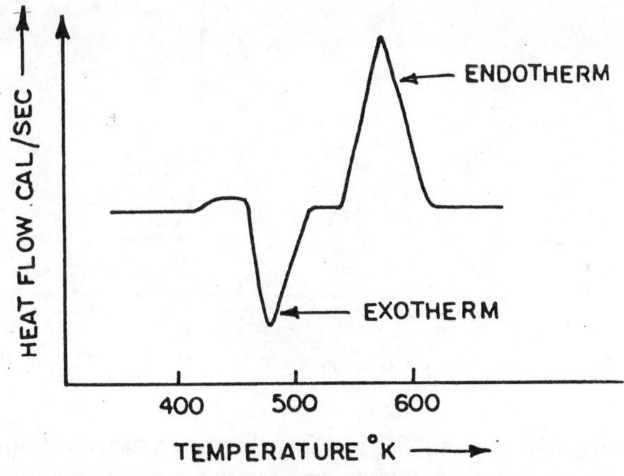

Fig. 25.3. DSC Thermogram.

A schematic representation of sample holders, sensors and heaters of a differential scanning calorimeter is shown in Fig. 25.4. Isothermal conditions i.e. $T_S = T_R$ are obtained by placing a platinum resistance thermometer in the sample with an identical sensor in the reference holder. The continuous and automatic adjustment of heater power i.e. energy per unit time produces a varying electrical signal. What is recorded is not ΔT, but heat flow into the sample to maintain isothermal conditions. Because phase changes occur in the sample during heating and cooling DSC can be used to detect polymorphic changes. Specific heats, heats of fusion, heats of dehydration and decomposition of samples can also be determined. Since the presence of impurity in a sample will affect the melting behaviour and therefore the shape of the thermogram, DSC can be used to assess the purity of substances especially those which are of high purity e.g. a DSC curve of carnauba wax (Fig. 25.5) shows three main peaks at 64°, 78° and 84°C.

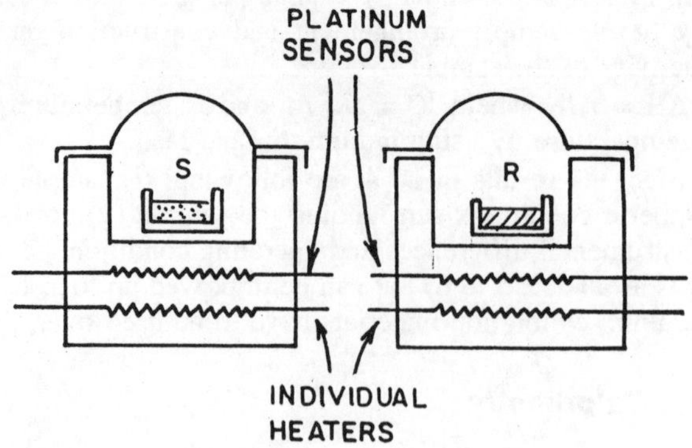

Fig. 25.4. Components for Differential scanning calorimetry.

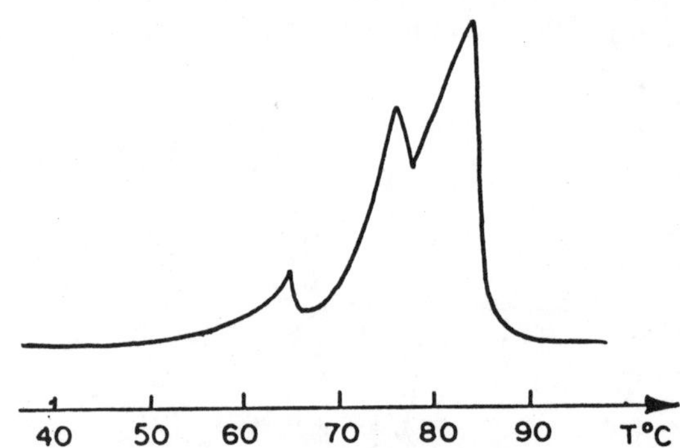

Fig. 25.5. DSC curve for carnauba Wax; Peaks at 64°, 78°, & 84°C; rate 10°/mint.

In general, each substance will give a DSC or DTA thermogram whose number, shape and position of various endothermic and exothermic features serve as a means of qualitative identification of the substance. When an endothermic change occurs the sample temperaure lags behind the reference temperature.. On the thermogram, the initiation point for a phase change or chemical reaction is the point at which the curve first deviates from baseline. When the transition is complete thermal diffusion brings the sample back to equilibrium quickly. The peak or minimum temperature indicates the temperature at which the reaction is completed. If the break is not sharp, a reproducible point can be obtained by drawing one line tangent to the baseline and another tangent to the initial slope of the curve.

A DSC thermogram of a hypothetical substance is shown in the Fig. 25.6. A broad endotherm indicates a slow change in heat capacity. A baseline shift i.e. T_1 denotes a decrease in order within the system or a second order transition. Sharp endotherms i.e. T_3 indicates crystalline rearrangement, fusion or solid-state transitions. Broader endotherms i.e. T_2 show behaviour like dehydration, temperature — dependent phase behaviour, or melting. Exothermic behaviour is associated with the decrease in enthalpy of a phase or chemical system. Narrow exotherms indicate crystallisation or ordering of a metastable system. Broad exotherms denote chemical reactions, polymerisation or curing of thermosetting resins.

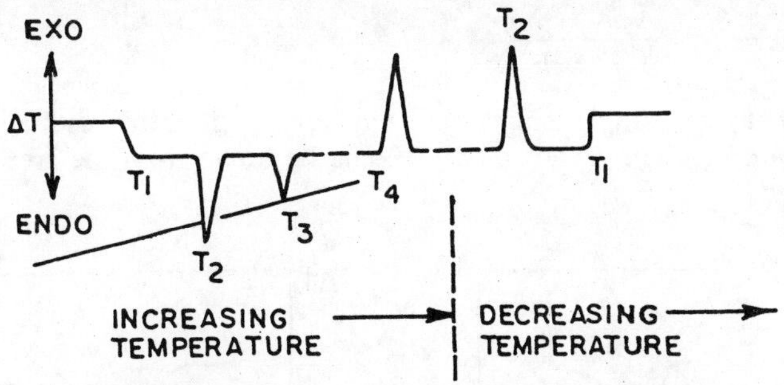

Fig. 25.6. DSC thermogram for a hypothetical substance.

25.4.2. Quantitative Aspects of DSC

Generally speaking, the presence of small amounts of an impurity in a substance will broaden its melting range and consequently lower the melting point by an amount of Δ T. The relationship between Δ T and the mole fraction (x_2) of the impurity is given by the Van't Hoffs equation shown below.

$$\Delta T = \frac{RT_0^2 X_2}{\Delta H_f} \qquad .....(2)$$

Where ΔH_f is the heat of fusion of the sample (J/mole).

T_0 is the melting point of the pure sample (^{0}K).

T_m is the melting point of the sample,

and $\Delta T = T_0 - T_m$.

By means of DSC, the thermal energy per unit of time i.e. dq/dt which is transferred to or from a sample as the sample holder is heated at a linear rate, dT/Dt is measured.

$$\therefore \quad \frac{dg}{dt} = \frac{dT}{dt} = \frac{dq}{dT} \qquad ....(3)$$

where dT/dt is the proportionality constant.

As per eq. (2) the melting point depression is directly proportional to X_2, the fraction of sample melting at any temperature T_s will be given by :

$$f = \frac{(T_o - T_m)}{(T_o - T_s)} \qquad ...... (4)$$

$$\text{But as } (T_o - T_m) = \Delta T = \frac{R T_0^2 X_2}{\Delta H_f}$$

$$\therefore \quad f = \frac{R T_0^2 X_z}{\Delta H_f(T_o - T_s)} \qquad ....(5)$$

$$\text{where } f = \frac{q}{\Delta q}$$

The aim is to find the percentage of sample that has melted at various temperatures and therefore the eq. (5) can be rearranged to :

$$T_s = T_o - \frac{1}{f}\,\frac{R\,T_o^2\,X_2}{\Delta H_f}. \qquad \text{....(6)}$$

If we plot a graph between sample temperature and 1/f, a straight line with a slope equal to — $RT_o^2 X_2/\Delta H_f$ and an intercept of T_o will be obtained. ΔH_f can be found from the area under the DSC curve and X_2 can be calculated.

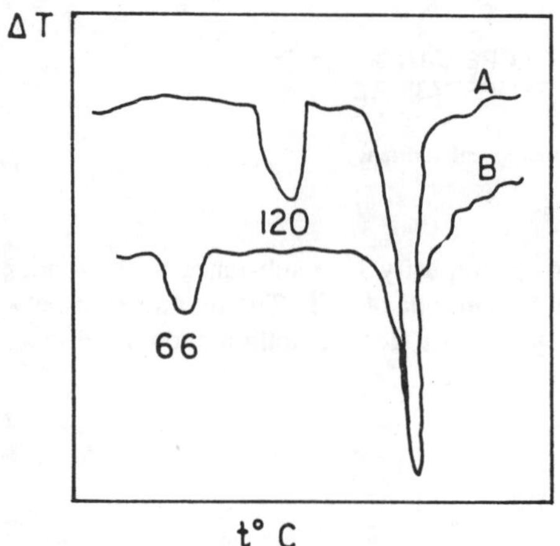

Fig. 25.7. DTA curve for sulphamonomethoxine; A in air at atmospheric pressure, B in Vacuo..

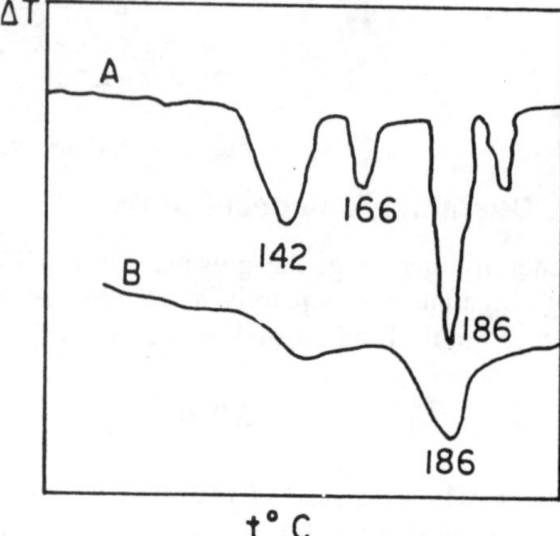

Fig. 25.8. DTA curve for Triamicinolone diacetate; A before drying B after drying.

25.4.3 Uses

Differential scanning calorimetry has a value for estimating the purity of drugs and pharmaceuticals. The basis for purity determination of DSC is that the melting of compound is of Ist order transition involving a characteristic heat of fusion and occuring at a characteristic temperature. The melting transition of a perfectly crystalline compound should therefore be infinitely sharp. The presence of impurity or of defects in crystal lattice broadens the melting range and lowers the final melting point.

EXERCISE 1. Familiarisation run and calibration of DTA/DSC.

As different models of DTA/DSC are commercially available operating manuals should be strictly followed.

Method: Weigh about 2—10 mg of sample and reference substances and place them in the corresponding dishes. Position the dishes in the sample chamber of the instrument and check that there is no contact between the two dishes. Ensure a satisfactory contact between the pan and the baseplate. Turn on the heater and allow the system to equilibrate for 5—10 min. Adjust the recorder and the baseline. Start the heating programme and record the DTA or DSC curve. A heating rate of 10°/min is generally sufficient. The instrument is calibrated with a reference material like indium or alumina which is heated from ambient to 100°C above the melting point of the sample substance. Thereafter in order to investigate the effects of rate of heating on the DTA or DSC curve, identical quantities of benzoic acid should be investigated at 2°. 10° and 25°C/min from ambient to 200°C.

EXERCISE 2. Determination of crystalline transition temperatures of Potassium Nitrate by DTA or DSC.

Method : As described in the previous experiment calibrate the instrument before a run is made with the unknown sample. Place the weighed sample in the sample chamber. Heat at 10°C/min at a temperature range form ambient to 350°C. After the temperature has touched 350°C, allow the sample chamber to cool to about 100°C and then repeat the run by heating up to 400°C. Read the peak melting temperature and compare with the literature. Note the crystalline transition temperature and observe the effect of cooling and reheating cycle.

EXERCISE 3. Demonstration of polymorphism in Triamicinolone by DTA or DSC.

It has been reported that triamicinolone exists in two forms, A and B. Form A is obtained by recrystallisation of triamicinolone from 60% aqueous isopropanol. Form B is obtained by recrystallisation from a mixture of dimethylformamide and water.

Method: Use samples of Form A and Form B and heat the instrument from ambient to 350°C. Now use a new sample of form A and heat up to 270° and then cool to ambient. Start again the cycle to 350 °C and compare the curve with previous one's. The most favoured form of the compound is the form to which the melt reverts on heating and cooling.

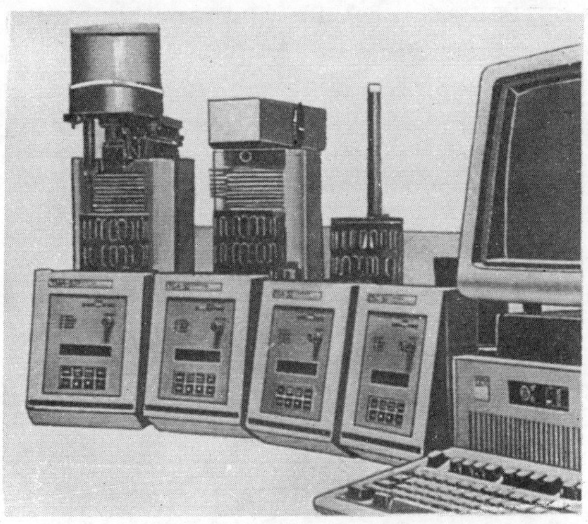

Fig. 25.9 Differential thermal Analyser Model — DTA-50 (Courtesy of Shimadzu)

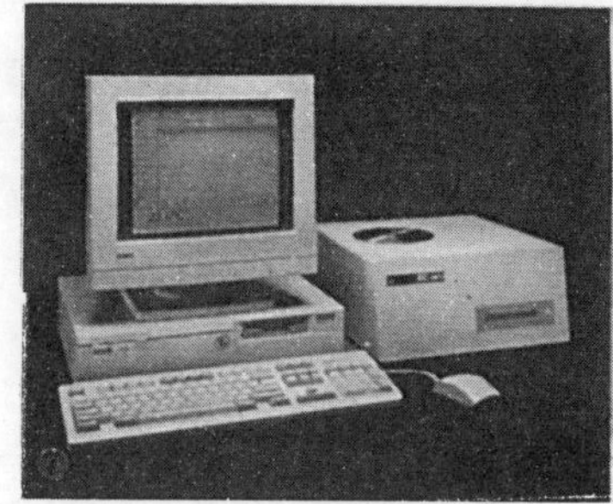

Fig. 25.10 Differential scanning calorimeter, Model — Heat Flux DSC6 (Courtesy of Perkin Elmer)

Appendices

Appendix –1

Results and Errors in Analysis

General

To be a successful analyst and quality control expert in the area of pharmaceuticals and drugs, one should not only possess fundamental knowledge on classical methods and instruments but also possess practical skills in executing such procedures and also be able to interpret the results or the data. The analyst should know the reactions on which a particular analysis is based or what is happening during an analysis. Similarly, he should understand the functional and operational working of the instruments and how to interpret the spectral data or elucidate the structure of molecules. Besides, an analyst should acquire patience and accuracy.

Drug Standards

The technology of drug standardization has undergone a remarkable change during the last two decades. Chemical analysis although has attained new levels of precision and sensitivity but inspite of its simplicity has given way to instrumental methods of analysis. There are also improvements in the techniques of isolation as well as refinements in the quantitation and thus instrumental measurements are replacing classical methods of analysis.

Honesty

As far as analytical and quality control work is concerned one should remember that absolute honesty is needed for controlling the purity and strength of substances used as medicaments. Every effort must be made to maintain accuracy and precision during the course of analysis and a full confidence must be established for interpretation of spectral data.

Source of Errors

Generally speaking it is observed that the numerical data obtained in quantitative determinations is subject to errors. Sometime it is difficult to obtain the same measurements when performed under identical conditions.

The errors can be classed into two types as (i) indeterminate or random errors and (ii) determinate errors. The indeterminate errors are errors which are beyond the control of the observer. Such type of errors are like fluctuations in temperature and pressure, inability to read marked divisions on a burets or pipette, general fatigue of the eyes and differences in individual judgement and skill of the analyst.

On the contrary determinate errors are errors that remain in a constant way and to a fixed degree in each of the determinations. Their nature and magnitude is such that they can be either eliminated or reduced. They include : (i) personal errors like inability to read colour change, faulty procedure, improper selection of indicators etc. (ii) instrumental errors like faulty balances, inaccurate pipetts or burets, incorrect weights etc. such types of errors can be detected and corrected.

Precision and Accuracy

The term "Precision" when applied to a numerical result means the degree of agreement between it and other values obtained under similar conditions. In pharmaceutical analysis there should be a high degree of agreement between the independently obtained results and therefore precision serves as a check on the values. On the other hand the term "accuracy" of a numerical result indicates the degree of agreement between it and the true value. In actual practice the "true value" of a determination is only known within certain limits therefore the accuracy will be known within those limits. This can be further elaborated by saying that in duplicate determinations there may be very close agreement between the two results but they may be far from the true value because an error of same magnitude is involved in each of the separate determinations performed. Hence in a quantitative result there may be a high degree of "precision" but not a high degree of "accuracy". If two different methods of analysis are followed and the results

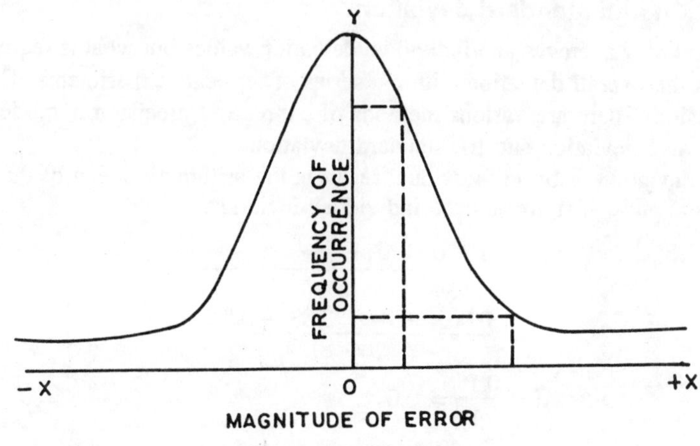

Fig. 1A. Probability Curve.

obtained are in close agreement the reliability of the results is very high.

Experimental Errors and Their Calculation

In order to recognize errors and to minimize their effect upon the final result the analyst must perform each determination a number of times either in triplicate or quadriplicate. The results from these repeated experiments are then combined to yield the final result for the determination. Statistical methods are applied to interpret these repeated experiments.

Average: The term average is understood as a measure of central tendency. It is also called arithmetic mean. It is obtained by adding replicate results and dividing by the number of those results.

Let us consider the following four results of the estimation of iron in an ore sample.

22.64 %
22.54 %
22.61 %
22.53 %

Sum = 90.32 %

The sum of the four determinations = 90.32 %. The arithmatic mean (x) or average is $\frac{90.32}{4}$ = 22.58 %

Deviation: Although average is important, but it does not indicate all the information which can be derived from a series of numerical results. The variation of a single value from the average is expressed as the difference between the two and this differences is termed as "deviation". If X_1, X_2, X_3 etc. represent various numerical values and X represents the arithmetic mean the several deviations (d_1, d_2, d_3 etc.) are represented as

$d_1 = X_1 - X$ (22.64 - 22.58) = + 0.06
$d_2 = X_2 - X$ (22.54 - 22.58) = – 0.04
$d_3 = X_3 - X$ (22.61 - 22.58) = – 0.03
$d_4 = X_4 - X$ (22.53 - 22.58) = – 0.05

The deviation is positive if the one experimental value is greater than the arithmetic mean and negative if arithmetic mean is greater. The algebraic sum of all the deviations in a set must equal zero.

Average deviation and standard deviation

It is not enough to know averages and individual deviation values but what is required is a single number that can represent the overall deviation within a series of replicate experiments. This overall deviation is actually the precision. There are various methods of expressing precision numerically, the two common ones are : (i). average deviation and (ii) standard deviation.

The average deviation, $\bar{d}$ of an individual result is the arithmetic mean of the individual deviations, disregarding the (+) and (–) signs on each individual deviation.

$$\bar{d} = \frac{d_1 + d_2 + d_3 + \text{-------}}{n}$$

$$= \frac{0.06 + 0.04 + 0.03 + 0.5}{4}$$

$$\bar{d} = \frac{0.18}{4} = 0.04$$

$$\text{Relative average deviation} = \frac{\bar{d}}{X} \times 1000$$

$$= \frac{0.04}{22.58} \times 1000 = 1.77$$

The standard deviation, S, of an individual result is the square root of the arithmetic mean of the squares of the individual deviations.

$$S = \sqrt{\frac{d_1^2 + d_2^2 + d_3^2 + d_4^2}{n - 1}}$$

$$= \sqrt{\frac{0.0036 + 0.0016 + 0.0009 + 0.0025}{4-1}}$$

$$= \sqrt{\frac{0.0086}{3}}$$

$$= 0.05$$

The relative standard deviation also called coefficient of variation is obtained by dividing the standard deviation by the mean and multiplying by 100.

$$\text{Relative standard deviation} = \frac{S}{x} \times 100$$

$$= \frac{0.05}{22.58} \times 100 = 0.22$$

The curve shown in the Fig. 1 represents the normal distribution of errors or deviations in a large number of runs for a determination. It is to be noted that small deviations are much more frequent than large deviations.

The curve also reveal that 68% of the X values fall within the range of X ± S, 95% within the range X ± 2S, and 99% within the range X ± 2.55.

Further, it is to be clearly understood that an analyst can never know with absolute certainly whether his arithmetic mean is the absolutely correct value unless he performs a large number of experiments. However, even with few determinations it is possible to specify a range of values centered upon the arithmetic mean and state that there is a 50-50 chance, 95 chances out of 100, 99 chances out of 100 that the true value lies within that range. That means, one can know and specify that the true value lies within a given range. This range can be indicated in terms of arithmetic mean and standard deviation. This range is termed "Confidence limit" and the likelihood that the true value lies within that range is called "probability".

Comparison of Averages: The aspect of comparison of average is of importance in statistics and helps in the interpretation of data on analytical experiments. The method is called the "t test" for comparing averages. It is represented by the formula shown below:

$$t = \frac{X - Y}{S}\sqrt{\frac{nm}{n + m}}$$

where X and Y are two averages, m and n are number of individual values averaged to obtain X and Y respectively.

- S is the overall standard deviation. X is taken as larger average Y is taken as smaller average.

Example : In an analysis on a particular sample four gravimetric estimations yielded the arithmetic mean of 20.44% and four volumetric determinations yielded the arithmetic mean of 20.54%. The standard deviation in both the case was 0.08. The question arises, are the results obtained in the gravimetric and volumetric methods different. The answer is obtained by using the t test formula :

$$t = \frac{X - Y}{S}\sqrt{\frac{nm}{n + m}}$$

$$t = \frac{20.54 - 20.44}{0.08}\sqrt{\frac{4 \times 4}{4 + 4}} = 1.77$$

The critical t values at 95% and 99% probability are found using the degree of freedom, (n + m - 2)

If an observed or calculated t exceeds the indicated critical t value the chances are 95 out of 100 or 99 out of 100 that the averages are significantly different.

Appendix 2

Electronics and Electrical Terminology

It is not the purpose of this text book to deal with electronics and devote a separate chapter on this subject. However, since these days a large number of analytical instruments contain integrated circuits, microprocessors and are also interfaced with personal computers, it becomes necessary that we should possess a preliminary or basic knowledge of electronics and computing capability. Therefore, these two aspects are being covered very briefly and that too in the form of terminology

Ampere (amp. A or I) : is a measure of the amount of electricity actually being drawn from the supply line i.e. it is the unit of current, gives rate per unit of time (1 ampere = 1 coulomb per second).

Ammeter : is a device to measure large currents in amperes. Similar to galvanometer equiped with a range selector permitting the measurement.

A.C. : A current that changes direction many times every second.

Analog Signals : Normally the signals processed by the electronic circuits are analog in nature i.e. they are permitted to assume any value over a wide range that will be limited only by the properties of the electronic devices involved.

Capacitor : Device used to store current in circuits. It has two metal surfaces separated by an insulator. One metal surface becomes positiviely charged and other negatively when it is connected to a battery.

D.C. : The flow of current with a fixed direction, e.g. a dry cell provides direct current because electron flow is always from one specific pole (electrode).

Diode : A valve which has two electrodes and electrons flow only from cathod to anode i.e. in only one direction.

Digital signals : These signals are operated with values restricted to two levels i.e. On and OFF. The two values usually used are 0 and 5V respectively. Digital signals are used to opearate computers which will not respond to intermediate levels like + 2 V, a negative voltage or a positive larger than + 5 V.

Electronics : It is simply the accurate control of electric currents using devices like transistors, resistors and capacitors.

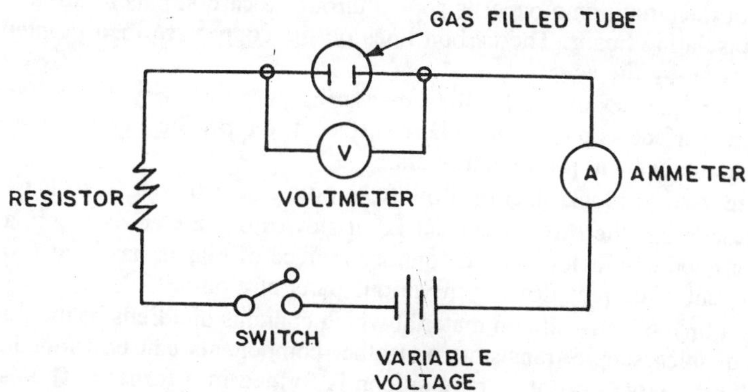

Fig. 2A.1. A Circuit diagram

Electric current : The overall flow of electrons from the negative end of the wire to the positive end. The process is repreated continuously along the wire.

Galvanometer : A device used to detect small amounts of current flow.

Impedance : This is the total resistance to current flow in A.C. circuits. It includes resistance due to resistors, capacitors and inductance. The unit is in ohms.

Imductance : It is the resistance to change in the amount of current flowing through a wire. It is usually achieved by placing a coil of wire in the circuit. The unit is Henry.

Interdomain Convertors : These are circuits and devices that are used to change digital to analog (D/A) signal and analog to a digital (A/D) signal. They usually consist of a binary counter, a converter, flip-plops and other components.

Light Emitting Diode (LED) : They glow like tiny bulbs when current passes through them. They are used to display letters as well as numbers.

Liquid crystals : The liquid crystals are made up of molecules. The arrangement of the molecules can be changed by electricity, altering the crystals shape. A liquid crystal display contains a number of these crystals, usually one for each segment. When there is no current passing through them, the crystals are twisted. Light from the display window passes through a transparent electrode and a polarizing sheet, which directs the light to the crystals.

Logic Gates : A gate is a device that controls the passage of a signal. There are three basic types, called AND, OR and INVERT. Their actions, are described by means of truth tables which give the output. The gates could be made up of one or two transistors and some ancillary components, but are genearally fabricated as ICs. The two widely used gates are (i) transistor-transistor logic (TTL) and complementary metal oxide semiconductor (CMOS).

Ohms (R) : is the degree of resistance to the flow of current or amount of resistance to electrical flow (I = V/R)

Operational Amplifiers : These devices have ability to perform mathematical operations when a signal is sent over to them. Thus external connections are provided to them so that the output voltage will be (i) algebric sum of two or more input voltages, (ii) product of a voltage and a constant factor, (iii) time integral of the input and (iv) time derivative of the input. Other mathematical functions like taking logarithms, squaring etc. can also be perfomed by the use of other components which can be hooked on to the amplifiers.

Oscilloscope : A measuring instrument that provides a visual image of electronic signals on a screen.

Printed ciruit : It consists of a network of copper strips attached to a board. In order to make a printed circuit, a plan of the circuit on a paper is copied through a carbon paper onto a clean copper plate which is glued to an insulating board. The carbon lines on the copper are then pointed with a material that will not be eaten away by the acid.

Photo Cells : They are devices useful for light-measuring purpose. They can be fabricated on a thin wafer of silicon with one surface as p type and othere surface as n type. Such cells act as photoconductive devices e.g. vacuum phototubes and photomultipliers.

Rictifier : A device used to block electron flow from pole converting A.C. to D.C.

Resistor : A resistor resists the flow of current i.e. it slowns down electrons. e.g. a piece of Cu has low resistance and is a good conductor, on the contrary a piece of plastic has high resistance. They are used to control the amount of current flowing in various parts of a circuit.

Silicon chip : It is a tiny silice of silicon material which contains hundreds or thousands of electronic components. Circuits of microscopic transistors and other components can be formed directly onto the surface of a silicon chip. A large crystal of pure silicon is formed in a furnace. This is then sliced into thin wafers which are made smooth or polished. The pattern of circuits are designed and these are printed onto the wafer and impurities are also added. The final wafer is cut into chips. The chips are fixed with fine wires to metal contacts which carry current to and from the chips.

Sine-Wave Oscillator : It is a source of alternating current.

Servo mechanisms : It is a device used whenever a mechanical effect has to be made proportinal to a varying signal. For example the control of slit width in spectrophotometers, where the beam of radiation passing through the reference cuvet serves as the signal to maintain the transmitted energy constant as the spectrum is scanned. Similarly, in case of a strip-chart recorder it is used in self-balacing the recording pen. It consists of a small motor, either dc or two phase ac, controlled in speed and direction by a amplifier.

Transformer : A device used to increase (step-up) or decrease (step-down) the voltage.

Thermoionic Valve : A device which works by passing a stream of electrons from negative electrode (heated cathode) to a positive electrode (anode).

Triode : It is like a diode but also contains a third electrode called the grid. Therefore it can be used to smitch the flow of current off or on in a circuit or to amplity it.

Transistor : A device to amplify very small currents. It is made up of a thin slice of semiconductor sandwitched between two thicker slices. An n-p-n-transistor has a layer of p-type material. The layers are known as collector, base and emitter.

Transducers : They are devices that can convert energy from one form to another and when applied to analytical instruments to convent information about a chemical system into electrical signals. The transducers can be based on the electrical quantity and is usually of three types (a) a variable resistor, (b) a source potential, and (c) a current source. Some of the examples of transducers are photoconductive cells, photovoltaic cells, thermocouple, photomultipliers, flame-ionization GC detectors etc.

Volt (Vor E) : is described as a unit of electrical pressure, potential or potential difference in a.wire e.g. 1.5 volt dry battery.

Valves : An electronic valve contains two metal conductors which are attached to a circuit at one end and either recieve or give out free electrons.

Watt (W) : is the unit of measure f electrical power . (W = V,I)

Appendix 3

Computer Terminology

As clearly spelled in the various chapters of this text book, in the last decade or so most of the analytical instruments have been incorporated with microprocessors, as well as interfaced with integraters/printers/plotters and personal computers. But, it will not serve any purpose to deal with computers exhaustively in this text book, therefore a simple terminology has been prepared for immediate reference.

Arithmetic operations : A computer is capable of performing complex mathematical operations which can be broken into simple arithmetic steps. Such important operations are addition, subtraction is a negative addition, multiplication is a repeated addition and division is a repeated negative addition. All that is needed is an automatic device which will cary out the addition of binary numerals in the form of electrical pulses.

Computer : A computer is an electronic device which can accept data, apply a series of logical operations and supply the results of these operations as information. Computers are used to perform complex series of mathematical calculations at very great speed. This enables them to be used for routine calculations, control industrial processes or guidance of satellites in space etc. There are three types of computers (i) analog computers (ii) digital computers and (iii) hybrid computers. There are relatively few hybrid computers in use. The digital computer is more versatile than the analog machine and is common.

Computer memory : The central processor unit contains a store or memory for holding numbers, results of calculations, instructions and other information. Various types of computer memories are (i) scratchpad memory (ii) main memory (iii) mass memory (iv) external memory.

Hardware : The computer is a machine which is capable of automatically executing a large number of instructions at very hard speed. The physical units or sub-systems are collectively called as hardware. These basically consist of elementary switches, amplifiers and gates.

Language in Computers : At present the most reliable electronic devices which can be used for represe ıting information in a machine are *flipflops* or *bistables*. These two devices are basically electronic switches possessing two stable states, an ON-state (yes) represented by 1, and an OFF-state (NO) represented by O. By assembling groups of bistables the information can be represented in combinations of Os and Is. The symbols 0 and 1 are the only ones necessary in the binary representation of numbers. They are called binary digits or *bits*. Two bistables can provide us with four combinations of bits each i.e. 00, 01, 10 and 11. Therefore, n bistables will give 2^n combinations. So with large set of bits. it is possible to represented all letters, symbols and digits that are required in computing. The central processor of a computer handles information in groups of *bits*. These may consist of 4, 8, 16 or 32 bits. Most of the microcomputers handle 8-bit groups known as *bytes*. A byte can be sent along a single wire in the form of pulses or spaces. A kilobyte (K) is 1024 bytes. Size of memory of a computer is described in terms of the number of kilobytes it can hold e.g. 16K, 32K, 64K etc.

Logic Gates : A digital computer contains sets of inter-connected electronic sub-systems. These sub-systems are constructed of simpler elements linked in such a way so that functions can be effectively carried out. The basic elements or fundamental building blocks are called logic gates. These are electronic circuits which can provide control of information flow, numerous logical and arithmetic functions, memory facility as well as timing circuitry.

Microprocessor : A microprocessor is a complete central processor etched on a single chip of silicon.

Structure of a Digital Computer : A digital computer consists of two electronic systems : (i) the central processor (CPU) and (ii) peripheral sub-system linked by a switching unit known as peripheral interface. Each system comprises of smaller sub units. The central processor contains : (a) an internal memory which is a high-speed storage device used to hold the immediately needed instructions or programme and data; (b) the arithmatic unit which can both temporarily hold and arithmetically process numbers fed into it, as well as carry out certain useful logic operations;

Software : All programmes which can be used on a particular computer system are called software. A digital computer has a high speed and capacity for manipulating large mass of data and perform complex actions. The early computers had to be programmed on a machine code. It was a coding system to which hardware would respond immediately but had no resemblance to a human languages. The various types of programming languages used in the computers today are (i) Fortran (ii) Algol (iii) cobol, (iv) Basic and time-sharing modes (v) Basic.

Appendix-4

Units

The system of units used in science is the metric system rather than the English system. The relation of the metric system of units to the English system of units is given in Table 1.

To relate large and small metric units systematically, the following usage has been adopted:

mega means *million* (1 megabar = 10^6 bars)
micro means *one millionth* (1 microgram = 10^6 gram)
kilo means *thousand* (1 kilogram = 10^3 grams)
milli means *one-thousandth* (1 millimeter = 10^3 meter)
centi means *one-hundredth* (1 centimeter = 10^2)

Table 1. The Metric System and the English System

	Metric System		*English System*
Length	1 meter (m)	=	39.37 inches
Mass	1 kilogram (kg)	=	2.205 pounds
Time	1 second (sec)	=	1 second
Volume	1 liter (l)	=	0.880 quart

Table 2 Useful Conversion Factors

Length 1 centimeter (cm)/10^4 microns (μ); 1 cm/10^8 Angstroms (Å)

Volume† $\frac{\text{1 litre}}{\text{1000 millilitres (ml)}}$; $\frac{\text{1.000028cm}^3}{\text{1 ml}} \approx \frac{\text{1 cmsup3}}{\text{1 ml}}$

Mass $\frac{\text{1atomic mass unit (amu)}}{1.66 \times 10^{-24} \text{ gram (gm)}}$

Pressure $\frac{\text{1 atmosphere (atm)}}{1.0133 \times 10^6 \text{ gm cm}^{-+} \text{ sec}^{-2} \text{ (dynes cm}^{-2})}$; $\frac{\text{1 atmosphere (atm)}}{\text{760 millimeters of mercury (mm Hg)}}$

Energy $\frac{\text{1 calorie (cal)}}{4.184 \times 10^7 \text{ gmcm}^2 \text{ sec}^{-2}\text{(ergs)}}$; $\frac{\text{1 electron volt (ev)}}{1.603 \times !10^{-12} \text{ erg}}$; $\frac{\text{1 ev}}{306 \times 10^4 \text{ cal}}$; $\frac{\text{1 litreatm}}{\text{24.22 cal}}$

Logarithms ln $x = 2.303 \log x$

Appendix - 5

Fundamental Constants

Symbol	*Name*	*Value*
c	Speed of light*	2.997925×10^{10} cm sec^{1}
h	Planck's constant*	$6.6256 \times$ 10=27 erg sec
k	Boltzmann's constant*	1.38054×10^{16} erg deg^{1} molecules
e	Charge on the electron*	4.80298×10^{10} eso
	Charge on the electron*	1.60210×10^{19} coulomb
m_r	Restmass of electron*	0.1091×10^{28} gm
m_p	Rest mass of proton*	1.67252×10^{24} gm
	Rest mass of proton*	1.00727663 a.m.u.
m_n	Rest mass of proton*	1.0086654 a.m.u.
N_0	Avogadro's number*	$6.02252 \times$ 10=23 molecules mole^{1}
R	Gas constant	82.055 atm cm^{3} deg^{1} mole^{1}
	Gas constant	0.082054 liter atm deg^{1} mole^{1}
	Gas constant*	8.3143 joule deg^{1} mole^{1}
	Gas constant	1.9872 def'd cal deg^{1} mole^{1}
V_a	Standard gas volume*	2.24136×10^{4} cm=3 mole^{1}
	Ice point ()°C)	273.15°K
	Triple point of H_2O (Base of International Temperature Scale)	273.16°K
g	Standard gravity	980.665 cm sec^{2}
F	Faraday constant*	$9.64870 \times$ 10=4 abs colomb equavalent^{1}
	Faraday constant	2.3060×10^{4} cal vol^{1} equivalent^{1}
ev	Electron volt*	1.60210×10^{12} erg molecule^{1}
	Electron volt	2.3060×10^{4} cal mole^{1}

Values of the physical constants are those recommended by the Committee on Fundamental Constants of the National Academy of Sciences-National Research Council and published in the *Technical News Bulletin* of the National Bureau of Standards, **47** 175 (1963).

Appendix - 6

Table of Atomic Weights

Element	*Symbol*	*Atomic Number*	*Atomic Weight*
Actinium	Ac	89	227
Aluminum	Al	13	26.9815
Americium	Am	95	243
Antimony	Sb	51	121.75
Argon	Ar	18	39.948
Arsenic	As	33	74.9216
Astatine	At	85	210
Barium	Ba	56	137.34
Berkelium	Bk	97	247
Baryllium	Be	4	9.0122
Bismuth	Bi	83	208.980
Boron	B	5	10.811
Bromine	Br	35	79.909
Cadmium	Cd	48	112.40
Calcium	Ca	20	40.08
Californium	Cf	98	251
Carbon	C	6	12.01115
Cerium	Ce	58	140.12
Cesium	Cs	55	132.905
Chlorine	Cl	17	35.453
Chromium	Cr	24	51.996
Cobalt	Co	27	58.9332
Copper	Cu	29	63.54
Curium	Cm	96	247
Dysprosium	Dy	66	162.50
Einsteinium	Es	99	254
Erbium	Er	68	167.26
Europium	Eu	63	151.96
Fermium	Fm	100	253
Fluorine	F	9	18.9984
Froncium	Fr	87	223
Godolinium	Gd	64	157.25
Gallium	Ge	31	69.72
Germanium	Ge	32	72.59
Gold	Au	79	196.967
Hafnium	Hf	72	178.49
Helium	He	2	4.0026
Holmium	Ho	67	164.930
Hydrogen	H	1	1.00797
Indium	In	49	114.82
Iodine	I	53	126.9044
Iridium	Ir	77	192.2
Iron	Fe	26	55.847
Krypton	Kr	36	83.80
Lanthanum	La	57	138.91
Lawrencium*	Lw	103	257
Lead	Pb	82	207.19
Lithium	Li	3	6.939

Element	*Symbol*	*Atomic Number*	*Atomic Weight*
Lithium	Li	3	6.939
Lutetium	Lu	71	174.97
Magnesium	Mg	12	24.312
Manganese	Mn	25	54.9381
Mendelevium	Md	101	256
Mercury	Hg	80	200.59
Molybdenum	Mo	42	95.94
Neodymium	Nd	60	144.24
Neon	Ne	10	20.183
Neptunium	Np	93	237
Nickel	Ni	28	58.71
Niobium	Nb	41	92.906
Nitrogen	N	7	14.0067
Nabelium	No	102	254
Osmium	Os	76	190.2
Oxygen	O	8	15.9994
Palladium	Pd	46	106.4
Phosphorus	P	15	30.9738
Platinum	Pt	78	195.09
Plutonium	Pu	94	242
Polonium	Po	84	210
Potassium	K	19	39.102
Proseodymium	Pr	59	140.907
Promethium	Pm	61	147
Protachnium	Po	91	231
Radium	Ra	88	226
Radon	Rn	86	222
Rhenium	Re	75	186.2
Rhodium	Rh	45	102.905
Rubidium	Rb	37	85.47
Ruthenium	Ru	44	101.07
Somarium	Sm	62	150.35
Scandium	Sc	21	44.956
Selenium	Se	34	78.96
Silicon	Si	14	28.086
Silver	Ag	47	107.870
Sodium	Na	11	22.9898
Strontium	Sr	38	87.62
Sulfur	S	16	32.064
Tontalum	Ta	73	180.948
Technetium	Tc	43	99
Tellurium	Te	52	127.60
Terbium	Tb	65	158.924
Thallium	Tl	81	204.37
Thorium	Th	90	232.038
Thulium	Tm	69	168.934
Tin	Sn	50	118.69
Titanium	Ti	22	47.90
Tungsten	W	74	183.85
Uranium	U	92	238.03
Vanadium	V	23	50.942
Xenon	Xe	54	131.30
Ytterbium	Yb	70	173.04
Yttrium	Y	39	88.905
Zinc	Zn	30	65.37
Zirconium	Zr	40	91.22

Index

B

C

E

F

G

H

I

K

L

Q

R

R

S